Gamuts in Nuclear Medicine

Gamuts in Nuclear Medicine

Third Edition

Frederick L. Datz, M.D.
Professor of Radiology
Director of Nuclear Medicine
University of Utah School of Medicine
Salt Lake City, Utah

 Mosby

St. Louis Baltimore Berlin Boston Carlsbad Chicago London Madrid
Naples New York Philadelphia Sydney Tokyo Toronto

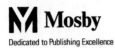

Mosby
Dedicated to Publishing Excellence

Executive Editor: Susan M. Gay
Senior Managing Editor: Lynne Gery
Project Manager: Linda Clarke
Production: Page Two Associates, Inc.
Manufacturing Manager: Theresa Fuchs

THIRD EDITION
Copyright © 1995 by Mosby–Year Book, Inc.

Printed in the United States of America
Composition by Page Two Associates, Inc.
Printing/binding by Malloy Lithographing, Inc.

Mosby–Year Book, Inc.
11830 Westline Industrial Drive
St. Louis, Missouri 63146

Library of Congress Cataloging-in-Publication Data
Gamuts in Nuclear Medicine
    Frederick L. Datz, M.D. — 3rd ed.
    Includes bibliographical references.
    ISBN 0-8016-8097-2
    1. Nuclear Medicine, Gamuts in — Handbooks, manuals, etc.
I. Datz, Frederick L.
    (DNLM: 1. Nuclear Medicine, Gamuts in — handbooks
DNLM/DLC
for Library of Congress

95 96 97 98 99 / 9 8 7 6 5 4 3 2 1

To Terry and Katie

Preface

This is an expanded version of the second edition of *Gamuts in Nuclear Medicine*, published in 1987. Since then, many changes have occurred in nuclear medicine.

This edition was written to incorporate those new studies as well as to expand the differential diagnoses of examinations covered in the previous two editions.

Gamuts is designed to help the busy practitioner determine the pathological cause of a finding on nuclear medicine scans. The book is divided into organ systems and includes gamuts of all of the major, and most of the less common, nuclear medicine studies. As in the previous two editions, references are provided at the end of each gamut. By scanning the references, the reader can quickly locate articles that provide an in-depth discussion of each subject.

I would like to thank those individuals who suggested additions to the book. I hope you find this new edition useful in your practice.

Frederick L. Datz

Contents

1. ENDOCRINE

2. CENTRAL NERVOUS SYSTEM

3. SKELETAL

4.   PULMONARY

Lung Imaging

5.   GASTROINTESTINAL

Hepatic Scintiangiography

Liver-Spleen Scan

Liver-Lung Scan

Liver-Spleen Scan

6. GENITOURINARY

7.   CARDIOVASCULAR

8.   HEMATOLOGY

Endocrine

THYROID IMAGING

Solitary Cold Nodule

COMMON: Adenoma
Adenomatous hyperplastia
Colloid cyst
Primary thyroid carcinoma

UNCOMMON: Hematoma
Hemiagenesis
Involution
Postoperative changes
Thyroiditis — acute, subacute, or chronic

RARE: Abscess
Amyloidosis
Artifact — metallic object
Bronchiogenic cyst
Caseating tuberculosis granuloma
Fibrosis following radiation
Lymph node enlargement, any cause
Lymphoma
Marine-Lenhart syndrome
Metastatic carcinoma
Nonchromaffin paragangliomatosis
Parathyroid adenoma

REFERENCES

1. Charkes ND: Graves' disease with functioning nodules (Marine-Lenhart syndrome). J Nucl Med 13:885, 1972

2. Farrer PA: Caseating tuberculous granuloma of the neck presenting as an avascular "cold" thyroid nodule. Clin Nucl Med 5:519, 1980

3. Freeman LM (ed): Nuclear Medicine Annual 1981. New York, Raven Press, 1981

4. Gottschalk A, Potchen EJ (eds): Diagnostic Nuclear Medicine. Baltimore, Williams and Wilkins, 1976

5. Lund RS, Shafer RB: Parathyroid adenoma presenting as a "cold nodule" on thyroid scan. Minn Med J 59:488, 1976

6. Miller TR, Abele JS, Greenspan FS: Fine-needle aspiration biopsy in the management of thyroid nodules. West J Med 134:198, 1981

7. Mailander JC, Graves VB: A thyroid nodule representing metastic renal carcinoma. Clin Nucl Med 10:650, 1985

8. Ram R: Cold nodule-thyroid scan. Semin Nucl Med 11:320, 1981

THYROID IMAGING

Multiple Cold Nodules

COMMON: Multinodular goiter

UNCOMMON: Following radiation — multiple neoplasms
Involution
Primary thyroid carcinoma
Thyroiditis acute, subacute or chronic

RARE: Abscess
Hematoma
Lymphoma
Marine-Lenhart syndrome
Metastatic carcinoma
Parathyroid cysts

REFERENCES

1. Charkes ND: Graves' disease with functioning nodules (Marine-Lenhart syndrome). J Nucl Med 13:885, 1972

2. Freeman LM (ed): Nuclear Medicine Annual 1981. New York, Raven Press, 1981

3. Gottschalk A, Potchen EJ (eds): Diagnostic Nuclear Medicine. Baltimore, Williams and Wilkins, 1976

4. Harada T, Shimaoka K, Okamura Y, et al: Nonfunctioning cystic disease of the parathyroid. Clin Nucl Med. 12:929, 1987

5. Kim E, Mattar AG: Primary and secondary carcinomata with focal nodular hyperplasia in a multinodular thyroid: Case report. J Nucl Med 17:938, 1976

6. Lester JW, Carter MP, Berens SV, et al: Colon carcinoma metastatic to the thyroid gland. Clin Nucl Med 10:634, 1985

7. Ram R: Cold nodule-thyroid scan. Semin Nucl Med 11:320, 1981

THYROID IMAGING

Hot Nodules

    COMMON: Adenoma — autonomous function

    UNCOMMON: Anatomic variant
                Hyperfunctioning normal tissue in a gland with previous injury such as thyroiditis, surgery, or other insult

    RARE: Carcinoma in region of hyperfunctioning tissue
          Following fine needle aspiration
          Hyperfunctioning thyroid carcinoma

REFERENCES

1. Becker F, Economou P, Schwartz TB: The occurrence of carcinoma in "hot" nodules. Ann Int Med 58:877, 1963

2. Burman, Warkel, Wartofsky: Hyperfunctioning thyroid nodules that become "cold." Med Ann DC 42:541, 1973

3. Freeman LM (ed): Nuclear Medicine Annual 1981. New York, Raven Press, 1981

4. Gottschalk A, Potchen EJ (eds): Diagnostic Nuclear Medicine. Baltimore, Williams and Wilkins Co., 1976

5. Harbert JC, Rocha AF (eds): Textbook of Nuclear Medicine: Clinical Applications. Philadelphia, Lea and Febiger, 1979

6. Landgarten S, Spencer RP: A study of the natural history of "hot" thyroid nodules. Yale J Biol Med 46:259, 1973

7. Meier DA, Hamburger JI: An autonomously functioning thyroid nodule, cancer, and prior radiation. Arch Surg 103:759, 1971

8. Miller JA, Hamburger JI: The thyroid scintiscan. I. The hot nodule. Radiology 84:66, 1965

9. Sandler MP, Fellmeth B, Salhany KE, Patton JA: Thyroid carcinoma masquerading as a solitary benign hyperfunctioning nodule. Clin Nucl Med 13:410, 1988

10. Shulkin BL: Hot nodule after fine-needle aspiration. Clin Nucl Med 13:131, 1988

THYROID IMAGING

Warm Nodules

COMMON: Adenoma — functioning nonautonomous or
autonomous

UNCOMMON: Anatomic variant
Cold nodule — anterior, posterior, or deep within
gland compressing normal tissue

RARE: Primary thyroid carcinoma

REFERENCES

1. Freeman LM (ed): Nuclear Medicine Annual 1981, New York, Raven Press, 1981
2. Gottschalk A, Pochen EJ (eds): Diagnostic Nuclear Medicine. Baltimore, Williams and Wilkins Co., 1976

THYROID IMAGING

Owl Eye Sign

      COMMON: Toxic nodular goiter

      RARE: Primary thyroid carcinoma

REFERENCES

1. Ashkar FS, Smoak WM: "Owl eye" sign of benign autonomous thyroid nodule. JAMA 214:1563, 1970
2. Ravel R: "Owl eye" sign in thyroid nodule of papillary carcinoma: Case report. J Nucl Med 17:985, 1976

THYROID IMAGING

Fish-Eye Sign

COMMON: Adenoma

UNCOMMON: Thyroid carcinoma

REFERENCE

1. Vaqueiro M, Gharib H, Wahner HW: "Fish-eye sign" in scintigraphy of benign thyroid nodule. Clin Nucl Med 10:817, 1985

THYROID IMAGING

Uptake in Only One Portion or One Lobe

COMMON: Following surgery
Hemiagenesis
Hyperfunctioning autonomous adenoma

UNCOMMON: Abscess
Thyroiditis — acute, subacute, or chronic

RARE: Adenoma
Adenomatous hyperplasia
Colloid cyst
Fibrosis following radiation
Following I-131 therapy
Lymphoma
Metastatic carcinoma
Primary thryoid carcinoma
Thyroiditis—traumatic (martial arts, seat belt)

REFERENCES

1. Abbassi V, Auth R: Hemiagenesis of the thyroid: Clinical and radiological presentation in the pediatric patient (letter to the editor). J Nucl Med 24:972, 1983

2. Avramides A, Vichayanrat A, Solomon N, et al: Thyroid hemiagenesis. Clin Nucl Med 2:310, 1977

3. Blum M, Schloss MF: Martial arts thyroiditis. N Engl J Med 311:199, 1984

4. Gottschalk A, Potchen EJ (eds): Diagnostic Nuclear Medicine. Baltimore, Williams and Wilkins Co., 1976

5. Leckie RG, Buckner AB, Bornemann ME: Seat belt-related thyroiditis documented with TC-99m pertechnetate scans. Clin Nucl Med 17:859, 1992

6. Lin DS: Thyroid imaging — Nonvisualization of one thyroid lobe. Semin Nucl Med 13:393, 1983

THYROID IMAGING

Disparate Results between Technetium and Iodine

COMMON: Adenomatous hyperplasia
Follicular adenoma
Primary thyroid carcinoma

UNCOMMON: Thyroiditis — subacute and chronic

RARE: Colloid cyst
Hürthle cell adenoma
Thyroglossal duct cyst

REFERENCES

1. Arnold JE, Pinsky S: Comparison of ^{99m}Tc and ^{123}I for thyroid imaging. J Nucl Med 17:261, 1976.

2. Athins HL, Lambrecht RM, Wolf AP: A comparison of technetium-99m and iodine-123 for thyroid imaging. AJR 117:195, 1973

3. Donoghue GD, Steinback JJ, Winterberger AR: Unusual Tc-99m and I-123 images in metastatic thyroid adenocarcinoma. Clin Nucl Med 4:468, 1979

4. Erjavec M, Movrin T, Auersperg M, et al: Comparative accumulation of Tc-99m and I-131 in thyroid nodules: Case report. J Nucl Med 18:346, 1977

5. Hirabayashi S, Koga Y, Kitahara T, et al: Inconsistent images of thyroid nodule scintigrams made with iodine and pertechnetate: Case report. J Nucl Med 16:918, 1975

6. Kim E, Kumar B: Discrepant imaging of nodular hyperplasia with pertechnetate and radioiodine. Clin Nucl Med 1:204, 1976

7. Massin JP, Planchon C, Perez R: Comparison of Tc-99m pertechnetate and I-131 in scanning of thyroid nodules. Clin Nucl Med 2:324, 1977

8. Miller JM, Kasenter MS, Marks DS: Disparate imaging of the autonomous functioning thyroid nodule with Tc-99m pertechnetate and radioiodine. Radiology 119:737, 1976

9. O'Connor MK, Cullen MJ, Malone JF: A kinetic study of I-131 and Tc-99m pertechnetate in thyroid carcinoma to explain a scan discrepancy: Case report. J Nucl Med 18:796, 1977

10. Patel BR, D'Cruz CA: Reverse discordant behavior in microfollicular adenoma of thyroid. Case Report. Clin Nucl Med 10:653, 1985

11. Remedios LV, Weber PW, Jasko IA: Thyroid scintiphotography in 1,000 patients: Rational use of Tc-99m and I-131 compounds. J Nucl Med 12:673, 1971

12. Ryo UY, Vardya P, Schneider A, et al: Histopathology of thyroid lesions that caused discrepant findings between Tc-99m scan and I-123 scan. J Nucl Med 20:678, 1979

13. Shambaugh GE, Quinn JL, Oyasu R, et al: Disparate thyroid imaging: Combined studies with sodium pertechnetate Tc-99m and radioactive iodine. JAMA 228:866, 1974

14. Steinberg M, Cavalieri RR, Choy SH: Uptake of technetium 99-pertechnetate in a primary thyroid carcinoma: Need for caution in evaluating nodules. J Clin Endocr 31:81, 1970

15. Strauss HW, Hurley PJ, Wagner HN: Advantages of ^{99m}Tc pertechnetate for thyroid scanning in patients with decreased radioiodine uptake. Radiology 97:307, 1970

16. Turner JW, Spencer RP: Thyroid carcinoma presenting as a pertechnetate "hot" nodule, but without I-131 uptake: Case report. J Nucl Med 17:22, 1976

17. Usher MS, Arzoumanian AY: Thyroid nodule scans made with pertechnetate may give inconsistent results. J Nucl Med 12:136, 1971

18. Wiener SN, Amiel-Fresen M, Genuth SM: Discordant imaging of a thyroglossal duct cyst. Clin Nucl Med 6:318, 1981

THYROID IMAGING

Reverse Discordant Results between Technetium and Iodine

COMMON AND
  UNCOMMON: Hashimoto's thyroiditis
                Microfollicular adenoma
                Thyroglossal duct cyst

REFERENCES

1. Arnold JE, Pinsky S: Comparison of ^{99m}Tc and ^{123}I for thyroid imaging. J Nucl Med 17:261, 1976
2. Huot D, Ton-That QT, LeBel L, et al: Reverse discordant behavior and progressive filling of a cold nodule on ^{99m}Tc pertechnetate thyroid imaging. Clin Nucl Med 15:5-7, 1990
3. Patel BR, D'Cruz Ca: Reverse discordant behavior in microfollicular adenoma of thyroid. Clin Nucl Med 10:653, 1985
4. Wiener SN, Aniel-Freson M, Genuth SM: Discordant imaging of a thyroglossal duct cyst. Clin Nucl Med 7:318, 1990

THYROID IMAGING

Diffusely Increased Activity

      COMMON: Hyperthyroidism

         RARE: Iodine deficiency
                   Recovery phase of thyroiditis.

REFERENCE

1. Freeman LM (ed): Nuclear Medicine Annual 1981. New York, Raven Press, 1981

THYROID IMAGING

Diffusely Decreased Activity or Nonvisualization

COMMON: Antithyroid medication
Increased iodine pool — recent contrast media study
or exogenous iodine
Thyroid suppression secondary to thyroid
replacement therapy

UNCOMMON: Hypothyroidism — primary, secondary, or tertiary
Thyroiditis

RARE: Ectopic thyroid tissue
Ingestion of goitrogens
Struma ovarii
Toxic intrathoracic goiter

REFERENCES

1. Freeman LM (ed): Nuclear Medicine Annual 1981. New York, Raven Press, 1981
2. Gottschalk A, Potchen EJ (eds): Diagnostic Nuclear Medicine. Baltimore, Williams and Wilkins Co., 1976
3. Prakash R, Lakshmipathi N, Jena A, et al: Hyperthyroidism caused by a toxic intrathoracic goiter with a normal-sized cervical thyroid gland. J Nucl Med 27:1423, 1986

THYROID IMAGING

Extrathyroidal Activity-I-123 or Tc-99m

COMMON: Ectopic thyroid — substernal, sublingual, pyramidal
lobe
Metastatic thyroid carcinoma
Pharynx/esophagus-swallowed secretions
Physiologic concentration — salivary glands, GI
tract, breasts, etc.

UNCOMMON
AND RARE: Achalasia
Adenoma on a stalk off thyroid
Barrett's esophagus
Contamination — saliva, sweat
Esophageal stricture
Gastric carcinoma
Gastric reflux
Hiatal hernia
Lung carcinoma
Papillary meningioma
Pulmonary fungal infection
Struma ovarii
Thymoma
Warthin's tumor
Zenker's diverticulum

REFERENCES

1. Abdel-Dayem HM, Halker K, El Sayed M: The radioactive wig in iodine-131 whole body imaging. Clin Nucl Med 9:454, 1984

2. Atmaram SH, Ganatra RD, Sharma SM, et al: Functioning metastases in liver from thyroid carcinoma: Case report. J Nucl Med 16:919, 1975

3. Bouvier J-F, You E, Peau J-Y, et al: Diffuse uptake of technetium-99m pertechnetate in a patient with metastases from thyroid carcinoma. Clin Nucl Med 11:728, 1986

4. Burt RW: Accumulation of ^{123}I in a Warthin's tumor. Clin Nucl Med 3:155, 1978

5. Chapman CN, Sziklas JJ, Spencer RP, et al: Hyperthyroidism with metastatic follicular thyroid carcinoma. J Nucl Med 25:466, 1984

6. Dhawan VM, Kaess KR, Spencer RP: False-positive thyroid scan due to Zenker's diverticulum. J Nucl Med 19:1231, 1978

7. Duong RB, Fernandez-Ulloa M, Planitz MK, et al: I-123 breast uptake in a young primipara with postpartum transient thyrotoxicosis. Clin Nucl Med 8:35, 1983

8. Feuerstein IM, Harbert JC: Hypertrophied thyroid tissue in a thyroglossal duct remnant. Clin Nucl Med 11:135, 1986

9. Gantra RD, Atmaram SH, Sharma SM: Unusual site of radionuclide concentration in patient with thyroid cancer. J Nucl Med 13:777, 1972

10. Grossman M: Gastroesophageal reflux: A potential source of confusion in technetium thyroid scanning: Case report. J Nucl Med 18:548, 1977

11. Lopez OL, Rodriguez Maisano E: Vascular retention of Tc-99m pertechnetate simulating ectopic or metastatic thyroid tissue. Clin Nucl Med 8:503, 1983

12. Park H-M, Tarver RD, Schauwecker DS, et al: Spurious thyroid cancer metastasis: Saliva contamination artifact in high dose iodine-131 metastases survey. J Nucl Med 27:634, 1986

13. Preisman RA, Halpern SE, Shishido R, et al: Uptake of ^{131}I by a papillary meningioma. AJR 129:349, 1977

14. Ryo UY, Stachura ME, Schneider AB, et al: Significance of extrathyroidal uptake of Tc-99m and I-123 in the thyroid scan: Concise communication. J Nucl Med 22:1039, 1981

15. Salvatore M, Gallo A: Accessory thyroid in the anterior mediastinum: Case report. J Nucl Med 16:1135, 1975

16. Sandler MP, Patton JA, Sacks GA, et al: Evaluation of intrathoracic goiter with I-123 scintigraphy and nuclear magnetic resonance imaging. J Nucl Med 25:874, 1984

17. Tyson JW, Wilkinson RH, Witherspoon LR, et al: False-positive I-131 total-body scans. J Nucl Med 15:1052, 1974

18. Vieras F: Preoperative scintigraphic detection of cervical metastases from thyroid carcinoma with technetium-99m pertechnetate. Clin Nucl Med 10:567, 1985

19. Woolfenden JM, Waxman AD, Wolfstein RS, et al: Scintigraphic evaluation of liver metastases from thyroid carcinoma. J Nucl Med 16:669, 1975

20. Wu S-Y, Kollin J, Coodley E, et al: I-131 total-body scan: Localization of disseminated gastric adenocarcinoma. Case report and survey of the literature. J Nucl Med 25:1204, 1984

21. Yeh E, Meade RC, Ruetz PP: Radionuclide study of struma ovarii. J Nucl Med 14:118, 1973

THYROID IMAGING

Elevated Uptake

COMMON: Geographic variation
Graves' disease
Toxic adenoma
Toxic multinodular goiter

UNCOMMON: Hashimoto's thyroiditis
Medications
Overtreatment with thyroid medications
Recovery phase of subacute thyroiditis

RARE: Chirrhosis
Contamination in room
Hereditary defects in hormone synthesis
Iodine deficiency goiter
Jod-Basedow phenomenon
Marine-Lenhart syndrome
Nephrosis
Renal failure
Retention of radioiodine from previous study
Thyroid carcinoma with hyperfunction
Zenker's diverticulum

REFERENCES

1. Freeman LM (ed): Nuclear Medicine Annual 1981. New York, Raven Press, 1981

2. Gottschalk A, Potchen EJ (eds): Diagnostic Nuclear Medicine. Baltimore, Williams and Wilkins Co., 1976

3. Hamberger JI: Application of the radioiodine uptake to the clinical evaluation of thyroid disease. Semin Nucl Med 1:281, 1971

4. Hayek A, Stanbury JB: The diagnostic use of radionuclides in the thyroid disorders of childhood. Semin Nucl Med 1:334, 1971

5. Keyes JW, Thrall JH, Carey JE: Technical considerations in in vivo thyroid studies. Semin Nucl Med 8:43, 1978

THYROID IMAGING

Decreased Uptake

COMMON: Hypothyroidism — primary, secondary, or tertiary
Medications other than thyroid medication
Recent iodine load including radiographic contrast
Thyroid medications
Thyroiditis — acute, subacute, or chronic

UNCOMMON: Exercise
Severe chronic illness
Thyrotoxicosis factitia

RARE: Congestive heart failure
Ectopic thyroid
Entire liquid dose not ingested
Goitrogens
Infectious hepatitis
Lack of absorption of capsule
Low serum chloride
Septicemia
Vomiting or diarrhea

REFERENCES

1. Desai KB, Ganatra RD, Sharma SM, et al: Thyroid uptake studies in infectious hepatitis. J Nucl Med 12:828, 1971

2. Halpern S, Alazraki N, Littenberg R, et al: ^{131}I thyroid uptakes: Capsule versus liquid. J Nucl Med 14:507, 1973

3. Hamberger JI: Application of the radioiodine uptake to the clinical evaluation of thyroid disease. Semin Nucl Med 1:287, 1971

4. Hamberger JI: Subacute thyroiditis: Diagnostic difficulties and simple treatment. J Nucl Med 15:81, 1974

5. Hankins JH, Heise CM, Cowan RJ: Iatrogenic hyperthyroidism secondary to dextrothyroxine administration. Clin Nucl Med 9:17, 1984

6. Hayek A, Stanbury JB: The diagnostic use of radionuclides in the thyroid disorders of children. Semin Nucl Med 1:334, 1971

7. Hooper PL, Rhodes BA, Conway MJ: Exercise lowers thyroid radioiodine uptake: Concise communication. J Nucl Med 21:835, 1980

8. Kan MK, Garcia JF, McRae J, et al: Marked suppression of thyroid function in rats with gram-negative septicemia. J Nucl Med 17:104, 1976

9. Keyes JW, Thrall JH, Carey JE: Technical considerations in in vivo thyroid studies. Semin Nucl Med 8:43, 1978

10. Leger AF, Fragu P, Rougier P, et al: Thyroid iodine content measured by x-ray fluorescence in amiodarone-induced thyrotoxicosis: Concise communication. J Nucl Med 24:582, 1983

11. Martino E, Aghini-Lombardi F, Lippi F, et al: Twenty-four hour radioactive iodine uptake in 35 patients with amiodarone associated thyrotoxicosis. J Nucl Med 26:1402, 1985

12. Robertson JS, Verhassett M, Wahner HW: Use of ^{123}I for thyroid uptake measurements and depression of ^{131}I thyroid uptakes by incomplete dissolution of capsule filler. J Nucl Med 15:770, 1974

13. Wong ET, Schultz AL: Changing values for the normal thyroid radioactive iodine uptake test. JAMA 238:1741, 1977

THYROID IMAGING

Medications Which Can Lower Iodine Uptake

COMMON: Antithyroid medications (e.g., propylthiouracil, tapazole)

Oral iodides and medications which contain iodine (e.g., Lugol's solution, potassium iodide, kelp preparations, many vitamin preparations, antiparasitic drugs)

Radiographic iodinated contrast media

Thyroid replacement medication (e.g., thyroid extract, triiodothyronine)

UNCOMMON: Adrenocorticosteroids

Aminobenzenes (e.g., paraaminosalicylic acid, paraaminobenzoic acid)

Amiodarone

Anticoagulants (e.g., heparin, coumarin)

Antihistamines

Bromides

Cobalt ion

Isoniazid

Mercurials

Nitrates

Perchlorate

Phenylbutazone

Progesterone

Resorcinol

Salicylates (large doses only)

Some sedatives (e.g., meprobamate, pentothal)

Sulfonamides

Sulfonylureas (e.g., tolbutamide)

Testosterone

Thiocyanate

Topical iodine compounds

Vitamin A

RARE: Epinephrine

Heavy metals

Morphine

Some antibiotics other than above (e.g., penicillin, chloramphenicol, chlortetracycline)

REFERENCES

1. Austen FK, Rubini ME, Meroney WH, et al: Salicylates and thyroid function. I. Depression of thyroid function. J Clin Invest 37:1131, 1958

2. Grayson R: Factors which influence the radioactive iodine thyroidal uptake test. Am J Med 24:397, 1960

3. Harbert JC, Rocha AF (eds): Textbook of Nuclear Medicine: Clinical Applications. Philadelphia, Lea and Febiger, 1984

4. Leger AF, Fragu P, Rougier P, et al: Thyroid iodine content measured by x-ray fluorescence in amiodarone-induced thyrotoxicosis: Concise communication, J Nucl Med 24:582, 1983

5. Martino E, Aghini-Lombardi F, Lippi F, et al: Twenty-four hour radioactive iodine uptake in 35 patients with amiodarone associated thyrotoxicosis. J Nucl Med 26:1402, 1985

6. Wolff J, Austen FK: Salicylates and thyroid function. I. The effect on the thyroid-pituitary interrelation. J Clin Invest 37:1144, 1958

THYROID IMAGING

Low T$_4$ and Elevated Uptake

COMMON: Overtreatment with antithyroid drugs
Thyroiditis — subacute and chronic

RARE: Hereditary defects in thyroid hormone synthesis
Iodine deficiency goiter

REFERENCE

1. Siegal BA, Alazraki NP, Alderson PO, et al (eds): Nuclear Radiology Syllabus, Second Series. Chicago, American College of Radiology, 1978

THYROID IMAGING

Elevated T_4 and Low or Normal Thyroid Uptake

COMMON: Exogenous iodine administration (contrast, medications, etc.)
Factitious
Thyroid medications
Thyroiditis — subacute, chronic, postpartum

UNCOMMON: Thyrotoxicosis with rapid turnover rate
Toxic adenoma
Toxic nodular goiter

RARE: Following head and neck irradiation
Metastatic thyroid carcinoma
Necrosis of hyperfunctioning adenoma
Nonthyroid medications (amiodarone)
Other metastatic carcinomas
Struma ovarii
Technical
Thyroiditis — acute, traumatic
Trapping defect with thyrotoxicosis

REFERENCES

1. Beierwaltes WH: The treatment of hyperthyroidism with iodine-131. Semin Nucl Med 8:95, 1978

2. Hamburger JI: Pitfalls in laboratory diagnosis of atypical hyperthyroidism. Arch Intern Med 139:96, 1979

3. Hayek A, Stanburg JB: The diagnostic use of radionuclides in the thyroid disorders of childhood. Semin Nucl Med 1:334, 1971

4. Keyes JW, Thrall JH, Carey JE: Technical considerations in in vivo thyroid studies. Semin Nucl Med 8:43, 1978

5. Klonecke A, Petersen MM, McDougall IR: Thyrotoxicosis with low thyroidal uptake of radioiodine. Semin Nucl Med XX:364, 1990

6. Leger AF, Fragu P, Rougier P, et al: Thyroid iodine content measured by x-ray fluorescence in amiodarone-induced thyrotoxicosis: Concise communication: J Nucl Med 24:582, 1983

7. Martino E, Aghini-Lombardi F, Lippi F, et al: Twenty-four hour radioactive iodine uptake in 35 patients with amiodarone associated thyrotoxicosis. J Nucl Med 26:1402, 1985

8. Ober KP, Cowan RJ, Sevier RE, Poole GJ: Thyrotoxicosis caused by functioning metastatic thyroid carcinoma. A rare and elusive cause of hyperthyroidism with low radioactive iodine uptake. Clin Nucl Med 12:345, 1987

9. Petersen M, Keeling CA, McDougall IR: Hyperthyroidism with low radioiodine uptake after head and neck irradiation for Hodgkin's disease. J Nucl Med 30:255, 1989

10. Yeh E, Meade RC, Ruetz PP: Radionuclide study of struma ovarii. J Nucl Med 14:118, 1973

THYROID IMAGING

T₃ Suppression Test — Failure to Suppress

COMMON: Euthyroid autonomous adenoma
Euthyroid Graves' disease
Graves' disease with hyperthyroid function
Toxic adenoma
Toxic multinodular goiter

RARE: Choriocarcinoma
Pituitary-induced hyperthyroidism
Thyroid carcinoma with hyperthyroid function

REFERENCES

1. Cassidy CE: Use of thyroid suppression test as a guide to prognosis of hyperthyroidism treated with antithyroid drugs. J Clin Endocrinol Metab 25:155, 1965

2. Gottschalk A, Potchen EJ (eds): Diagnostic Nuclear Medicine. Baltimore, Williams and Wilkins Co., 1976

3. Hales I, Steil J, Reeve T, et al: Prediction of the long term result of antithyroid drug therapy for thyrotoxicosis. J Clin Endocrinol Metab 29:998, 1969

4. Hamberger JI: Application of the radioiodine uptake to the clinical evaluation of thyroid disease. Semin Nucl Med 1:281, 1971

5. Tamai H, Nakagawa T, Takahashi H, et al: Triiodothyronine suppression tests and TSH-releasing hormone tests before and after I-131 therapy for Graves' disease. J Nucl Med 21:240, 1980

THYROID IMAGING

Positive Perchlorate Discharge Test

COMMON: Congenital organification defects
                        Hashimoto's thyroiditis

UNCOMMON: Antithyroid medications

REFERENCES

1. DeGroot LJ, Stanbury JB: The Thyroid and Its Diseases. New York, John Wiley and Sons, 1975
2. Gottschalk A, Potchen EJ (eds): Diagnostic Nuclear Medicine. Baltimore, Williams and Wilkins Co., 1976
3. Harbert JC, Rocha AF (eds): Textbook of Nuclear Medicine: Clinical Applications. Philadelphia, Lea and Febiger, 1984

THYROID IMAGING

Clinical Syndromes Associated with Hyperthyroidism

COMMON: Graves' disease
Toxic multinodular goiter

UNCOMMON: Thyroiditis — subacute or chronic
Toxic adenoma

RARE: Choriocarcinoma
Factitious hyperthyroidism
Iodine-induced hyperthyroidism
Pituitary-induced hyperthyroidism
Primary thyroid carcinoma with hyperfunction
Struma ovarii

REFERENCES

1. Jubiz W: Endocrinology: A Logical Approach for Clinicians. New York, McGraw-Hill, 1979

2. Kirchner PT (ed): Nuclear Medicine Review Syllabus. New York, Society of Nuclear Medicine, 1980

3. Leger AF, Fragu P, Rougier P, et al: Thyroid iodine content measured by x-ray fluorescence in amiodarone-induced thyrotoxicosis: Concise communication. J Nucl Med 24:582, 1983

4. Martino E, Aghini-Lombardi F, Lippi F, et al: Twenty-four hour radioactive iodine uptake in 35 patients with amiodarone associated thyrotoxicosis. J Nucl Med 26:1402, 1985

THYROID IMAGING

Iodine-131 Whole-body Imaging for Metastatic Thyroid Carcinoma — Uptake

COMMON: Gastrointestinal and genitourinary activity (normal)
Liver activity (functioning thyroid remnants or functioning metastases)
Nose (normal)
Thyroid carcinoma
Thyroid remnants

UNCOMMON
AND RARE: Chronic inflammatory lung disease
Disseminated gastric cancer
Dressings
Following acupuncture therapy
Fungal infection
Intrathoracic stomach
Large-cell bronchogenic carcinoma
Left colon graft
Lung infections
Meckel's diverticulum
Nonmalignant periocardial effusion
Pectus excavatum
Pericardial effusion
Periodontal disease
Postpartum or lactating breasts
Pulmonary adenocarcinoma
Saliva- or mucus-contaminated handkerchief
Sialadenitis
Struma ovarii
Sweat underneath a wig
Teratoma
Tracheostomy
Zenker's diverticulum

REFERENCES

1. Baeumler GR, Joo KG: Radioactive iodine uptake by breasts. J Nucl Med 27:149, 1986
2. Bakheet S, Hammami MM: Spurious lung metastases on radioiodine thyroid and whole-body imaging. Clin Nucl Med 18:307, 1993

3. Boulahdour H, Meignan M, Melliere D, et al: False-positive ^{131}I scan induced by Zenker's diverticulum. Clin Nucl Med 17:243, 1992

4. Boxen I, Zhang M: Nasal secretion of [131]I. Clin Nucl Med 15:610, 1990

5. Caplan RH, Gundersen GA, Abellera RM, Kisken WA: Uptake of ^{131}I by a Meckel's diverticulum mimicking metastatic thyroid cancer. Clin Nucl Med 12:760, 1987

6. Ceccarelli C, Pacini F, Lippi F, Pinchera A: Unusual case of false-positive ^{131}I whole-body scan in patient with papillary thyroid cancer. Clin Nucl Med 13:192, 1988

7. Chandramouly BS, Scagnelli T, Burgess CK: Artifact on ^{131}I whole-body scan due to contaminated handkerchief. Clin Nucl Med 14:301, 1989

8. Herzog G, Kisling G, Bekerman C: Diagnostic significance of dental history in the clinical evaluation of patients with thyroid carcinoma — Periodontal surgery mimicking a metastasis on ^{131}I whole-body survey. Clin Nucl Med 17:589, 1992

9. Hoschl R, Choy DHL, Gandevia B: [131]I uptake in inflammatory lung disease: A potential pitfall in treatment of thyroid carcinoma. J Nucl Med 29:701, 1988

10. Kolla IS, Alazraki NP, Watts NB: Sialadenitis mimicking metastatic thyroid carcinoma. Clin Nucl Med 14:564, 1989

11. Lakshmanan M, Reynolds JC, DelVecchio S, et al: Pelvic radioiodine uptake in a rectal wall teratoma after thyroidectomy for papillary carcinoma. J Nucl Med 10:1848, 1992

12. March DE, Desai AG, Park CH, et al: Struma ovarii: Hyperthyroidism in a postmenopausal woman. J Nucl Med 29:263, 1988

13. Maslack MM, Wilson CA: [131]I accumulation in a pericardial effusion. J Nucl Med 28:133, 1987

14. Muherji S, Ziessman HA, Earll JK, Keyes JW: False-positive ^{131}I whole-body scan due to pectus excavatum. Clin Nucl Med 13:207, 1988

15. Norby EH, Neutze J, VanNostrand D, et al: Nasal radioiodine activity: A prospective study of frequency, intensity, pattern. J Nucl Med 31:52, 1990

16. Otsuka N, Fukunaga M, Morita K, et al: [131]I uptake in patient with thyroid cancer and rheumatoid arthritis during acupuncture treatment. Clin Nucl Med 15:29, 1990

17. Park HM, Tarver RD, Schauwecker DS, Burt R: Spurious thyroid cancer metastases: Saliva contamination artifact in high-dose ^{131}I metastases survey. J Nucl Med 27:634, 1986

18. Park HM, Wellman HN: Hot nose after ^{131}I sodium iodide thyroablation therapy. Clin Nucl Med 17:130, 1992

19. Pochis WT, Krasnow AZ, Isitman AT, et al: Radioactive handkerchief sign — A contamination artifact in ^{131}I imaging for metastatic thyroid carcinoma. Clin Nucl Med 15:491, 1990

20. Rosenbaum RC, Johnston GS, Valente WA: Frequency of hepatic visualization during ^{131}I imaging for metastatic thyroid carcinoma. Clin Nucl Med 13:657, 1988

21. Schober B, Cohen P, Lyster D, et al: Diffuse liver uptake of [131]I. J Nucl Med 31:1575, 1990

22. Thomas RD, Batty VB: Metastatic malignant struma ovarii. Clin Nucl Med 17:577, 1992

23. White JE, Flickinger FW, Morgan ME: [131]I accumulation in gastric pull-up simulating pulmonary metastases on total-body scan for thyroid cancer. Clin Nucl Med 15:809, 1990

24. Ziessman HA, Bahar H, Fahey FH, Dubiansky V: Hepatic visualization on ^{131}I whole-body thyroid cancer scans. J Nucl Med 28:1408, 1987

THYROID IMAGING

Iodine-131 Whole-body Imaging for Thyroid Carcinoma — Head and Neck Uptake

COMMON: Metastatic thyroid carcinoma
Normal salivary or nasal gland uptake
Primary thyroid carcinoma
Swallowed secretions in esophagus
Thyroid remnant following surgery or ablation

UNCOMMON
AND RARE: Ectopic thyroid
External contamination from saliva or mucus
Periodontal disease
Sialadenitis
Tracheostomy
Zenker diverticulum

REFERENCES

1. Boulahdour H, Meignan M, Melliere D, et al: False-positive ^{131}I scan induced by Zenker's diverticulum. Clin Nucl Med 17:243, 1992

2. Boxen I, Zhang ZM: Nasal secretion of [131]I. Clin Nucl Med 15:610, 1990

3. Herzog G, Kisling G, Beckerman C: Diagnostic significance of dental history in clinical evaluation of patients with thyroid carcinoma — Periodontal survery mimicking a metastasis on ^{131}I whole-body survey. Clin Nucl Med 17:589, 1992

4. Kolla IS, Alazraki NP, Watts NB: Sialadenitis mimicking metastatic thyroid carcinoma. Clin Nucl Med 14:564, 1989

5. Norby EH, Neutze J, VanNostrand D, et al: Nasal radioiodine activity: A prospective study of frequency, intensity, pattern. J Nucl Med 31:52, 1990

6. Park HM, Tarver RD, Schauwecker DS, Burt R: Spurious thyroid cancer metastases: Saliva contamination artifact in high-dose ^{131}I metastases survey. J Nucl Med 27:634, 1986

7. Park HM, Wellman HN: Hot nose after ^{131}I sodium iodide thyroablation therapy. Clin Nucl Med 17:130, 1992

8. Thomas RD, Batty VB: Metastatic malignant struma ovarii. Clin Nucl Med 17:577, 1992

THYROID IMAGING

Iodine-131 Whole-body Imaging for Metastatic Thyroid Carcinoma — Pulmonary Uptake

COMMON: Thyroid carcinoma metastases

COMMON AND
UNCOMMON: Colonic graft
Disseminated gastric cancer
External contamination via coughing
Fungal infection
Inflammatory pulmonary infection
Intrathoracic stomach
Large-cell brochogenic carcinoma
Pectus excavatum
Pericardial effusion
Pulmonary adenocarcinoma
Salivary- or mucus-contaminated handkerchief in
    shirt pocket
Uptake by postpartum or lactating breasts

REFERENCES

1. Baeumler GR, Joo KG: Radioactive iodine uptake by breasts. J Nucl Med 27:149, 1986

2. Bakheet S, Hammami MM: Spurious lung metastases on radioiodine thyroid and whole-body imaging. Clin Nucl Med 18:307, 1993

3. Ceccarelli C, Pacini F, Lippi F, Pinchera A: Unusual case of false-positive ^{131}I whole-body scan in a patient with papillary thyroid cancer. Clin Nucl Med 13:192, 1988

4. Chandramouly BS, Scagnelli T, Burgess CK: Artifact on ^{131}I whole-body scan due to contaminated handkerchief. Clin Nucl Med 14:301, 1989

5. Hoschl R, Choy DHL, Gandevia B: [131]I uptake in inflammatory lung disease: A potential pitfall in treatment of thyroid carcinoma. J Nucl Med 29:701, 1988

6. Maslack MM, Wilson CA: [131]I accumulation in a pericardial effusion. J Nucl Med 28:133, 1987

7. Muherji S, Ziessman HA, Earll JM, Keyes JW: False-positive ^{131}I whole-body scan due to pectus excavatum. Clin Nucl Med 13:207, 1988

8. White JE, Flickinger FW, Morgan ME: [131]I accumulation in gastric pull-up simulating pulmonary metastases on total-body scan for thyroid cancer. Clin Nucl Med 15:809, 1990

THYROID IMAGING

Iodine-131 Whole-body Imaging for Thyroid Carcinoma — Abdominal Activity

COMMON: Liver uptake (See Gamut)
Normal gastrointestinal or genitourinary excretion

UNCOMMON
AND RARE: Contaminated handkerchief
Contamination with sweat or secretions
Meckel's diverticulum
Ovarian cyst
Ovarian adenoma
Rectal wall teratoma
Struma ovarii
Surgical drains or dressings

REFERENCES

1. Caplan RH, Gundersen GA, Abellera RM, Kisken WA: Uptake of ^{131}I by a Meckel's diverticulum mimicking metastatic thyroid cancer. Clin Nucl Med 12:706, 1987

2. March DE, Desai AG, Park CH, et al: Struma ovarii: Hyperthyroidism in a postmenopausal woman. J Nucl Med 29:263, 1988

3. Lakshmanan M, Reynolds JC, DelVecchio S, et al: Pelvic radioiodine uptake in a rectal wall teratoma after thyroidectomy for papillary carcinoma. J Nucl Med 33:1848, 1992

4. Zwas ST, Heyman Z, Lieberman LM: [131]I ovarian uptake in a whole-body scan for thyroid carcinoma. Semin Nucl Med XIX:340, 1989

THYROID IMAGING

Iodine-131 Whole-body Imaging for Metastatic Thyroid Carcinoma — Diffuse Liver Uptake

COMMON AND
UNCOMMON: Functioning metastases outside of liver
             Hepatic metastases
             Presence of residual functioning normal thyroid
             tissue

REFERENCES

1. Rosenbaum RC, Johnston GS, Valente WA: Frequency of hepatic visualization during ^{131}I imaging for metastatic thyroid carcinoma. Clin Nucl Med 13:657, 1988

2. Schober B, Cohen P, Lyster D, et al: Diffuse liver uptake of ^{131}I. J Nucl Med 31:1575, 1990

3. Ziessman HA, Bahar H, Fahey FH, Dubiansky V: Hepatic visualization on ^{131}I whole-body thyroid cancer scans. J Nucl Med 28:1408, 1987

THYROID IMAGING

Iodine-131 Whole-Body Imaging for Metastatic Thyroid Carcinoma — Bone Uptake

COMMON: Thyroid carcinoma metastases

UNCOMMON
AND RARE: Acupuncture sites
Contamination — saliva, sweat
Rheumatoid arthritis

REFERENCES

1. Otsuka N, Fukunaga M, Morita K, et al: [131]I uptake in a patient with thyroid cancer and rheumatoid arthritis during acupuncture treatment. Clin Nucl Med 15:29, 1990
2. Pochis WT, Krasnow AZ, Isitman AT, et al: Radioactive handkerchief sign — A contamination artifact in ^{131}I imaging for metastatic thyroid carcinoma. Clin Nucl Med 15:491, 1990

PARATHYROID IMAGING

Positive Tl-201 and Tc-99m Study

COMMON: Parathyroid adenoma
Parathyroid hyperplasia

UNCOMMON
AND RARE: Brown tumor in bone
Chronic thyroiditis
Colloid cyst
Hodgkin's lymphoma
Lymph node involvement-sarcoid
Lymph node metastases (thyroid carcinoma and other carcinomas)
Parathyroid carcinoma
Pyramidal lobe
Subtraction artifact
Thyroid adenoma
Thyroid adenomateous hyperplasia
Thyroid carcinoma

REFERENCES

1. Basarab RM, Manni A, Harrison TS: Dual isotope subtraction parathyroid scintigraphy in the preoperative evaluation of suspected hyperparathyroidism. Clin Nucl Med 10:300, 1985

2. Conte FA, Orzel JA, Weiland FL, Borchert RD: Prevention of motion artifacts on dual isotope subtraction parathyroid scintigraphy. J Nucl Med 28:1335, 1987

3. Ferlin G, Borsato N, Camerani M, et al: New perspectives in localizing enlarged parathyroids by technetium-thallium subtraction scan. J Nucl Med 24:438, 1983

4. Intenzo C, Park CH: Coexistent parathyroid adenoma and thyroid carcinoma: Nonspecificity of dual tracer parathyroid imaging for parathyroid lesions. Clin Nucl Med 10:560, 1985

5. Maslack MM, Brosbe RJ: Dual isotope parathyroid imaging. Clin Nucl Med 11:622, 1986

6. Okerlund MD, Sheldon K, Corpuz S, et al: A new method with high sensitivity and specificity for localization of abnormal parathyroid glands. Ann Surg 200:381, 1984

7. Park CH, Intenzo C, Cohn HE: Dual tracer imaging for localization of parathyroid lesions. Clin Nucl Med 11:237, 1986

8. Punt CJA, De Hooge P, Hoekstra JBL: False-positive subtraction scintigram of the parathyroid glands due to metastatic tumor. J Nucl Med 26:155, 1985

9. Winzelberg GG, Hydovitz JD: Radionuclide imaging of parathyroid tumors: Historical perspectives and newer techniques. Semin Nucl Med 15:161, 1985

10. Winzelberg GG, Hydovitz JD, O'Hara KR, et al: Parathyroid adenomas evaluated by Tl-201/Tc-99m pertechnetate subtraction scintigraphy and high-resolution ultrasonography. Radiology 155:231, 1985

11. Winzelberg GG, Melada GA, Hydovitz JD: False-positive thallium-201 parathyroid scan of the mediastinum in Hodgkin's lymphoma. AJR 147:819, 1986

12. Yang CJC, Seabold JE, Gurll NJ: Brown tumor of bone: A potential source of false-positive ^{201}Tl localization. J Nucl Med 30:1264, 1989

PARATHYROID IMAGING

False-negative Parathyroid Subtraction Scan

COMMON AND
UNCOMMON: Attenuation of activity from ectopic glands located
deep in mediastinum
Parathyroid hyperplasia
Patient motion
Small-size of lesion

REFERENCES

1. Basarab RB, Manni A, Harrison TS: Dual isotope subtraction parathyroid scintigraphy in the preoperative evaluation of suspected hyperparathyroidism. Clin Nucl Med 10:300, 1985

2. Blue PW, Crawford G, Dydek GJ: Parathyroid subtraction imaging: Pitfalls in diagnosis. Clin Nucl Med 14:47, 1989

3. Chen CC, Irony I, Jaffe GS, Norton JA: ^{99m}Tc uptake in a parathyroid adenoma potential pitfall in ^{99m}Tc/^{201}Tl subtraction imaging. Clin Nucl Med 17:539, 1992

4. Sandrock D, Dunham RG, Neumann RD: Simultaneous dual-energy acquisition for ^{201}Tl/^{99m}Tc parathyroid subtraction scintigraphy: Physical and physiological considerations. Nucl Med Comm 11:503, 1990

PARATHYROID IMAGING

MIBI Uptake

COMMON: Parathyroid adenoma
Parathyroid hyperplasia

UNCOMMON
AND RARE: Astrocytoma
Hyperactive bone secondary to hyperparathyroidism
Metastatic thyroid cancer
Parathyroid carcinoma

REFERENCES

1. Kitapci MT, Tastekin G, Turgut M, et al: Preoperative localization of parathyroid carcinoma using ^{99m}Tc MIBI. Clin Nucl Med 18:217, 1993
2. Park CH, Kim SM, McEwan JE, et al: Small parathyroid adenoma associated with hyperactive bone demonstrated by ^{99m}Tc MIBI scintiscan. Clin Nucl Med 19:160, 1994

MIBG IMAGING

Positive Uptake

COMMON: Adrenal medullary hyperplasia
MEN 2a and b
Normal adrenal medulla
Pheochromocytoma
Physiologic (liver, spleen, bladder, bowel, salivary,
heart, thyroid; etc.)

UNCOMMON
AND RARE: Acute focal pyelonephritis
Adrenal adenoma
Carcinoid
Cavernous hemangioma
Chemodactoma
Choriocarcinoma
Dilated renal pelvis
Gastrinoma
Infantile myofibromatosis
Insulinoma
Medullary thyroid carcinoma
Merkel cell skin tumor
Neuroblastoma
Paraganglioma
Parathyroid adenoma
Retinoblastoma   .
Schwannoma
Small cell carcinoma of lung
Uterus-menses

REFERENCES

1. Ansari AN, Siegel ME, DeQuattro V, Gazarian LH: Imaging of medullary thyroid carcinoma and hyperfunctioning adrenal medulla using Iodine-131 metaiodobenzylguanidine. J Nucl Med 27:1858, 1986

2. Bahar RH, Mahmoud S, Ibrahim A, Al-Gazzar AH: False-positive I-131 MIBG due to dilated renal pelvis. Clin Nucl Med 13:900, 1988

3. Beierwaltes WH: Endocrine imaging: Parathyroid, adrenal cortex and medulla, and other endocrine tumors. Part II. J Nucl Med 32:1627, 1991

4. Bomanji J, Britton KE: Uterine uptake of I-123 metaiodobenzylguanidine during the menstrual phase of uterine cycle. Clin Nucl Med 12:601, 1987

5. Feldman JM, Blinder RA, Lucas KJ, Coleman RE: I-131 metaiodobenzylguanidine scintigraphy of carcinoid tumors. J Nucl Med 27:1691, 1986

6. Geatti O, Shapiro B, Barillari B: Scintigraphic depiction of an insulinoma by I-131 metaiodobenzylguanidine. Clin Nucl Med 14:903, 1989

7. Geatti O, Shapiro B, Sisson JC, et al: Iodine-131 metaiodobenzylguanidine scintigraphy for the location of neuroblastoma: Preliminary experience in ten cases. J. Nucl Med 26:736, 1985

8. Hanson MW, Feldman JM, Blinder RA, et al: Carcinoid tumors: I-131 MIBG scintigraphy. Radiol 172:699-703, 1989

9. Hayward RS, Bowering CK, Warshawski RS: I-131 metaiodobenzylguanidine uptake in a parathyroid adenoma. Clin Nucl Med 13:632, 1988

10. Hoefnagel CA, Den Hartog Jager FCA, Van Gennip AH: Diagnosis and treatment of a carcinoid tumor using iodine-131 metaiodobenzylguanidine. Clin Nucl Med 11:149, 1986

11. Horne T, Glaser B, Krausz Y, et al: Unusual causes of I-131 metaiodobenzylguanidine uptake in nonneural crest tissue. Clin Nucl Med 16:239, 1991

12. Jacobs A, Lenior P, Delree M, et al: Unusual Tc-99m and I-123 MIBG images in focal pyelonephritis. Clin Nucl Med 15:821, 1990

13. Lynn MP, Shapiro B, Sisson JC, et al: Portrayal of pheochromocytoma and normal human adrenal medulla by m-[123I]iodobenzylguanidine: Concise communication. J Nucl Med 25:436, 1984

14. Mangner TJ, Tobes MC, Wieland DW, et al: Metabolism of iodine-131 metaiodobenzylguanidine in patients with metastatic pheochromocytoma. J Nucl Med 27:37, 1986

15. McEwan AJ, Shapiro B, Sisson JC, et al: Radio-iodobenzylguanidine for the scintigraphic location and therapy of adrenergic tumors. Semin Nucl Med 15:132, 1985

16. Munkner T: 131I-metaiodobenzylguanidine scintigraphy of neuroblastomas. Semin Nucl Med 15:154, 1985

17. Nakajo M, Shapiro B, Copp J, et al: The normal and abnormal distribution of the adrenomedullary imaging agent in m-[I-131]iodobenzylguanidine (I-131 MIBG) in man: Evaluation by scintigraphy. J Nucl Med 24:672, 1983

18. Nakajo M, Shapiro B, Glowniak J, et al: Inverse relationship between cardiac accumulation of meta-[131I]iodobenzylguanidine (I-131 MIBG) and circulating catecholamines in suspected pheochromocytoma. J Nucl Med 24:1127, 1983

19. Nakajo M, Shapiro B, Sisson JC, et al: Salivary gland accumulation of meta-[131I]iodobenzylguanidine. J Nucl Med 25:2, 1984

20. Nakajo M, Taguchi M, Shimabukuro K, et al: I-131 MIBG uptake in a small-cell carcinoma of the lung. J Nucl Med 27:1785, 1986

21. Shapiro B, Copp JE, Sisson JC, et al: Iodine-131 metaiodobenzylguanidine for the locating of suspected pheochromocytoma: Experience in 400 cases. J Nucl Med 26:576, 1985

22. Smit AJ, van Essen LH, Hollema H, et al: Meta-[I131]iodobenzylguanidine uptake in a nonsecreting paraganglioma. J Nucl Med 25:984, 1984

23. Sone T, Fukunaga M, Otsuka N, et al: Metastatic medullary thyroid cancer: Localization with iodine-131 metaiodobenzylguanidine. J Nucl Med 26:604, 1985

24. Stadalnik RC: Biodistribution of metaiodobenzylguanidine. Semin Nucl Med XXII: 46, 1992

25. Stewart RE, Grossman DM, Shulkin BL, Shapiro B: I-131 metaiodobenzyl-guanidine uptake in infantile myofibromatosis. Clin Nucl Med 14:344, 1989

26. VanGils APG, VanDerMey AGL, Hoogma RPLM, et al: I-123-metaio-dobenzylguanidine scintigraphy in patients with chemodectomas of the head and neck region. J Nucl Med 31: 1147, 1990

27. VonMoll L, McEwan AJ, Shapiro B, et al: I-131 MIBG scintigraphy of neu-roendocrine tumors other than pheochromocytoma and neuroblastoma. J Nucl Med 28:979 1987

28. Wieland DM, Wu J-I, Brown LE, et al: Radiolabeled adrenergic neuron-block-ing agents: Adrenomedullary imaging with [131I] iodobenzylguanidine. J Nucl Med 21:349, 1980

MIBG IMAGING

False-Negative

COMMON AND
UNCOMMON: Chemotherapy
Interfering medications
Metabolic alteration of tumor cells
Obscured by normal gastrointestinal or
    genitourinary activity

REFERENCES

1. Gordon I, Peters AM, Gutman A, et al: Skeletal assessment in neuroblastoma — The pitfalls of ^{123}I-MIBG scans. J Nucl Med 31:129, 1990

2. Gross MD, Shapiro B: Scintigraphic studies in adrenal hypertension. Semin Nucl Med XIX:122, 1989

3. Hoefnagel CA, Voute PA, DeKraker J, et al: Radionuclide diagnosis and therapy of neural crest tumors using ^{131}I metaiodobenzylguanidine. J Nucl Med 15:154, 1985

4. Khafagi FA, Shapiro B, Fig LM, et al: Labetalol reduces ^{131}I MIBG uptake by pheochromocytoma and normal tissues. J Nucl Med 30:481, 1989

5. Nakajo M, Shapiro B, Copp B, et al: The normal and abnormal distribution of the adrenal medullary imaging agent m-(^{131}I) iodobenzylguanidine (^{131}I MIBG) in man: Evaluation by scintigraphy. J Nucl Med 24:672, 1983

MIBG IMAGING

Drugs That Might Interfere with MIBG Imaging

Adrenergic neuron blockers, e.g. guanethidine
Antipsychotics (major tranquilizers)
    Butyrophenones
        Droperidol
        Haloperidol
        Pimozine
    Phenothiazines
        Chlorpromazine, triflupromazine, promethazine
        Fluphenazine, acetophenazine, perphenazine
        Prochlorperazine, thiethylperazine, trifluoperazine
        Thioridazine, mesoridazine
    Thioxanthines
        Chlorprothixene
        Thiothixene
Atypical antidepressants
    Maprotiline
    Trazolone
Bethanidine
Bretylium
Calcium-channel blockers
    Diltiazem
    Nifedipine
    Verapamil
Cocaine
Debrisoquine
Labetalol
Reserpine
Sympathomimetics
    Known
        Phenylephrine
        Phenylpropanolamine
        Pseudoephedrine, ephedrine
    Expected
        Amphetamine and related compounds
        Amphetamine and derivatives
        Diethylpropion
        Fenfluramine
        Mazindol
        Methylphenidate

Phenmetrazine and derivatives
Phentermine and derivates
Beta-sympathomimetics
Albuterol (salbutamol)
Isoetharine
Isoproterenol
Metaproterenol
Terbutaline
Dopamine
Metaraminol
Tricyclic antidepressants
Amitriptyline and derivatives
Amoxapine
Doxepin
Imipramine and derivatives
Loxapine (antipsychotic agent)

REFERENCES

1. Gross MD, Shapiro B: Scintigraphic studies in adrenal hypertension. Semin Nucl Med XIX:122, 1989

2. Khafagi FA, Shapiro B, Fig LM, et al: Labetalol reduces ^{131}I MIBG uptake by pheochromocytoma and normal tissues. J Nucl Med 30:481, 1989

MIBG IMAGING

Drugs Known Not to Significantly Affect MIBG Imaging

Alpha adrenergic blockers, e.g. phenoxybenzamine,
    phentolamine, prazosin, clonidine
Alpha methyldopa
Alpha methylparatyrosine
Angiotensin-converting enzyme inhibitors, e.g. captopril,
    enalapril
Barbiturates
Benzodiazepines
Beta adrenergic blockers (nonspecific and cardioselective)
Digitalis glycosides
Diuretics
Minor analgesics (nonsteroidals and acetaminophen)

REFERENCES

1. Gross MD, Shapiro B: Scintigraphic studies in adrenal hypertension. Semin Nucl Med XIX:122, 1989
2. Khafagi FA, Shapiro B, Fig LM, et al: Labetalol reduces ^{131}I MIBG uptake by pheochromocytoma and normal tissues. J Nucl Med 30:481, 1989

ADRENAL IMAGING

Symmetrical Visualization of the Adrenals

COMMON: Adrenal hyperplasia secondary to Cushing's disease
(increased glucocorticoids)
Bilateral hyperplasia — hyperaldosteronism
Normal

UNCOMMON: Ectopic adrenocorticotropic hormone excess
syndromes

RARE: Adrenogenital syndrome secondary to
21-hydroxylase deficiency

REFERENCES

1. Chatal JF, Charbonnel B, Guihard D: Radionuclide imaging of the adrenal glands. Clin Nucl Med 3:71, 1978
2. Freeman LM (ed): Nuclear Medicine Annual 1980. New York, Raven Press, 1980
3. Thrall JH, Freitas JE, Beierwaltes WH: Adrenal scintigraphy. Semin Nucl Med 8:23, 1978
4. Wahner HW, Northcutt RC, Salassa RM: Adrenal scanning: Usefulness in adrenal hyperfunction. Clin Nucl Med 2:253, 1977

ADRENAL IMAGING

Asymmetrical Visualization of the Adrenals

COMMON: Macronodular hyperplasia — hyperaldosteronism
Normal — right greater than left
Small aldosteronomas

UNCOMMON: Carcinoma — aldosterone or androgen producing
Micronodular hyperplasia — hyperaldosteronism
Prior adrenal surgery

RARE: Coexistence of Cushing's adenoma and hyperplasia
Confusion with gallbladder activity
Paraganglioma
Pheochromocytoma

REFERENCES

1. Freeman LM (ed): Nuclear Medicine Annual 1980. New York, Raven Press, 1980
2. Freitas JE, Thrall JH, Swanson DP, et al: Normal adrenal asymmetry: Explanation and interpretation. J Nucl Med 19:149, 1978
3. Thrall JH, Freitas JE, Beierwaltes WH: Adrenal scintigraphy. Semin Nucl Med 8:23, 1978

ADRENAL IMAGING

Unilateral Visualization

COMMON: Ademona — Cushing's disease (excess
glucocorticoids)
Unilateral remnant — following "total"
adrenalectomy

UNCOMMON: Adrenal infarction
Carcinoma — aldosterone or androgen producing

RARE: Carcinoma — Cushing's disease
Gallbladder visualization simulating unilateral
adrenal visualization
Nonbiochemically functioning adrenal tumor
(normal glucocorticoids)

REFERENCES

1. Chatal JF, Charbonnel B, Buihard D: Radionuclide imaging of the adrenal glands. Clin Nucl Med 3:71, 1978

2. Freeman LM (ed): Nuclear Medicine Annual 1980. New York, Raven Press, 1980

3. Ryo UY: Unilateral visualization of the adrenal gland. Semin Nucl Med 11:224, 1981

4. Thrall JH, Freitas JE, Beierwaltes WH: Adrenal scintigraphy. Semin Nucl Med 8:23, 1978

5. Wahner HW, Northcutt RC, Salassa RM: Adrenal scanning: Usefulness in adrenal hyperfunction. Clin Nucl Med 2:253, 1977

ADRENAL IMAGING

Bilateral Nonvisualization

COMMON: Adrenal carcinoma — Cushing's disease (excess
glucocorticoids)

UNCOMMON: Incorrect patient positioning
Unknown exogenous hormone administration

RARE: Extravasation of injected dose
Hyperlipidemia
Idiopathic
Late visualization
Poor radiolabeling

REFERENCES

1. Freeman LM (ed): Nuclear Medicine Annual 1980. New York, Raven Press, 1980
2. Gordon L, Mayfield RK, Levine JH, et al: Failure to visualize adrenal glands in a patient with bilateral adrenal hyperplasia. J Nucl Med 21:49, 1980
3. Thrall JH, Freitas JE, Beierwaltes WH: Adrenal scintigraphy. Semin Nucl Med 8:23, 1978
4. Valk TW, Gross MD, Freitas JE, et al: The relationship of serum lipids to adrenal-gland uptake of 6B-I-131 Iodomethyl-19-Norcholesterol in Cushing's syndrome. J Nucl Med 21:1069, 1980
5. Wahner HW, Northcutt RC, Salassa RM: Adrenal scanning: Usefulness in adrenal hyperfunction. Clin Nucl Med 2:253, 1977

ADRENAL IMAGING

Nonvisualization on Dexamethasone Suppression

COMMON: Normal

UNCOMMON: Low renin "essential" hypertension

REFERENCES

1. Rifai A, Beierwaltes WH, Freitas JE: Adrenal scintigraphy in low renin "essential" hypertension. J Nucl Med 18:599, 1977
2. Thrall JH, Freitas JE, Beierwaltes WH: Adrenal scintigraphy. Semin Nucl Med 8:23, 1978
3. Wahner HW, Northcutt RC, Salassa RM: Adrenal scanning: Usefulness in adrenal hyperfunction. Clin Nucl Med 2:253, 1977

ADRENAL IMAGING

Unilateral Visualization on Dexamethasone Suppression

COMMON: Aldosteronoma

UNCOMMON: Adenoma-adrenal hyperandrogenism
Adrenal cortical carcinoma
Adrenal hyperplasia
Low renin "essential" hypertension

REFERENCES

1. Chatal JF, Charbonnel B, Guihard D: Radionuclide imaging of the adrenal glands. Clin Nucl Med 3:71, 1978

2. Freeman LM (ed): Nuclear Medicine Annual 1980. New York, Raven Press, 1980

3. Gross M, Freitas J, Swansen D, et al: Dexamethasone suppression adrenal scintigraphy in hyperandrogenism. J Nucl Med 20:621, 1979

4. Gross MD, Shapiro B, Freitas JE: Limited significance of asymmetric adrenal visualization on dexamethasone-suppression scintigraphy. J Nucl Med 26:43, 1985

5. Kazerooni EA, Sisson JC, Shapiro B, et al: Diagnostic accuracy and pitfalls of [Iodine-131] 6-beta-iodomethyl-19-norcholesterol (NP-59) imaging. J Nucl Med 31:526, 1990

6. Rifai A, Beierwaltes WH, Freitas JE: Adrenal scintigraphy in low renin "essential" hypertension. J Nucl Med 18:599, 1977

7. Thrall JH, Freitas JE, Beierwaltes WH: Adrenal scintigraphy. Semin Nucl Med 8:23, 1978

8. Wahner HW, Northcutt RC, Salassa RM: Adrenal scanning: Usefulness in adrenal hyperfunction. Clin Nucl Med 2:253, 1977

ADRENAL IMAGING

Bilateral Visualization on Dexamethasone Suppression

COMMON: Macronodular hyperplasia — hyperaldosteronism
Micronodular hyperplasia — hyperaldosteronism

UNCOMMON: Adenoma plus hyperplasia
Drugs (oral contraceptives, diuretics)
Hyperplasia — adrenal hyperandrogenism
Low renin "essential" hypertension

RARE: Patient stops taking dexamethasone before the end
of the study
Renal artery stenosis

REFERENCES

1. Freeman LM (ed): Nuclear Medicine Annual 1980. New York, Raven Press, 1980

2. Gross M, Freitas J, Swansen D, et al: Dexamethasone suppression adrenal scintigraphy in hyperandrogenism. J Nucl Med 20:621, 1979

3. Gross MD, Valk TW, Swanson DP, et al: The role of pharmacologic manipulation in adrenal cortical scintigraphy. Semin Nucl Med 11:128, 1981

4. Juni JE, Gross MD: Bilateral visualization on adrenal cortical scintigraphy. Semin Nucl Med 13:168, 1983

5. Rifai A, Beierwaltes WH, Freitas JE: Adrenal scintigraphy in low renin "essential" hypertension. J Nucl Med 18:599, 1977

6. Thrall JH, Freitas JE, Beierwaltes WH: Adrenal scintigraphy. Semin Nucl Med 8:23, 1978

7. Wahner HW, Northcutt RC, Salassa RM: Adrenal scanning: Usefulness in adrenal hyperfunction. Clin Nucl Med 2:253, 1977

ADRENAL IMAGING

Cold Defect

COMMON: Pheochromocytoma

UNCOMMON
AND RARE: Cyst
Other tumors
Paraganglionoma

REFERENCES

1. Chatal JF, Charbonnel B, Guihard D: Radionuclide imaging of the adrenals. Clin Nucl Med 3:71, 1978
2. Gross MD, Freitas JE, Silver TM: Documentation of adrenal cyst by adrenal scanning techniques. J Nucl Med 19:1092, 1978
3. Thrall JH, Freitas JE, Beierwaltes WH: Adrenal scintigraphy. Semin Nucl Med 8:23, 1978
4. Wahmer HW, Northcutt RC, Salassa RM: Adrenal scanning: Usefulness in adrenal hyperfunction. Clin Nucl Med 2:253, 1977

ADRENAL IMAGING

Drugs That May Affect the Adrenal Scan

Adrenocorticoids
4-Aminopyrazolopyrimidine
Antagonists
    Diuretics
    Spironolactone
Antihypertensives
    Propranolol
Cholesterol-lowering agents
Dexamethasone
Hypercholesterolemia (any cause)
Metabolic inhibitors
    Aminoglutethimide
    Exogenous ACTH
    Metyrapone
    Op' DDD
Oral contraceptives

REFERENCES

1. Gross MD, Shapiro B: Scintigraphic studies in adrenal hypertension. Semin Nucl Med XIX:122, 1989

2

Central Nervous System

BRAIN IMAGING

SPECT — Decreased Focal HMPAO Uptake

COMMON: Alzheimer's disease
Brain death (diffuse)
Cerebrovascular disease — TIA, RIND
Epilepsy — interictal
Infarction
Neonates
Posttrauma
Tumor
Vasospasm — posthemorrhage, migraine, etc.

UNCOMMON: Acetazolamide enhancement with cerebrovascular disease
AIDS — dementia complex
Alcoholism
Arteriovenous malformation
Balloon occlusion
Cocaine users
Encephalopathy
Primary and metastatic tumor
Schizophrenia

RARE: Binswanger's disease
Child abuse

Congenital dysphasia
Huntington's disease
Hypoxia
Landau-Kleffner syndrome
MELAS syndrome
Mood disorders
Moyamoya
Multiple sclerosis
Parkinson's disease
Progressive supranuclear palsy
Rasmussen's syndrome
Sneddon syndrome
Subdural hematoma
Tuberous sclerosis
Wilson's disease

REFERENCES

1. Abdel-Dayem HM, El-Hilu S, Sehweil A, et al: Cerebral perfusion changes in schizophrenic patients using ^{99m}Tc hexamethylpropylene amineoxime (HMPAO). Clin Nucl Med 15:468, 1990

2. Abdel-Dayem HM, Sadek SA, Kouris K, et al: Changes in cerebral perfusion after acute head injury: Comparison of CT with ^{99m}Tc HMPAO SPECT. Radiology 165:221, 1987

3. Biersack HJ, Grunwald F, Kropp J: Single-photon emission computed tomography imaging of brain tumors. Semin Nucl Med XXI:2, 1991

4. Bonte FJ, Hom J, Tintner R, Weiner MF: Single-photon tomography in Alzheimer's disease and the dementias. Semin Nucl Med XX:342, 1990

5. Burke GJ, Fifer SA, Yoder J: Early detection of Rasmussen's syndrome by brain SPECT imaging. Clin Nucl Med 17:730, 1992

6. Burt RW, Reddy RV, Mock BM, et al: Acetazolamide enhancement of HPDM brain flow distribution imaging. J Nucl Med 27:1627, 1986

7. Burt RW, Witt RM, Cikrit DF, Reddy RV: Carotid artery disease: Evaluation with acetazolamide-enhanced ^{99m}Tc HMPAO SPECT. Radiology 182:461, 1992

8. Cleto EM, Holmes RA, Singh A, et al: Radiographic and neuro-SPECT imaging in an immature third ventricle teratoma. J Nucl Med 33:435, 1992

9. Cohen MB, Graham LS, Lake R, et al: Diagnosis of Alzheimer's disease and multiple infarct dementia by tomographic imaging of ^{123}I IMP. J Nucl Med 27:769, 1986

10. Coupland D, Lentle B: Bilateral subdural hematomas diagnosed with ^{99m}Tc HMPAO brain SPECT. J Nucl Med 32: 1915, 1991

11. de la Riva A, Gonzalez FM, Llamas-Elvira JM, et al: Diagnosis of brain death: Superiority of perfusion studies with ^{99m}Tc HMPAO over conventional radionuclide cerebral angiography. Br J Radiol 65:289, 1992

12. Denays R, VanPachterbeke TM, Tondeur M, et al: Brain single-photon emission computed tomography in neonates. J Nucl Med 30:1337, 1989

13. Devous MD, Leroy RF, Homan RW: Single-photon emission computed tomography in epilepsy. Semin Nucl Med XX:325, 1990

14. DiPiero V, Caneschi S, Bosisio CB, et al: Cerebral arterial spasm after subarachnoid hemorrhage — A case report with SPECT and ^{123}I HIPDM. Clin Nucl Med 12:395, 1987

15. Erbas B, Bekdik C, Erbengi G, et al: Regional cerebral blood flow changes in chronic alcoholism using ^{99m}Tc HMPAO SPECT — Comparison with CT parameters. Clin Nucl Med 17:123, 1992

16. Gzesh D, Goldstein S: Complex partial epilepsy: Role of neuroimaging in localizing a seizure focus for surgical intervention. J Nucl Med 31:1839, 1990

17. Hellman RS, Tikofsky RS: Overview of contribution of regional cerebral blood flow studies in cerebrovascular disease: Is there a role for single-photon emission computed tomography? Semin Nucl Med XX:303, 1990

18. Holman BL. Carvalho PA, Mendelson J, et al: Brain perfusion is abnormal in cocaine-dependent polydrug users: A study using ^{99m}Tc HMPAO and SPECT. J Nucl Med 32:1206, 1991

19. Johnson KA, Sperling RA, Holman BL, et al: Cerebral perfusion in progressive supranuclear palsy. J Nucl Med 33:704, 1992

20. Kao CH, Wang SJ, Liao SQ, Yeh SH: [99m]Tc HMPAO brain SPECT findings in Creutzfeldt-Jakob disease. Clin Nucl Med 18:234, 1993

21. Lee A, Mena IG, Miller B: Cerebral hypoxic injury detected by Tc-HMPAO SPECT. Clin Nucl Med 14:482, 1989

22. Masdeu JC, Yudd A, VanHeertum RL, et al: Single-photon emission computed tomography in human immunodeficiency virus encephalopathy. J Nucl Med 32:1471, 1991

23. Matsuda H, Higashi S, Tsuji S, et al: High-resolution ^{99m}Tc HMPAO SPECT in a patient with transient global amnesia. Clin Nucl Med 1846, 1993

24. Menzel C, Reinhold U, Grunwald F, et al: Cerebral blood flow in Sneddon syndrome. J Nucl Med 35:461, 1994

25. Nagel JS, Ichise M, Holman BL: Scintigraphic evaluation of Huntington's disease and other movement disorders using single-photon emission computed tomography perfusion brain scans. Semin Nucl Med XXI:11, 1991

26. Nagel JS, Johnson KA, Ichise M, et al: Decreased ^{123}I IMP caudate nucleus uptake in patients with Huntington's disease. Clin Nucl Med 13:486, 1988

27. Ohashi K, Fernandez-Ulloa M, Hall LC: SPECT, magnetic resonance and angiographic features in a moyamoya patient before and after external-to-internal carotid artery bypass. J Nucl Med 33:1692, 1992

28. O'Tauma LA, Urion DK, Janicek MJ, et al: Regional cerebral perfusion in Landau-Kleffner syndrome and related childhood aphasias. J Nucl Med 33:1758, 1992

29. Perani D, DiPiero V, Vallar G, et al: [99m]Tc HMPAO SPECT study of regional cerebral perfusion in early Alzheimer's disease. J Nucl Med 29:1507, 1988

30. Peterman SB, Taylor A, Hoffman JC: Improved detection of cerebral hypoperfusion with internal carotid balloon test occlusion and ^{99m}Tc HMPAO cerebral perfusion SPECT imaging. AJNR 12:1035, 1991

31. Pohl P, Vogl G, Fill H, et al: Single-photon emission computed tomography in AIDS dementia complex. J Nucl Med 29:1382, 1988

32. Rubinstein M, Denays R, Ham HR, et al: Functional imaging of brain maturation in humans using ^{123}I iodoamphetamine and SPECT. J Nucl Med 30:1982, 1989

33. Sackeim HA, Prohovnik I, Moeller JR, et al: Regional cerebral blood flow in mood disorders. II. Comparison of major depression and Alzheimer's disease. J Nucl Med 34:1090, 1993

34. Seto H, Shimizu M, Futatsuya R, et al: Basilar artery migraine — Reversible ischemia demonstrated by ^{99m}Tc HMPAO brain SPECT. Clin Nucl Med 19:215, 1994

35. Shih WJ, Loh F, Domstad PA, DeLand FH: Absent-decreased perfusion in cerebral SPECT study using ^{123}I HIPDM. Semin Nucl Med XVIII:169, 1988

36. Sieg KG, Harty JR, Simons M, et al: [99m]Tc HMPAO SPECT imaging of the central nervous system in tuberous sclerosis. Clin Nucl Med 16:665, 1991

37. Soucy JP, McNamara D, Mohn G, et al: Evaluation of vasospasm secondary to subarachnoid hemorrhage with ^{99m}Tc hexamethyl-propyleneamine oxime HMPAO tomoscintigraphy. J Nucl Med 31:972, 1990

38. Suess E, Malessa S, Ungersbock K, et al: [99m]Tcm-d, 1-hexamethylpropyleneamine oxime HMPAO uptake and glutathione content in brain tumors. J Nucl Med 32:1675, 1991

39. Takahashi N, Nishihara N, Odano I, et al: Regional cerebral blood flow measured with ^{123}I IMP SPECT in a case of subcortical arteriosclerotic encephalopathy (Binswanger's disease). Clin Nucl Med 17:882, 1992

40. VanHeertum RL, O'Connell RA: Functional brain imaging in evaluation of psychiatric illness. Semin Nucl Med XXI:24, 1991

BRAIN IMAGING

SPECT — Increased Focal HMPAO Uptake

COMMON: Encephalitis
Epilepsy — ictal
Tumor, e.g. gliomas, meningiomas

UNCOMMON: Luxury perfusion

RARE: Acute disseminated encephalitis
MELAS syndrome
Noisy imaging room
Photic stimulation
Schizophrenia and alcoholics with auditory
hallucinations
Skull metastasis
Transient global amnesia
Tumors

REFERENCES

1. Biersack HJ, Grunwald F, Kropp J: Single-photon emission computed tomography imaging of brain tumors. Semin Nucl Med XXI:2, 1991
2. Broich K, Horwich D, Alavi A: HMPAO-SPECT and MRI in acute disseminated encephalomyelitis. J Nucl Med 32:1897, 1991
3. Bushnell DL, Gupta S, Mlcoch AG, et al: Demonstration of focal hyperemia in acute cerebral infarction with [123I] iodoamphetamine. J Nucl Med 28:1920, 1987
4. Launes J, Nikkinen P, Lindroth L, et al: Diagnosis of acute herpes simplex encephalitis by brain perfusion single-photon emission computed tomography. Lancet May 28:1188, 1988
5. Matsuda H, Gyobu T, Li M, Hisada K: [123I] iodoamphetamine brain scan in patient with auditory hallucination. J Nucl Med 29:558, 1988
6. Matsuda H, Gyobu T, Li M, Hisada K: Increased accumulation of N-isopropyl ([123I]) p-iodoamphetamine in left auditory area in schizophrenic patient with auditory hallucinations. Clin Nucl Med 13:53, 1988
7. Meyer MA: Focal high uptake of HMPAO in brain perfusion studies: A clue in diagnosis of encephalitis: J Nucl Med 31:1094, 1990
8. Nakano S, Kinoshita K, Jinnouchi S, et al: Dynamic SPECT with [99mTc] HMPAO in meningiomas — A comparison with [123I] IMP. J Nucl Med 30:1101, 1989
9. Notardonato H, Gonzalez-Avilez A, VanHeertum RL: Potential value of serial cerebral SPECT scanning in evaluation of psychiatric illness. Clin Nucl Med 14:319, 1989

10. Park CH, Kim SM, Zhang JJ, et al: ^{99m}Tc MIBI brain SPECT in diagnosis of recurrent glioma. Clin Nucl Med 19:57, 1994

11. Ramsay SC, McLaughlin AF, Greenough R, et al: Comparison of independent aura, ictal and interictal cerebral perfusion. J Nucl Med 33:438, 1992

12. Strashun A, Dun EK, Sarkar SS, et al: Reversible increased ^{99m}Tc HMPAO cerebral cortical activity: A scintigraphic reflection of luxuriant hyperperfusion. J Nucl Med 33:117, 1992

13. VanHeertum RL, O'Connell RA: Functional brain imaging in evaluation of psychiatric illness. Semin Nucl Med XXI:24, 1991

14. Woods SW, Hegeman IM, Zubal IG, et al: Visual stimulation increases ^{99m}Tc HMPAO distribution in human visual cortex. J Nucl Med 32:210, 1991

BRAIN IMAGING

SPECT — Bilateral Parietal Abnormalities

COMMON: Alzheimer's disease
Encephalitis (usually increased uptake)
Parkinson's disease

UNCOMMON
AND RARE: Carbon monoxide intoxication
Hypoglycemia
Mitochondrial encephalopathy
Multiinfarct dementia
Other causes of increased or decreased uptake (See Gamuts)

REFERENCES

1. Holman BL, Devous MD: Functional brain SPECT: The emergence of a powerful clinical method. J Nucl Med 33:1888, 1992
2. Kuwabara Y, Ichiya Y, Otsuka M, et al: Differential diagnosis of bilateral parietal abnormalities in ^{123}I IMP SPECT imaging. Clin Nucl Med 15:893, 1990

BRAIN IMAGING

SPECT — Asymmetrical Cerebellar Uptake

COMMON AND
  UNCOMMON: Crossed cerebellar diaschisis (See Gamut)
                        Unilateral cerebellar infarct

REFERENCE

1. Shih WJ, Schleenbaker RE: Asymmetrical cerebellar uptake in brain single-photon emission computed tomography. Semin Nucl Med XXII:51, 1992

BRAIN IMAGING

SPECT — Crossed Cerebellar Diaschisis

COMMON: Brain tumor
            Cerebral hemorrhage
            Infarction

UNCOMMON
AND RARE: Alzheimer's disease
            Progressive supranuclear palsy
            Spinocerebellar degeneration
            Sturge-Weber syndrome
            TIA
            Tuberous sclerosis
            Wada test

REFERENCES

1. Brott TG, Gelfant MJ, Williams CC, et al: Frequency and patterns of abnormality detected by ^{123}I amine emission CT after cerebral infarction. Radiology 158:729, 1986

2. DeKosky ST, Shih WJ, Schmitt FA, et al: Assessing utility of single-photon emission computed tomography (SPECT) scan in Alzheimer disease: Correlation with cognitive severity. Alzheimer Dis & Assoc Disorders 4:14, 1990

3. Kushner M, Alavi A, Reivich M, et al: Contralateral cerebellar hypometabolism following cerebral insult: A positron emission tomographic study. Ann Neurol 15:425, 1984

4. Matsuda H, Tsuji S, Sumiya H, et al: Acetazolamide effect on vascular response in areas with diaschisis as measured by ^{99m}Tc HMPAO brain SPECT. Clin Nucl Med 17:581, 1992

5. Pantano P, Baron JC, Samson Y, et al: Crossed cerebellar diaschisis. Brain 109:677, 1986

6. Shih WJ, Coupal JJ, Magoun S, et al: [123]I HIPDM planar brain images demonstrating crossed cerebellar diaschisis. Clin Nucl Med 15:34, 1990

7. Yamauchi H, Fukuyama H. Yamaguchi S, et al: Crossed cerebellar hypoperfusion in unilateral major cerebral artery occlusive disorders. J Nucl Med 33:1632, 1992

BRAIN IMAGING

SPECT — Reverse Crossed Cerebellar diaschsis

COMMON AND
UNCOMMON: Epilepsy — ictal

REFERENCES

1. Park CH, Kim SM, Streletz LJ, et al: Reverse crossed cerebellar diaschisis in partial complex seizures related to herpes simplex encephalitis. Clin Nucl Med 17:732, 1992

BRAIN IMAGING

SPECT — HMPAO — Extracranial

COMMON AND
UNCOMMON: Fetus
Lungs — smokers
Normal — liver, kidneys, lacrimal glands
Tumor

REFERENCES

1. Hoshi H, Jinnouchi S, Sameshima M, et al: ^{99m}Tc hexamethylpropylene-amine oxime (HMPAO) uptake in bone metastasis. Clin Nucl Med 13:595, 1988

2. Maguire C, Florence S, Powe JE, et al: Hepatic uptake of ^{99m}Tc HMPAO in a fetus. J Nucl Med 31:237, 1990

3. Morita K, Ono S, Fukunaga M, et al: Accumulation of N-isopropyl-p[^{123}I] iodoamphetamine and [^{99m}Tc] hexamethyl propylene amine oxime in metastatic hepatocellular carcinoma. J Nucl Med 29:1460, 1988

4. Ohnishi T, Noguchi S, Murakami N, et al: Early and delayed imaging of ^{99m}Tc HMPAO vs ^{201}Tl in benign and malignant thyroid tumors — Similar uptake but different retention. Clin Nucl Med 17:806, 1992

5. Shih WJ, Gruenwald F, Biersack HJ, et al: ^{99m}Tc HMPAO diffuse pulmonary uptake demonstrated in cigarette smokers. Clin Nucl Med 16:668, 1991

6. Shih WJ, Rehm SR, Frunwald F, et al: Lung uptake of ^{99m}Tc HMPAO in cigarette smokers expressed by lung/liver activity ratio. Clin Nucl Med 18:227, 1993

RADIONUCLIDE ANGIOGRAPHY

Unilaterally Decreased Flow

COMMON: Cerebrovascular disease, including stroke
Subdural fluid collections other than blood —
    empyema, effusion, hydroma
Subdural hematoma — acute or chronic

UNCOMMON: Aneurysm
Cerebral contusion
Intracranial cysts — leptomeningeal, arachnoid,
    porencephalic, etc.
Tumor — especially if cystic
Unilateral hydrocephalus
Vasospasm secondary to subarachnoid hemorrhage

RARE: Abscess
Arteriovenous malformation on the contralateral
    side
Carotid cavernous fistula
Cerebral cysticercosis
Epidural hematoma
Moyamoya
Sturge-Weber syndrome (arterial phase)

REFERENCES

1. DeLand FH, Garcia F: Perfusion studies in the diagnosis of cerebral aneurysms. J Nucl Med 15:358, 1974

2. Fish MB, Barnes B, Pollycove M: Cranial scintiphotographic blood flow defects in arteriographically proven cerebrovascular disease. J Nucl Med 14:558, 1973

3. Gates GF, Fishman LS; Segall HD: Scintigraphic detection of congenital intracranial vascular malformations. J Nucl Med 19:235, 1978

4. Gilday DL, Ash J, Milne N: Dural fluid collections in infants and children. A successful nuclear medicine approach. Radiology 114:367, 1975

5. Goodman SJ, Hayes M: Value of cerebral isotope flow studies in timing of surgery for ruptured aneurysms when there is vasospasm and neurologic deficit. J Nucl Med 15:1113, 1974

6. Holman LB: Concepts and clinical utility of the measurement of cerebral blood flow. Semin Nucl Med 6:233, 1976

7. Hopkins GB, Kristensen KA: Rapid sequential scintiphotography in the radionuclide detection of subdural hematomas. J Nucl Med 14:288, 1974

8. Kuhl DE, Bevilacqua J, Mishkin MN, et al: The brain scan in Sturge-Weber syndrome. Radiology 103:621, 1972

9. Matin P, Shafer RB, Tully TE, et al: A review of carotid cavernous fistula including diagnosis and evaluation by nuclear medicine angiography. Clin Nucl Med 3:9, 1978

10. Mori H, Maeda T, Suguki Y, et al: Brain scan in cerebrovascular disease. AJR 124:583, 1975

11. O'Brien MJ, Ash JM, Gilday DL, Radionuclide brain scanning in perinatal hypoxia/ischemia. Develop Med Child Neurol 21:161, 1979

12. Rockett JF, Moinuddin M: Dynamic cerebral imaging. Clin Nucl Med 1:166, 1976

13. Sy WM: Manifestations of subdural and epidural hematomas on gamma imaging. CRC Crit Rev Clin Radiol Nucl Med 8:381, 1977

14. Yum HA, Ryo UR, Patel D, et al: Radionuclide brain imaging in cerebral cysticercosis. Clin Nucl Med 1:10, 1976

15. Zilkha A. Irwin GA: The rim sign in epidural hematoma: Case report. J Nucl Med 17:977, 1976

RADIONUCLIDE ANGIOGRAPHY

Bilaterally Decreased Flow

COMMON: Bilateral cerebrovascular disease
Bilateral fluid collections other than blood —
effusions, hygromas, empyemas
Bilateral subdural hematomas
Brain death
Congestive heart failure
Faulty injection
Superficial cortical atrophy

UNCOMMON: Hydrocephalus
Increased intracranial pressure — any cause
Obstruction of venous return
Perinatal hypoxia/ischemia
Pressure of head against collimator
Reflux into internal jugular veins

RARE: Arteriovenous malformation — deep midline
Carotid cavernous fistula
Epidural hematoma
Fibromuscular dysplasia
Moyamoya
Superior saggital sinus thrombosis
Vasospasm secondary to subarachnoid hemorrhage

REFERENCES

1. Aita JF, Keyes JW: Radionuclide studies in vascular infantile hemiplegia. J Nucl Med 15:300, 1974

2. Buozas DJ, Barrett IR, Mishkin FS: Diagnosis of epidural hematoma by brain scan and perfusion study: Case report. J Nucl Med 17:975, 1976

3. Fish MB, Barnes B, Pollycove M: Cranial scintiphotographic blood flow defects in arteriographically proven cerebrovascular disease. J Nucl Med 14:558, 1973

4. Gates GF, Fishman LS, Segall HD: Scintigraphic detection of congenital intracranial vascular malformation. J Nucl Med 19:235, 1978

5. Gilday DL, Ash J, Milne N: Dural fluid collections in infants and children: A successful nuclear medicine approach. Radiology 114:367, 1975

6. Goodman JM, Mishkin FS, Dyken M: Determination of brain death by isotope angiography. JAMA 209:1869, 1969

7. Hopkins GB, Kristensen KA: Rapid sequential scintiphotography in the radionuclide detection of subdural hematomas. J Nucl Med 14:288, 1974

8. Maeda T, Mori H, Hisada K, et al: Radionuclide cerebral angiography in moyamoya disease. Clin Nucl Med 4:513, 1979

9. Matin P, Shafer RB, Tully TE, et al: A review of carotid cavernous fistula including diagnosis and evaluation by nuclear medicine angiography. Clin Nucl Med 3:9, 1978

10. Stein MA, Winter J: Delayed appearance of anterior cerebral arteries on isotopic cerebral flow study: A sign of bleeding anterior communicating artery aneurysm. J Nucl Med 15:1217, 1974

11. Steinbach JJ, Mattar AG, Makin DT: Alteration of the cerebral blood flow study due to reflux in internal jugular veins. J Nucl Med 17:61, 1976

12. Sy WM: Manifestations of subdural and epidural hematomas on gamma imaging. CRC Crit Rev Clin Radiol Nucl Med 8:391, 1977

13. Teates CD, Allen DM: Superficial cortical atrophy simulating bilateral subdural hematomas. Clin Nucl Med 1:156, 1976

14. Williamson BR, Teates CD, Bray ST, et al: Radionuclide brain scan findings in superior sagittal sinus thrombosis. Clin Nucl Med 3:184, 1978

RADIONUCLIDE ANGIOGRAPHY

Unilaterally Increased Flow

COMMON: Arteriovenous malformation
Intracranial abscess
Intracranial tumor (especially glioblastoma,
meningiomas, and some metastatic lesions)
Luxury perfusion following a cerebrovascular
accident
Meningitis
Meningoencephalitis
Postsurgical

UNCOMMON: Carotid cavernous fistula
Fibrous dysplasia
Osteomyelitis
Paget's disease
Recent seizure
Scalp infection
Subdural empyema

RARE: Congenital dilation of cerebral veins
Following subarachnoid hemorrhage
Intracranial aneurysm
Subdural hematoma

REFERENCES

1. Fitzer PM: Nuclide angiography in Paget's disease of the skull: Case report. J Nucl Med 16:619, 1975

2. Fitzer PM: Radionuclide angiography— brain and bone imaging in craniofacial fibrous dysplasia (CFD): Case report. J Nucl Med 18:709, 1976

3. Gelmers HJ, Beko JW, Journee HL: Regional cerebral blood flow in patients with subarachnoid hemorrhage. Acta Neurochirugica 47:245, 1979

4. Karlin CA, Robinson RG, Hinthorn DR, et al: Radionuclide imaging in herpes simplex encephalitis. Radiology 126:181, 1978

5. Matin P, Goodwin DA, Nayyar SN: Radionuclide cerebral angiography in diagnosis and evaluation of carotid cavernous fistula. J Nucl Med 15:1105, 1974

6. Moore JS, Kieffer SA, Goldberg ME, et al: Intracranial tumors: Correlation of angiography with dynamic radionuclide studies. Radiology 115:393, 1975

7. Rujanavech N, Mattar AG, Coleman RE: Abnormal rapid sequence imaging in a patient with subdural empyema: Case report. J Nucl Med 17:980, 1976

8. Siddiqui A, Ryo UY, Yum HY, et al: Increased blood flow on radionuclide cerebral flow studies in subdural hematoma. Clin Nucl Med 2:436, 1977

9. Snow RM, Keyes JW Jr: The "luxury-perfusion syndrome" following a cerebrovascular accident demonstrated by radionuclide angiography. J Nucl Med 15:907, 1974

10. Stevens JS, Mishkin FS: Abnormal radionuclide cerebral angiograms and scans due to seizures. Radiology 117:113, 1975

11. Williamson BR, Teates CD: Value of routine flow studies in nuclear brain scanning. South Med J 71:1082, 1978

12. Witherspoon LR, Tyson JW, Goodrich JK: The appearance of peripheral postsurgical activity on cerebral dynamic studies. J Nucl Med 15:709, 1974

RADIONUCLIDE ANGIOGRAPHY

Bilaterally Increased Flow

COMMON: Meningitis
           Meningoencephalitis

UNCOMMON: Bilateral abscesses
           Bilateral metastatic tumor
           Fibrous dysplasia
           Osseous metastases to skull
           Osteomyelitis
           Paget's disease
           Postsurgical
           Scalp infection

RARE: Bilateral arteriovenous malformations
           Bilateral subdural empyemas
           Congenital dilation of cerebral veins
           Following seizures

REFERENCES

1. Fitzer PM: Nuclide angiography in Paget's disease of the skull: Case report. J Nucl Med 16:619, 1975

2. Fitzer PM: Radionuclide angiography — brain and bone imaging in craniofacial fibrous dysplasia (CFD): Case report. J Nucl Med 18:709, 1976

3. Gelmers HJ. Beko JW, Journee HL: Regional cerebral blood flow in patients with subarachnoid hemorrhage. Acta Neurochirugica 47:245, 1979

4. Karlin CA, Robinson RG, Hinthorn DR, et al: Radionuclide imaging in herpes simplex encephalitis. Radiology 126:181, 1978

5. Matin P, Goodwin DA, Nayyar SN: Radionuclide cerebral angiography in diagnosis and evaluation of carotid cavernous fistula. J Nucl Med 15:1105, 1974

6. Moore JS, Kieffer SA, Goldberg ME, et al: Intracranial tumors: Correlation of angiography with dynamic radionuclide studies. Radiology 115:393, 1975

7. Rujanavech N, Mattar AG, Coleman RE: Abnormal rapid sequence imaging in a patient with subdural empyema: Case report. J Nucl Med 17:980, 1976

8. Siddiqui A, Ryo UY, Yum HY, et al: Increased blood flow on radionuclide cerebral flow studies in subdural hematoma. Clin Nucl Med 2:436, 1977

9. Snow RM, Keyes JW Jr: The "luxury-perfusion syndrome" following a cerebrovascular accident demonstrated by radionuclide angiography. J Nucl Med 15:907, 1974

10. Stevens JS, Mishkin FS: Abnormal radionuclide cerebral angiograms and scans due to seizures. Radiology 117:113, 1975

11. Williamson BR, Teates CD: Value of routine flow studies in nuclear brain scanning. South Med J 71:1082, 1978

12. Witherspoon LR, Tyson JW, Goodrich JK: The appearance of peripheral postsurgical activity on cerebral dynamic studies. J Nucl Med 15:709, 1974

RADIONUCLIDE ANGIOGRAPHY

"Hot Nose"

> COMMON: Cerebrovascular disease

> UNCOMMON: Increased intracranial pressure — any cause
> Psychotropic drugs
> Sinusitis

> RARE: Cerebral atrophy
> Hyperthyroidism
> Subdural hematoma

REFERENCES

1. Brucer M: Cerebral Perfusion, A Routine Adjunct to the Brain Scan. St. Louis, Mallincknodt, 1975
2. Joe SH, Watts G. Mena I: The significance of increased nasopharyngeal flow in cerebral radionuclide angiogram: "Hot nose" phenomenon. Clin Nucl Med 2:221, 1977

RADIONUCLIDE ANGIOGRAPHY

Jugular Reflux

COMMON: Left antecubital injection
Mediastinal tumor
Normal variant — secondary to incompetent or
absent venous valves
Valsalva maneuver

UNCOMMON: Congestive heart failure
Mediastinal infection
Mediastinal irradiation
Trauma

RARE: Aortic aneurysm
Compton scatter
Patent ductus arteriosus
Substernal goiter
Tricuspid regurgitation

REFERENCES

1. Friedman BH, Lovegrove FT, Wagner HN: An unusual variant in cerebral circulation studies. J Nucl Med 15:363, 1974

2. Hayt DB, Perez LA: Cervical venous reflux in dynamic brain scintigraphy. J Nucl Med 17:9, 1976

3. Murray IP, Hoschl R, Choy D: The jugular venous reflux. Clin Nucl Med 3:56, 1978

4. Ogawa TK, So SK, Gerberg E, et al: Jugular-dural sinuses, jugular reflux in dynamic brain flow imaging as a sign of unilateral innominate vein obstruction: Case report. J Nucl Med 18:39, 1977

5. Peart RA, Dreidger AA: Effect of obstructed mediastinal venous return on dynamic brain flow studies: Case report. J Nucl Med 16:622, 1975

6. Steinbach JJ, Mattar AG, Mahin DT: Alteration of the cerebral blood flow study due to reflux in internal jugular veins. J Nucl Med 17:61, 1976

RADIONUCLIDE ANGIOGRAPHY

Focal Area of Increased Activity in the Neck

COMMON: Contralateral arterial stenosis
            Jugular reflux

UNCOMMON: Arteriovenous malformation
            Carotid artery aneurysm
            Carotid body tumors
            Glomus jugulare tumors
            Postsurgical

RARE: Any other type of vascular tumor
            Cervical adenitis
            Metastatic thyroid carcinoma

REFERENCES

1. Laird JD, Ferguson WR, McIlrath EM, et al: Radionuclide angiography as the primary investigation in chemodectoma: Concise communication. J Nucl Med 24:475, 1983

2. Makhija M: Demonstration of a glomus tumor on a dynamic nuclear angiogram. Clin Nucl Med 4:247, 1979

3. Makler PT, Charles D, Malmud LS: Metastatic thyroid carcinoma presenting as a hypervascular neck lesion. Clin Nucl Med 2:192, 1977

4. Rockett JF, Moinuddin M: Dynamic cerebral imaging. Clin Nucl Med 1:166, 1976

5. Rockett JF, Moinuddin M, Robertson JT, et al: Vertebral artery fistula detected by radionuclide angiography: Case report. J Nucl Med 17:24, 1976

6. Serafini AN, Weinstein MB: Radionuclide evaluation of a carotid body tumor. J Nucl Med 13:640, 1972

7. Stevens JS, Mishkin FS: Abnormal radionuclide angiogram in cervical lymphadenitis: Case report. J Nucl Med 16:26, 1975

8. Sty JR, Babbitt DP, Geiss DM: Arteriovenous malformation of the vertebral artery in a child. Clin Nucl Med 3:36, 1978

9. Zwas ST, Kronenberg J. Tadmor R, et al: Diagnosis of jugular paraganglioma by radionuclide angiography: Concise communication. J Nucl Med 24:1005, 1983

RADIONUCLIDE ANGIOGRAPHY

Vascular Blush on Dynamic Imaging Followed by Intense Uptake on Static Imaging

COMMON: Meningioma
Vascular metastasis (especially renal, thyroid)

UNCOMMON: Glioma
Large arteriovenous malformation without washout

RARE: Arteriovenous fistula
Hemangiopericytoma
Plasmacytoma

REFERENCES

1. Front D: Distinctive imaging characteristics of different types of brain tumors. Clin Nucl Med 4:211, 1979
2. Gates GF, Fishman LS, Segall HD: Scintigraphic detection of congenital intracranial vascular malformations. J Nucl Med 19:235, 1978
3. Sostre S: Vein of Galen malformation. Clin Nucl Med 1:211, 1976
4. Wakat MA, Cowan RJ: Plasmacytoma simulating meningioma on brain scan. Clin Nucl Med 4:327, 1979

STATIC PLANAR IMAGING

Solitary Focus of Uptake

COMMON: Abscess
Cerebrovascular accident — ischemic or
  hemorrhagic
Ear artifact
Meningitis
Neoplasm — primary or metastatic
Perinatal asphyxia
Postcraniotomy
Scalp contusion
Sinusitis
Subdural fluid collections other than blood —
  empyema, effusion, hygroma, etc.
Subdural hematoma — acute or chronic
Temporal muscle uptake

UNCOMMON: Arteriovenous malformation
Blood pool in superficial vessels
Brain contusion
Cephalohematoma
Choroid plexus uptake — fourth ventricle
Fibrous dysplasia
Following renal dialysis
Following seizures
Hemangioma of the skull
Infiltrated scalp vein injection
Intracerebral hematoma
Intraventricular hemorrhage
Multiple sclerosis
Occipital sinus activity (simulating posterior fossa
  lesion)
Osseous metastases to the skull
Osteomyelitis
Paget's disease
Radiation necrosis
Scalp abscess or cellulitis
Sebaceous cyst
Secondary to recent EEG lead placement
Skull fracture
Subarachnoid hemorrhage
Superior sagittal sinus thrombosis

RARE: Adrenoleukodystrophy
Amyloidoma
Bullet track
Carotid cavernous fistula
Cerebral cysticerocosis
Cerebral venous angioma
Chemotherapeutic neurotoxicity
Coronal suture
Epidural hematoma
Following contrast injection during cerebral
   angiography
Hemiatrophy causing a pseudoparasagittal mass
Intracerebral sarcoidosis
Intracerebral systemic lupus erythematosis
Intracranial cavernous hemangioma
Moyamoya
Neurosyphilis
Scalp tumors
Subacute sclerosing panencephalitis
Unilateral pyogenic ventriculitis
Vein of Galen malformation

REFERENCES

1. Aita JF, Keyes Jr JW: Radionuclide studies in vascular infantile hemiplegia. J Nucl Med 15:300, 1974

2. Baker HL, Houser WO, Campbell JK: National Cancer Institute study: Evaluation of computed tomography in the diagnosis of intracranial neoplasms. Radiology 136:91, 1980

3. Brill DR, Shoop JD: Sensitivity of radionuclide isotope brain scan in cerebral meliodosis: Case report. J Nucl Med 18:987, 1977

4. Buell U, Niendorf HP, Kazner E, et al: Computerized transaxial tomography and cerebral serial scintigraphy in intracranial neoplasms — rates of detection and tumor-type identification: Concise communication. J Nucl Med 19:476, 1978

5. Burt RW: Brain scan abnormalities produced by electroencephalographic procedures. J Nucl Med 15:369, 1974

6. Carrier L, Chartrans R, Picard D: Brain scan: A useful tool in detection of neurosyphilis (letter to the editor). J Nucl Med 26:209, 1985

7. Chin LC, McWilliams FE, Christie JH: Comparison of radionuclide and computed tomography scanning in nonneoplastic intracranial disease. CT: J Comput Tomog 2:295, 1978

8. Christie JH, Go RT, Suzuki T: The occipital sinus and posterior fossa lesions. Boston, Scientific exhibit presented Soc Nucl Med Meeting July, 1972

9. Dodson WE, Prensky AL, Siegal BA: Radionuclide imaging in subacute sclerosing panencephalitis. Neurology 29:749, 1979

10. Fitzer PM: Radionuclide angiography — brain and bone imaging in craniofacial fibrous dysplasia (CFD): Case report. J Nucl Med 18:709, 1976

11. Gilday DL: Various radionuclide patterns of cerebral inflammation in infants and children. AJR 120:247, 1974

12. Go RT, Ptack JJ: Localization of ^{99m}Tc in the choroid plexus of the fourth ventricle. J Nucl Med 14:352, 1973

13. Klingensmith WC, Datu J, Tuberculomeningitis of the sylvian fissure. Clin Nucl Med 3:315, 1978

14. Lee HK: Unilateral pyogenic ventriculitis. J Nucl Med 18:403, 1977

15. Lentle BC, Scott JR, Noujaim AD, et al: Iatrogenic alterations in radionuclide biodistribution. Semin Nucl Med 9:131, 1979

16. Lloyd TV, Antonmattei S: Intracranial subdural chondrosarcoma. Clin Nucl Med 4:208, 1979

17. McCartney WH, Lendner LE, Prather JL, et al: Brain scan abnormalities in intracerebral sarcoidosis. Clin Nucl Med 4:32, 1979

18. Moreno AJ, Brown JM, Brown TJ, et al: Scintigraphic findings in a primary cerebral amyloidoma. Clin Nucl Med 8:528, 1983

19. O'Brien MJ, Ash JM, Gilday DL: Radionuclide brain scanning in perinatal hypoxia/ischemia. Develop Med Child Neurol 21:161, 1979

20. Patton DD, Brasfield DL: Ear artifact in brain scans. J Nucl Med 17:305, 1976

21. Penning L, Front D: Scintigraphic demonstration of a bullet track in the brain. J Nucl Med 15:140, 1974

22. Puri S, Spencer RP, Gordon ME: Positive brain scan in toxoplasmosis. J Nucl Med 15:641, 1974

23. Rockett JF, Mournudden M: Dynamic cerebral imaging. Clin Nucl Med 1:166, 1976

24. Savocardo M, Passerini A: CT, angiography, and RN scans in intracranial cavernous hemangiomas. Neuroradiology 16:256, 1978

25. Sherkow LH: Chemotherapeutic neurotoxicity on brain scintigraphy. Clin Nucl Med 4:439, 1979

26. Silberstein EB: Brain scintigraphy in the diagnosis of the sequelae of head trauma. Semin Nucl Med 13:153, 1983

27. Sostre S: Vein of Galen malformation. Clin Nucl Med 1:211, 1976

28. Soucek CD: Sinusitis demonstrated by brain scanning. J Nucl Med 16:89, 1975

29. Tan RF, Gladman DD, Urowitz MB, et al: Brain scan diagnosis of central nervous system involvement in systemic lupus erythematosis. Annal Rheum Dis 37:357, 1978

30. Teplick SK, Van Heertum RL, Clark RE, et al: Pseudoparasagittal masses caused by displacement of the falx and superior sagittal sinus. J Nucl Med 15:1047, 1974

31. Wolfstein RS, Tanasescu DE, Waxman AD, et al: Transient brain scan abnormalities in renal dialysis patients. J Nucl Med 17:6, 1977

32. Yum HA, Ryo UR, Patel D, et al: Radionuclide brain imaging in cerebral cysticerosis. Clin Nucl Med 1:10, 1976

33. Zwas ST, Czerniak P: Head and brain scan findings in rhinocerebral mucormycosis: Case report. J Nucl Med 16:925, 1975

STATIC PLANAR IMAGING

Multiple Foci of Uptake

COMMON: Bilateral fluid collections other than blood —
empyema, effusion, hygroma, etc.
Bilateral subdural hematomas
Cerebritis
Cerebrovascular accident — especially embolic
Lateral ventrical visualization (choroid plexus)
Meningitis
Multifocal abscesses
Multiple metastases
Multiple osseous metastases to the skull
Perinatal asphyxia
Sinusitis

UNCOMMON: Blood pool in superficial vessels
Chemotherapeutic neurotoxicity
Fibrous dysplasia
Following renal dialysis
Following seizures
Multifocal abscesses
Multiple brain contusions
Multiple intracerebral hematomas
Multiple sclerosis
Paget's disease
Postcraniotomy
Scalp contusions
Secondary to recent EEG lead placement

RARE: Adrenoleukodystrophy
Central nervous system
Central nervous system involvement by acute
lymphocytic cell leukemia
Cerebral cysticercosis
Herpes zoster
Intracerebral sarcoidosis
Intracerebral systemic lupus erythematosis
Moyamoya
Multifocal leukodystrophy
Multifocal osteomyelitis
Multiple arteriovenous malformations

Multiple primary tumors
Multiple scalp tumors
Radiation necrosis
Schilder's disease
Subacute sclerosing panencephalitis

REFERENCES

1. Aita JF, Keyes JW, Jr: Radionuclide studies in vascular infantile hemiplegia. J Nucl Med 15:300, 1974

2. Baker HL, Houser WO, Campbell JK: National Cancer Institute study: Evaluation of computed tomography in the diagnosis of intracranial neoplasms. Radiology 136:91, 1980

3. Brill DR, Shoop JD: Sensitivity of radionuclide isotope brain scan in cerebral melioidosis: Case report. J Nucl Med 18:987, 1977

4. Buell U, Niendorf HP, Kazner E, et al: Computerized transaxial tomography and cerebral serial scintigraphy in intracranial neoplasms — rates of detection and tumor-type identification: Concise communication. J Nucl Med 19:476, 1978

5. Burt RW: Brain scan abnormalities produced by electroencephalographic procedures. J Nucl Med 15:369, 1974

6. Catterton BE: Progressive abnormalities in the brain scan in adrenal leukodystrophy. AJR 129:939, 1977

7. Chin LC, McWilliams FE, Christie JH: Comparison of radionuclide and computed tomography scanning in nonneoplastic intracranial disease. CT: J Comput Tomog 2:295, 1978

8. Christie JH, Go RT, Suzuki T: The occipital sinus and posterior fossa lesions. Boston, Scientific exhibit presented Soc Nucl Med Meeting, July, 1972

9. Dodson WE, Prensky AL, Siegal BA: Radionuclide imaging in subacute sclerosing panencephalitis. Neurology 29:749, 1979

10. Fitzer PM: Radionuclide angiography — brain and bone imaging in craniofacial fibrous dysplasia (CFD): Case report. J Nucl Med 18:709, 1976

11. Gilday DL: Various radionuclide patterns of cerebral inflammation in infants and children. AJR 120:247, 1974

12. Go RT, Ptack JJ: Localization of ^{99m}Tc in the choroid plexus of the fourth ventricle. J Nucl Med 14:352, 1973

13. Klingensmith WC, Datu J, Tuberculomeningitis of the sylvian fissure. Clin Nucl Med 3:315, 1978

14. Lee HK: Unilateral pyogenic ventriculitis. J Nucl Med 18:403, 1977

15. Lentle BC, Scott JR, Noujaim AD, et al: Iatrogenic alterations in radionuclide biodistribution. Semin Nucl Med 9:131, 1979

16. Lloyd TV, Antonmattei S: Intracranial subdural chondrosarcoma. Clin Nucl Med 4:208, 1979

17. McCartney WH, Lendner LE, Prather JL, et al: Brain scan abnormalities in intracerebral sarcoidosis. Clin Nucl Med 4:32, 1979

18. Miller SW, Potsaid MS: Focal brain scan abnormalities in multiple sclerosis. J Nucl Med 15:131, 1974

19. Moreno AJ, Brown JM, Waller SF, et al: The complementary roles of brain scintigraphy and computed tomography in multiple sclerosis. Clin Nucl Med 8:618, 1983

20. O'Brien MJ, Ash JM, Gilday DL: Radionuclide brain scanning in perinatal hypoxia/ischemia. Develop Med Child Neurol 21:161, 1979

21. Patton DD, Brasfield DL: Ear artifact in brain scans. J Nucl Med 17:305, 1976

22. Penning L, Front D: Scintigraphic demonstration of a bullet track in the brain. J Nucl Med 15:140, 1974

23. Puri S, Spencer RP, Gordon ME: Positive brain scan in toxoplasmosis. J Nucl Med 15:641, 1974

24. Rockett JF, Mournudden M: Dynamic cerebral imaging. Clin Nucl Med 1:166, 1976

25. Savocardo M, Passerini A: CT, angiography, and RN scans in intracranial cavernous hemangiomas. Neuroradiology 16:256, 1978

26. Sherkow LH: Chemotherapeutic neurotoxicity on brain scintigraphy. Clin Nucl Med 4:439, 1979

27. Shih W-J, Domstad PA, DeLand FH: Opportunistic intracranial infection in AIDS detection by technetium-99m DTPA brain scintigraphy. J Nucl Med 27:498, 1986

28. Silberstein EB: Causes of abnormalities reported in nuclear medicine testing. J Nucl Med 17:229, 1976

29. Sostre S: Vein of Galen malformation. Clin Nucl Med 1:211, 1976

30. Soucek CD: Sinusitis demonstrated by brain scanning. J Nucl Med 16:89, 1975

31. Sty J, Kun L, Throp S: Scintigraphy in acute lymphocytic cell leukemia. J Nucl Med 20:1101, 1979

32. Tan RF, Gladman DD, Urowitz MB, et al: Brain scan diagnosis of central nervous system involvement in systemic lupus erythematosis. Annal Rheum Dis 37:357, 1978

33. Teplick SK, Van Heertum RL, Clark RE, et al: Pseudoparasagittal masses caused by displacement of the falx and superior sagittal sinus. J Nucl Med 15:1047, 1974

34. Weisbaum SD, Garnett ES: Brain scan in Schilder's disease. J Nucl Med 14:291, 1973

35. Wolfstein RS, Tanasescu DE, Waxman AD, et al: Transient brain scan abnormalities in renal dialysis patients. J Nucl Med 17:6, 1977

36. Yum HA, Ryo UR, Patel D, et al: Radionuclide brain imaging in cerebral cysticercosis. Clin Nucl Med 1:10, 1976

37. Zwas ST, Czerniak P: Head and brain scan findings in rhinocerebral mucormycosis: Case report. J Nucl Med 16:925, 1975

STATIC PLANAR IMAGING

Suprasellar Uptake

COMMON: Craniopharyngioma
Meningioma
Pituitary adenoma

UNCOMMON: Chordoma
Glioma
Metastasis

RARE: Aneurysm
Arachnoiditis

REFERENCE

1. Theros EG (ed): Nuclear Radiology Syllabus, Set Seven. Chicago, American College of Radiology, 1974

STATIC PLANAR IMAGING

Anterior Midline Lesions

COMMON: Glioblastoma

UNCOMMON: Aneurysm
Astrocytoma
Metastatic malignant melanoma (and other
metastases)

RARE: Arteriovenous malformation
Cerebrovascular accident
Focal encephalitis
Lipoma of the corpus callosum
Multiple sclerosis

REFERENCES

1. Addlestone R, Workman JB: Lipoma of the corpus callosum. J Nucl Med 15:714, 1974
2. DeLand FH, Garcia F: Perfusion studies in the diagnosis of cerebral aneurysms. J Nucl Med 15:358, 1974
3. Makler T, Gutowicz MF: Focal encephalitis presenting as a dumbbell-shaped lesion crossing midline. Clin Nucl Med 1:8, 1976
4. Ucmackli AU: The pathogenic significance of corpus callosum involvement in brain scans. J Nucl Med 13:510, 1972
5. Veluvolu P, Collier BD, Isitman AT, et al: "Butterfly" pattern of uptake in posterior brain scan in diffuse histiocytic lymphoma. Clin Nucl Med 10:50, 1985

STATIC PLANAR IMAGING

Doughnut Sign

COMMON: Abscess
Neoplasm — primary (especially glioblastoma) and
metastatic

UNCOMMON: Cerebrovascular accident
Intracerebral hematoma
Osseous metastasis to the skull
Subdural hematoma

RARE: Adrenoleukodystrophy
Arteriovenous malformation
Cephalohematoma
Cranial cholesteatoma
Craniotomy flap with granulation tissue
Osteomyelitis
Radionecrosis
Scalp abscess
Sebaceous cyst of the scalp
Subdural effusion

REFERENCES

1. Beauchamp JM, Belanger MA, Neitzschman HR: An unusual cause of "doughnut" sign in brain scanning. J Nucl Med 16:432, 1975

2. Gottschalk A, Abatie JD, Petasnick P, et al: The comparison between sensitivity and resolution based on a clinical evaluation with the ACRH brain scanner in medical radioisotopes scintigraphy. In Medical Radioisotope Scintigraphy. II. Vienna, IAEA, 1969

3. Holloway W, Elgammal T, Pool WH: Doughnut sign in subdural hematomas. J Nucl Med 13:630, 1971

4. Kuhl DE, Sanders TP: Characterizing brain lesions with use of transverse section scanning. Radiology 198:595, 1971

5. O'Mara RE, McAfee JG, Chodos RD: The "doughnut" sign in cerebral radioisotope images. Radiology 92:581, 1969

6. Polga JP, Dann RH: Sebaceous cysts of the scalp presenting as doughnut lesions on radionuclide brain imaging. Clin Nucl Med 3:300, 1978

7. Rockett JF, Freedman BI, Kaplan ES: Significance of "doughnut" sign. J Nucl Med 13:777, 1972

8. Sty JR, Swick H: "Doughnut" sign in adrenoleukodystrophy. Clin Nucl Med 3:158, 1978

9. Sutherland JB, Hill N, Banerjee AK, et al: Brain scanning and brain abscesses. J Can Assoc Radiol 23:176, 1972

10. Sy WM, Klateb R, Bay R: Rim and "doughnut" signs and variants: Review and reappraisal. Clin Nucl Med 1:186, 1976

11. Tarcan TA, Fajman W, Marc J, et al: "Doughnut" sign in brain scanning. AJR 126:842, 1976

12. Theros EG (ed): Nuclear Radiology Syllabus. Chicago, American College of Radiology, 1978

13. Trackler RT, Miller KE, Cohen ML: The "doughnut" sign in subdural effusion. Am J Dis Child 129:373, 1975

STATIC PLANAR IMAGING

Increased Peripheral Uptake (Rim Sign)

COMMON: Cephalohematoma
Motion artifact
Postsurgical
Scalp contusion, laceration or hematoma
Scalp vein injection
Subdural fluid collections other than blood —
   effusion, empyema, hygroma
Subdural hematoma
Subgaleal hematoma

UNCOMMON: Cerebral abscess
Cerebral contusion
Cerebral neoplasm
Fibrous dysplasia
Following subdural taps
Hyperostosis frontalis interna
Infarct
Meningitis
Paget's disease
Skull fracture

RARE: Arteriovenous malformation
Asymmetrical superficial veins
Epidural abscess
Epidural hematoma
Fetal molding
Hemiatrophy
Leptomeningeal cyst
Osteomyelitis
Plagiocephaly
Porencephaly
Postural molding
Reticulosis
Scalp cellulitis or abscess
Scalp tumors (e.g., hemangioma)
Scaphocephaly
Sturge-Weber syndrome
Subarachnoid cyst
Systemic lupus erythematosis
Unilateral hydrocephalus

REFERENCES

1. Conway JJ, Vollert JM: The accuracy of radionuclide imaging in detecting pediatric dural fluid collections. J Nucl Med 105:77, 1972

2. Gilday DL: Various radionuclide patterns of cerebral inflammation in infants and children. AJR 120:247, 1974

3. Martin TR, Moore JS, Shafer RB: Evaluation of the posterior flow study in brain scintigraphy. J Nucl Med 17:13, 1976

4. Preimesberger KF, Loken MK, Shafer RB: Abnormal brain scan in Paget's disease of bone contusion with subdural hematoma. J Nucl Med 15:880, 1974

5. Rujanavech N, Mattar AG, Coleman RE: Abnormal rapid sequence imaging in a patient with subdural empyema: Case report. J Nucl Med 17:980, 1976

6. Shih W-J, Domstad PA, DeLand FH: Crescent sign on radionuclide static brain imaging. Semin Nucl Med 15:67, 1985

7. Sy WM, Khatib R, Bary R: Rim and "doughnut" signs and variants: Review and reappraaisal. Clin Nucl Med 1:186, 1976

8. Sy WM, Weinberger G, Weinberger G, Ngo N, et al: Imaging patterns of subdural hematoma — a proposed classification. J Nucl Med 15:693, 1973

9. Tan RF, Gladman DD, Urowitz MB, et al: Brain scan diagnosis of central nervous system involvement in systemic lupus erythematosis. Ann Rheum Dis 37:357, 1978

10. Teates CD, Allen DM: Superficial cortical atrophy simulating bilateral subdural hematomas. Clin Nucl Med 4:156, 1976

11. Teplick SK, Van Heestum RL, Clark RE, et al: Pseudoparasagittal masses caused by displacement of the falx and superior sagittal sinus. J Nucl Med 15:1047, 1974

12. Ter Brugge KG, Meindok H: Rim sign in brain scintigraphy of epidural hematoma. J Nucl Med 14:709, 1973

13. Witherspoon LR, Tyson JW, Goodrich JK: The appearance of peripheral postsurgical activity on cerebral dynamic studies. J Nucl Med 15:709, 1974

14. Zilkha A, Irwin GA: The rim sign in epidural hematoma: Case report. J Nucl Med 17:977, 1976

STATIC PLANAR IMAGING

Decreased Uptake

COMMON: Brain death
Metallic plate in skull
Surgical defect in skull

UNCOMMON: Avascular tumors
Fingers of technologist holding head, especially
wearing a ring
Hair clips
Hydrocephalus
Intracerebral hematoma
Intracranial cysts — porencephalic, arachnoid
Subdural collections other than blood — large
Subdural hematoma — large
Subgaleal hematoma
Superior sagittal sinus thrombosis

RARE: Complete occlusion of one internal carotid
Epidural hematoma
Scalp pressing against the collimator

REFERENCES

1. Anderson PO, Gilday DL, Mikhael M, et al: Value of routine cerebral angiography in pediatric brain imaging. J Nucl Med 17:780, 1976

2. Conway JJ: The hole in the head: An artifact of early brain imaging. J Nucl Med 15:485, 1974

3. Goodman JM, Mishkin FS, Dyken M: Determination of brain death by isotope angiography. JAMA 209:1869, 1969

4. Mishkin F, Truska J: The diagnosis of intracranial cysts by means of the brain scan. Radiology 90:740, 1968

5. Silberstein EB: Causes of abnormalities reported in nuclear medicine testing. J Nucl Med 17:229, 1976

6. Silberstein EB: Epidural hematoma with decreased radionuclide uptake. J Nucl Med 15:712, 1974

7. Sy WM: Manifestations of subdural and epidural hematomas on gamma imaging. CRC Crit Rev Clin Radio Nucl Med 8:391, 1977

STATIC PLANAR IMAGING

Choroid Plexus Visualization

COMMON: Lack of previous perchlorate administration

UNCOMMON: Choroid plexus papilloma
Following intrathecal methotrexate
Infection
Intraventricular hemorrhage

RARE: Anoxia

REFERENCES

1. Daly MJ, Patton DP: Ventriculitis: Diagnosis with technetium-99m DTPA. J Nucl Med 19:1233, 1978

2. Fulmer LR, Sfakianakis GN: Cerebral ventricle visualization during brain scanning with 99m-Tc pertechnetate. J Nucl Med 15:202, 1974

3. Lee HK: Unilateral pyogenic ventriculitis. J Nucl Med 18:403, 1977

4. Lentle BC, Scott JR, Noujaim AA, et al: Iatrogenic alterations in radionuclide biodistributions. Semin Nucl Med 9:131, 1979

5. Logic JR, Dubousky EV, Harsh GR: Visualization of the cerebral ventricular system in an adult with 99m-Tc-DTPA. Clin Nucl Med 1:97, 1976

6. Makler PT, Gutowicz MF, Kuhl DE: Methotrexate-induced ventriculitis: Appearance on routine radionuclide scan and emission computed tomography. Clin Nucl Med 3:22, 1978

7. Moinuddin M, Rockett JF: Intraventricular hemorrhage demonstrated on brain scan. Clin Nucl Med 2:433, 1977

8. Silver L, Sham R, Klein HA: Cerebral hematoma with intraventricular bleeding. J. Nucl Med 15:639, 1974

STATIC PLANAR IMAGING

Falsely Normal

COMMON: Deeply located lesion
Lack of sufficient abnormal vascular permeability
(e.g., low grade glioma)
Lesion size smaller than resolving power of system

UNCOMMON: Corticosteroids
Improper timing of examination relative to injection
Improper timing of examination relative to the
disease process (e.g., cerebrovascular accident)
Recent administration of tin (e.g., prior bone scan)

RARE: Hyperaluminumemia
Inability to flex head to demonstrate posterior fossa

REFERENCES

1. Fletcher JW, George EA, Henry RE, et al: Brain scans, dexamethasone therapy, and brain tumors. JAMA 232:1261, 1975

2. Khentigari A, Garrett M, Lum D, et al: Effects of prior administration of Sn(II) complexes on in vivo distribution of 99m-Tc-sodium pertechnetate. J Nucl Med 17:380, 1976

3. Lentle BC, Scott JR, Noujaim AA, et al: Iatrogenic alterations in radionuclide biodistributions. Semin Nucl Med 9:131, 1979

4. Lewis SE, Hickey DC, Parkey RW: Radionuclide brain imaging — its role and relation to CT scanning computerized tomography. Comput Tomogr 2:155, 1978

5. McRae J, Sugar RM, Shipley B, et al: Alterations in tissue distribution of 99m-Tc-pertechnetate in rats given stannous tin. J Nucl Med 15:157, 1974

6. Silberstein EB: Causes of abnormalities reported in nuclear medicine testing. J Nucl Med 17:229, 1976

7. Wang TST, Famwaz RA, Erser PD, et al: Altered body distribution of 99m-Tc-pertechnetate in iatrogenic hyperaluminumemia. J Nucl Med 19:381, 1978

STATIC PLANAR IMAGING

CNS Uptake of Bone Agents

COMMON: Cerebral infarction
Meningiomas (especially sphenoid wing and convexity)

UNCOMMON: Intracranial primary and metastatic lesions

RARE: Amyloidoma
Intracranial abscess
Subdural hematoma

REFERENCES

1. Fisher KC, McKusick KA, Pendergrass HP, et al: Improved brain scan specificity utilizing 99m-Tc-pertechnetate and 99m-Tc(Sn)-diphosphonate. J Nucl Med 16:705, 1975

2. Lee K, Tanaka T, Ohi T: Focally accentuated uptake in an area of increased activity in Tc-99m-HEDP brain scans. J Nucl Med 19:290, 1978

3. McQuade S, Higgins HP: 99m-Tc-polyphosphonate in diagnosing meningiomas of the sphenoid wing. J Nucl Med 15:1205, 1974

4. Moreno AJ, Brown JM, Brown TJ, et al: Scintigraphic findings in a primary cerebral amyloidoma. Clin Nucl Med 8:528, 1983

5. Mori H, Maeda T, Hisada K, et al: Cerebral infarction: A disparity between Tc-99m-pertechnetate and Tc-99m-EHDP images. Clin Nucl Med 5:310, 1980

6. Wenzel W, Heasty RG: Uptake of 99m-Tc-stannous polyphosphate in an area of cerebral infarction. J Nucl Med 15:207, 1974

CISTERNOGRAPHY

Focal Accumulation

COMMON: Arachnoid cyst
Cerebrospinal fluid extravasation
Focal atrophy secondary to surgery, trauma,
cerebrovascular accident
Meningocele and myelomeningocele
Porencephalic cyst

UNCOMMON: Cerebellar degeneration
Dandy-Walker malformation
Large cisterna magna
Leptomeningeal cyst
Subdural hematoma
Subdural injection of radionuclide

RARE: Achondroplasia
Arteriovenous malformation
Embolic vascular disease
Following decompression of Arnold-Chiari
malformation
Intravenous injection
Paget's disease
Sturge-Weber syndrome
Subdural hygroma

REFERENCES:

1. Black P, Cooper M: Posterior fossa cyst demonstrated by isotope cisternography. J Nucl Med 14:944, 1973

2. Chang JC, Jackson GL, Baltz R: Isotopic cisternography in Sturge-Weber syndrome. J Nucl Med 11:551, 1970

3. Front D, Penning L: Subcutaneous extravasation of CSF demonstration by scinticisternography. J Nucl Med 15:200, 1974

4. Gelfand MJ, Walus M, Tomsick T, et al: Nasoethmoidal encephalomeningocele demonstrated by cisternography: Case report. J Nucl Med 18:706, 1977

5. Goluboff LG: Arachnoid cyst of the posterior fossa demonstrated by isotope cisternography. J Nucl Med 14:61, 1973

6. Lusins J: Stasis of ^{111}In-DTPA in the posterior fossa in patients with cerebellar degeneration. J Nucl Med 17:349, 1976

7. Lusins J, Hiroshi N, Sorek M, et al: Cisternography and CT scanning with ^{111}In-DTPA in evaluation of posterior fossa arachnoid cysts. Clin Nucl Med 4:161, 1979

8. Maki Y, Kokubo Y, Nose T, et al: Some characteristic findings of isotope cisternograms in children. J Neurosurg 45:56, 1976

9. McClelland RR: Focally increased activity on scinticisternography: Report of two cases. J Nucl Med 17:626, 1976

10. McKusick KA: The diagnosis of traumatic cerebrospinal fluid rhinorrhea. J Nucl Med 18:1234, 1977

11. Schlesinger A, Lee VW, Fisher E, et al: Asymmetrical ventricular enlargement secondary to recent cerebrovascular accident as demonstrated by cisternography. Clin Nucl Med 10:103, 1985

12. Shreiner DP: Focally increased activity on scinticisternography. J Nucl Med 18:95, 1977

13. So SK, Ogawa T, Gerberg E, et al: Tracer accumulation in a subdural hygroma: Case report. J Nucl Med 17:119, 1976

14. Sty JR, Babbitt DP, D'Souza B: Pediatric radionuclide ventriculography. Clin Nucl Med 4:417, 1979

3

Skeletal

BONE IMAGING

Solitary Site of Uptake

COMMON: Benign primary tumor
Dental disease (e.g., pulpitis, periodontitis, recent
    tooth extraction or root canal treatments, ill-
    fitting dentures)
Fracture
Hyperostosis frontalis
Lower neck uptake on anterior view — normal
Malignant primary tumor
Metastases
Osteoarthritis
Osteomyelitis
Postsurgical changes
Shoulder uptake corresponding to handedness
Sinusitis
Uptake around orthopedic devices recently
    implanted

UNCOMMON: Abscess
Angle of Louis
Biopsy site
Calvarial foci due to cartilaginous rests
Calyx activity superimposed on a rib

Cellulitis
Cruciate ligament tear
Cyst
Fibrous dysplasia — monostotic
Flare phenomenon
Infarct
Ischiopubic synchondrosis
Prosthesis — infected
Prosthesis — loose
Radiation
Reflex sympathetic dystrophy
Sacral tubercle — normal
Shin splints
Sterile osteitis (e.g., osteitis pubis)
Stress fracture
Stroke
Sympathectomy
Urine contamination
Viable bone graft

RARE: Bone graft
Bone island
Bursitis
Caisson disease
Calcific discitis
Condensing osteitis
Costochondritis
Deltoid tuberosity — asymmetrical
Faulty electronics
Herniation pit of the femoral neck
Improper photopeak
Lyme disease
Most causes of multiple uptake not listed above
Multiple hereditary exostoses with benign or
   malignant growth
Peripheral neuropathy (e.g., alcohol, diabetes)
Plantar fasciitis
Prosthesis foreign body reaction
Schmorl's node
Scurvy
Spondylolysis
Systemic mastocytosis
Talocalcaneal coalition
Tampon simulating uptake

REFERENCES

1. Aburano T, Yokoama K, Taki J, et al: ^{99m}Tc MDP bone imaging in inflammatory enthesopathy. Clin Nucl Med 15:105, 1990

2. Aitasalo K, Ruotsalainen P: Effects of irradiation on mandibular scintigraphy. J Nucl Med 26:1263, 1985

3. Amundsen TR, Siegel MJ, Siegel BA: Osteomyelitis and infarction in sickle cell hemoglobinopathies: Differentiation by combined technetium and gallium scintigraphy. Radiology 153:807, 1984

4. Baron NW, Davis LP, Flaherty LE, et al: Scintigraphic findings in patients with shoulder pain caused by Interleukin-2. AJR 154:327, 1990

5. Bellah RD, Summerville DA, Treves ST, Micheli LJ: Low-back pain in adolescent athletes: Detection of stress injury to pars interarticularis with SPECT. AJR 180:509, 1991

6. Blie L, Cano RA, Jones E, et al: Hot spots on bone scan. Clin Nucl Med 3:351, 1978

7. Bobba RV, Fink-Bennett D: A dural calcification presenting as a solitary lesion on radionuclide bone scan. Clin Nucl Med 3:35, 1978

8. Bomanji J, Nagaraj N, Jewkes R, et al: Pachydermoperiostosis: ^{99m}Tc methylene diphosphonate scintigraphic pattern. J Nucl Med 32:1907, 1991

9. Bray ST, Partain CL, Teates CD, et al: The value of the bone scan in idiopathic regional migratory osteoporosis. J Nucl Med 20:1268, 1979

10. Brown WT, Lyons KP, Winer RL: Changing manifestations of Brown tumors on bone scan in renal osteodystrophy. J Nucl Med 19:1146, 1978

11. Cawley KA, Dvorak AD, Wilmot MD: Normal anatomic variant: Scintigraphy of the ischiopubic synchondrosis. J Nucl Med 24:14, 1983

12. Charkes ND: Mechanisms of skeletal tracer uptake. J Nucl Med 20:794, 1979

13. Coleman RE, Mashiter G, Whitaker KB, Rubens RD: Bone scan flare predicts successful systemic therapy for bone metastases. J Nucl Med 29:1354, 1988

14. Corcoran RJ, Thrall JK, Kyle RW, et al: Solitary abnormalities in bone scans of patients with extraosseous malignancies. Radiology 121:663, 1976

15. Delpassand ES, Barron BJ, Gundzik JM: Bone scintigraphy in calcific discitis of childhood. J Nucl Med 31:234, 1990

16. DeNef JJEM, VanDerVis-Melsen M: Bone scan abnormalities in child with Lyme disease. Clin Nucl Med 15:727, 1990

17. DuCret RP, Boudreau RJ, Maguire FP, Althaus SJ: Sigmoid augmentation artifact in skeletal imaging. Clin Nucl Med 13:375, 1988

18. Epstein DA, Levin EJ: Bone scintigraphy in hereditary multiple exostoses. AJR 130:331, 1978

19. Fink-Bennett DM, Benston MT: Unusual exercise-related stress fractures: Two case reports. Clin Nucl Med 9:430, 1984

20. Fink-Bennett DM, Shapiro EE: The angle of Louis: A potential pitfall ("Louie's Hot Spot") in bone scan interpretation. Clin Nucl Med 9:352, 1984

21. Fink-Bennett D, Vicuna-Rios J: The deltoid tuberosity — a potential pitfall (the "delta sign") in bone scan interpretation: Concise communication. J Nucl Med 21:211, 1980

22. Fitzer PM: Radionuclide angiography — brain and bone imaging in craniofacial fibrous dysplasia (CFD): Case report. J Nucl Med 18:709, 1977

23. Front D, Hardoff R, Levy J, et al: Bone scintigraphy in scurvy. J Nucl Med 19:916, 1978

24. Front D, Israel O: Nuclear medicine in monitoring response to cancer treatment. J Nucl Med 30:1731, 1989

25. Gallini C, DeCicco CD, Legnaioli M, Cavaciocchi A: Potential pitfall in bone scan by transcutaneous nitroglycerin. Clin Nucl Med 15:920, 1990

26. Goergen TG, Resnick D, Lomonaco A, et al: Radionuclide bone scan abnormalities in leprosy: Case reports. J Nucl Med 17:788, 1976

27. Goris ML, Gross DM, Jones HH: Variable correlation between x-ray and scintigraphy in caisson disease. Clin Nucl Med 2:55, 1977

28. Greyson ND, Kassel EE: Serial bone scan changes in recurrent bone infarction. J Nucl Med 17:184, 1976

29. Greyson ND, Tepperman PS: Three-phase bone studies in hemiplegia with reflex sympathetic dystrophy. J Nucl Med 25:423, 1984

30. Harbert J, Desai R: Small calvarial bone scan foci — normal variations. J Nucl Med 26:1144, 1985

31. Harcke HT: Bone imaging in infants and children: A review. J Nucl Med 19:324, 1978

32. Holder LE, Mackinnon SE: Reflex sympathetic dystrophy in the hands: Clinical and scintigraphic criteria. Radiology 152:517, 1984

33. Holder LE, Michael RH: The specific scintigraphic pattern of "shin splints in the lower leg": Concise communication. J Nucl Med 25:865, 1984

34. Hubner KF, Andrews GA, Hayes RL, et al: The use of rare earth radionuclides and other bone seekers in the evaluation of bone lesions in patients with multiple myeloma or solitary plasmocytoma. Radiology 125:171, 1977

35. Jap TB, Lipschutz H, Meyers C, et al: Melorheostosis. Clin Nucl Med 3:450, 1978

36. Kagen S, Rafii M, Kramer EL: Focal uptake on bone imaging in asymptomatic Schmorl's node. Clin Nucl Med 13:615, 1988

37. Lee HK, Skarzynski J: Bladder herniation in inguinal hernia detected during bone imaging. Clin Nucl Med 11:740, 1986

38. Lentle BC, Glazebrook GA, Percy JS, et al: Sympathetic denervation and the bone scan. Clin Nucl Med 2:276, 1977

39. Lisbona R, Rennie WRJ, Daniel RK: Radionuclide evaluation of free vascularized bone graft viability. AJR 134:387, 1980

40. Lisbona R, Rosenthall L: Role of radionuclide imaging in osteoid osteoma. AJR 122:77, 1979

41. McNeil BJ: Rationale for the use of bone scans in selected metastatic and primary bone tumors. Semin Nucl Med 8:336, 1978

42. Machida K, Makita K, Nishikawa J, et al: Scintigraphic manifestation of fibrous dysplasia. Clin Nucl Med 11:426, 1986

43. Mandell GA, Harcke HT: Scintigraphy of persistent vertebral transverse process epiphysis. Clin Nucl Med 12:359, 1987

44. Mandell GA, Harcke HT, Hugh J, et al: Detection of talocalcaneal coalitions by magnification bone scintigraphy. J Nucl Med 31:1797, 1990

45. Massoud M, Frankel RS: Radionuclide imaging in skeletal inflammatory and ischemic disease in children. AJR 126:382, 1976

46. Martin P: The appearance of bone scans following fractures, including immediate and long term studies. J Nucl Med 20:1227, 1979

47. Miller SW, Castronovo FP, Pendergrass HP, et al: Technetium-99m-labeled diphosphonate bone scanning in Paget's disease. AJR 121:177, 1974

48. Moreno AJ, Reeves TA, Turnbull GL: Hemangioma of bone. Clin Nucl Med 13:768, 1988

49. Moskowitz GW, Lukash F: Evaluation of bone graft viability. Semin Nucl Med XVIII:246, 1988

50. Murray IPC, Bass S: False-positive artifact in investigation of osteitis pubis. Clin Nucl Med 16:597, 1991

51. Murray IPC, Dixon J. Kohan L: SPECT for acute knee pain. Clin Nucl Med 15:828, 1990

52. Oppenheim BE, Cantez S: What causes lower neck uptake in bone scans? Radiology 124:749, 1977

53. Outwater E, Oates E: Condensing osteitis of clavicle. J Nucl Med 29:1122, 1988

54. Papanicolaou N, Wilkinson RH, Emans JB: Bone scintigraphy and radiography in young athletes with low back pain. AJR 145:1039, 1985

55. Park HM, Hunt-Reimann A, Appledorn CR, Siddiqui A: Comet-tail imaging artifact due to hot point source and faulty electronics. Clin Nucl Med 18:341, 1993

56. Pennell RG, Maurer AH, Bonakdarpour A: Stress injuries of the pars interarticularis: Radiologic classification and indications for scintigraphy. AJR 145:763, 1985

57. Prakash V, Kamel JN, Lin MS, et al: Increased skeletal localization of ^{99m}Tc-diphosphonate in paralyzed limbs. Clin Nucl Med 1:48, 1976

58. Rosenthall L, Losbona R: Role of radionuclide imaging in benign bone and joint diseases of orthopedic interest. In Freeman LM (ed): Nuclear Medicine Annual 1981. New York, Raven Press, 1981

59. Rosenthall L: Radiophosphate visualization of foreign body reaction to wear debris from total knee prosthesis. J Nucl Med 28:915, 1987

60. Sain AK: Bone scan in Tietze's syndrome. Clin Nucl Med 3:470, 1978

61. Sewell JR, Black CM, Chapman AH, et al: Quantitative scintigraphy in diagnosis and management of plantar fasciitis (calcaneal periostitis): Concise communication. J Nucl Med 21:633, 1980

62. Silberstein EB: Causes of abnormalities reported in nuclear medicine testing. J Nucl Med 17:229, 1976

63. Silberstein EB, Schneider HJ, Khodadad G, et al: Laminectomy: Effects on postoperative technetium and gallium scintigraphy. Radiology 151:785, 1984

64. Stewart CA, Siegal ME, King D, Moser L: Radionuclide and radiographic demonstration of condensing osteitis of clavicle. Clin Nucl Med 13:177, 1988

65. Sweeney DC, Greenberg JS, McAfee JG, Jacobs ER: Benign bone lesions simulating metastases on ^{99m}Tc diphosphonate imaging. Clin Nucl Med 17:134, 1992

66. Teates CD, Brower AC, Williamson BRJ, et al: Bone scan in condensing osteitis of clavicle. South Med J 71:736, 1978

67. Thomason CB, Silverman ED, Walter RD, et al: Focal bone tracer uptake associated with a herniation pit of the femoral neck. Clin Nucl Med 8:304, 1983

68. Thrall JH, Nassar G, Geslien GE, et al: Pitfalls in Tc-99m-polyphosphate skeletal imaging. AJR 121:739, 1974

69. Tong ECK, Samii M, Tchang F: Bone imaging as aid for diagnosis of osteopoikilosis. Clin Nucl Med 13:816, 1988

70. Towe DE, Garcia DA, Jansons D, et al: Bone scan in dental diseases. J Nucl Med 19:845, 1978

71. Utz JA, Lull RJ, Galvin EG: Asymptomatic total hip prosthesis: Natural history determined using Tc-99m MDP bone scans. Radiology 161:509, 1986

72. VanValenberg P, Corstens FH: Hunter's shoulder in bone imaging. Clin Nucl Med 13:62, 1988

73. Vieras F, Boyd CM: Focal renal activity in bone scans (letter to editor). J Nucl Med 17:426, 1976

74. Weiss PE, Mall JC, Hoffer PB, et al: 99m-Tc-methylene diphosphonate bone imaging in the evaluation of total hip prostheses. Radiology 133:727, 1979

75. Whyte MP, Murphy WA, Siegel BA: 99m-Tc-pyrophosphate bone imaging in osteopoikilosis, osteopathia striata, and melorheostosis. Radiology 127:439, 1978

76. Woolfenden JM, Pitt MJ, Durie BGM, et al: Comparison of bone scintigraphy and radiography in multiple myeloma. Radiology 134:723, 1980

BONE IMAGING

Multiple Sites of Uptake

COMMON: Dental disease (e.g., pulpitis, periodontitis, recent
tooth extractions, or root canal treatments, ill-
fitting dentures)
Fractures
Metastases
Osteoarthritis
Paget's disease
Postsurgical
Rheumatoid arthritis
Urine contamination

UNCOMMON: Aseptic necrosis
Bladder diverticula
Deltoid tuberosity — normal variant
Discitis
Fibrous dysplasia — polyostotic
Flare phenomenon
Hyperparathyroidism
Hypertrophic pulmonary osteoarthropathy
Insertion of iliocostalis (stippled ribs)
Lymphoma
Multiple myeloma
Myelofibrosis
Osteomalacia
Osteomyelitis
Other arthritides
Reflex sympathetic dystrophy
Renal osteodystrophy
Shin splints
Sinus disease
Stippled ribs — back muscle insertion

RARE: Acne — clavicular hyperostosis
Bone abscesses
Caisson disease
Chester-Erdheim disease
Craniometaphyseal dysplasia
Englemann's disease
Gaucher's disease

Hereditary multiple exostoses — children
Hereditary onychoosteodysplasia
Histiocytosis X
Hyperthyroidism
Hypoparathyroidism
Infantile cortical hyperostosis
Leprosy
Lyme disease
Melorheostosis
Migratory osteoporosis
Multiple primary tumors
Neurofibromatosis
Osteogenesis imperfecta
Osteopetrosis
Osteopoikilosis
Pachydermoperiostitis
Polycythemia vera
Progressive systemic sclerosis
Pseudofractures
Sarcoidosis
Scheuermann's disease
Schmorl's nodes
Sickle cell disease
Sternoclavicular hyperostosis
Systemic mastocytosis
Unilateral pulmonary hypovascularity
Waldenstrom's macroglobulinemia

REFERENCES

1. Atkins HL, Klopper JF, Ansari AN, et al: Lipid (cholesterol) granulomatosis (Chester-Erdheim disease) and congenital megacalices. Clin Nucl Med 3:324, 1978

2. Bergstedt HF, Carenfelt C, Lind MG, et al: Facial bone scintigraphy V: Differentiation of purulent from nonpurulent inflammation of the maxillary sinus. Acta Radiol Diagn 20:458, 1979

3. Charkes ND: Mechanisms of skeletal tracer uptake. J Nucl Med 20:794, 1979

4. Charkes ND, Fordham EF: Sympathetic nervous system disorders of bone: Scintigraphic detection. J Nucl Med 21:55, 1980

5. Cheng TH, Holman BL: Radionuclide assessment of Gaucher's Disease. J Nucl Med 19:1333, 1978

6. Cinti DC, Hawkins HB, Slavin JD: Radioisotope bone scanning in a case of sarcoidosis. Clin Nucl Med 10:192, 1985

7. Cooper KL, Beabout JW, Swee RG: Insufficiency fractures of the sacrum. Radiology 156:15, 1985

8. DeGeeter F: Rib lesions on bone scan after thoracotomy. Clin Nucl Med 15:40, 1990

9. Epstein DA, Alter AA, Levin EJ, et al: Bone scintigraphy in myelofibrosis. Clin Nucl Med 1:51, 1976

10. Epstein DA, Levin EJ: Bone scintigraphy in hereditary multiple exostoses. AJR 130:331, 1978

11. Fink-Bennett D, Vicuna-Rios J: The deltoid tuberosity — a potential pitfall (the "delta sign") in bone scan interpretation: Concise communication. J Nucl Med 21:211, 1980

12. Fink-Bennett D, Johnson J: Stippled ribs: A potential pitfall in bone scan interpretation. J Nucl Med 27:216, 1986

13. Fogelman I, McKillop JH, Greig WR, et al: Pseudofracture of the ribs detected by bone scanning. J Nucl Med 18:1236; 1977

14. Freeman LM (ed): Nuclear Medicine Annual 1981. New York, Raven Press, 1981

15. Gates GF: Scintigraphy of discitis. Clin Nucl Med 2:20, 1977

16. Goergen TG, Resnick D, Lomonaco A, et al: Radionuclide bone scan abnormalities in leprosy: Case reports. J Nucl Med 17:788, 1976

17. Goris ML, Gross DM, Jones HH: Variable correlation between x-ray and scintigraphy in Caisson's disease. Clin Nucl Med 2:55, 1977

18. de Graaf P, Schict EK, Pauwels KJ, et al: Bone scintigraphy in renal osteodystrophy. J Nucl Med 19:1289, 1978

19. Greene GS: Polyostotic fibrous displasia. Clin Nucl Med 9:600, 1984

20. Greyson ND, Kassel EE: Serial bone scan changes in recurrent bone infarction. J Nucl Med 17:184, 1976

21. Hudson TM: Sternocostoclavicular hyperostosis. Clin Nucl Med 9:105, 1984

22. Hudson TM, Chew FS, Manaster BJ: Scintigraphy of benign exostoses and exostotic chondrosarcomas. AJR 140:581, 1983

23. Harcke TH: Bone imaging in infants and children: A review. J Nucl Med 19:324, 1978

24. Hermann G, Goldblatt J, Levy RN, et al: Gaucher's disease type 1: Assessment of bone involvement by CT and scintigraphy. AJR 147:943, 1986

25. Helfgott S, Tannerbaum H, Rosenthall L: Radiophosphate imaging of regional migratory osteoporosis. Clin Nucl Med 3:330, 1979

26. Hisada K, Suzuki Y, Iimori M: Technetium-99m-pyrophosphate bone imaging in the evaluation of trauma. Clin Nucl Med 1:18, 1976

27. Holder LE, MacKinnon SE: Reflex sympathetic dystrophy in the hands: Clinical and scintigraphic criteria. Radiology 152:517, 1984

28. Kramer EL, Rafii M, Fazzini E, et al: Bone scan appearance of osteogenesis imperfecta in an adult. Clin Nucl Med 11:331, 1986

29. McNeil B: Rationale for the use of bone scans in selected metastatic and primary bone tumors. Semin Nucl Med 8:336, 1978

30. Madsen JL: Scintigraphic detection of clavicular hyperostosis in patient with fulminant acne. Clin Nucl Med 13:345, 1988

31. Marino GG, Robinson WL: Acute myelofibrosis: Correlation of radiographic, bone scan and biopsy findings. J Nucl Med 30:251, 1989

32. Marks MA, Tow DE, Jay M: Bone scanning in Waldenstrom's macroglobulinemia. J Nucl Med 26:1412, 1985

33. Meurman KO, Elfving S: Stress fracture in soldiers: A multifocal bone disorder. Radiology 134:483, 1980

34. Meyer JR, Shulkin BL: Flar response in Ewing's sarcoma. Clin Nucl Med 16:807, 1991

35. Miller SW, Castronovo FP, Pendergrass HP, et al: Technetium-99m-labeled diphosphonate bone scanning in Paget's disease. AJR 121:177, 1974

36. Moreno AJ, Billingsley JL, Lundy MN, et al: Scintigraphy in disseminated coccidioidomycosis. Clin Nucl Med 8:88, 1983

37. Mungovan JA, Tung GA, Lambiase RE, et al: ^{99m}Tc MDP uptake in osteopoikilosis. Clin Nucl Med 19:6, 1994

38. Nail-Patella syndrome: Hereditary onchyoosteodysplasia — diagnosis by ^{99m}Tc MDP bone scan. Clin Nucl Med 15:53, 1990

39. Namey TC, Rosenthall L: Generalized periarticular uptake of 99m-Tc-pyrophosphate in progressive systemic sclerosis. Clin Nucl Med 2:26, 1977

40. Otsuka N, Fukunaga M, Sone T, et al: Usefulness of bone imaging in diagnosis of sternocostoclavicular hyperostosis. Clin Nucl Med 11:651, 1986

41. Parker M, Cowan RJ: Symmetrical osteomyelitis of the lower extremities. Clin Nucl Med 4:303, 1979

42. Preisman R, Halpern SE: Effect of unilateral pulmonary hypovascularity on the bone scan: Case report. J Nucl Med 17:27, 1976

43. Ramseyer LTH, Leonard JC, Stacy TM: Bone scan findings in craniometaphyseal dysplasia. Clin Nucl Med 18:137, 1993

44. Reichter RE, Park H-M, Hall D: Skull defects due to Mayfield head stabilizer. Clin Nucl Med 8:553, 1983

45. Rosenbaum RC, Frieri M, Metcalfe DD: Patterns of skeletal scintigraphy and their relationship to plasma and urinary histamine levels in systemic mastocytosis. J Nucl Med 25:859, 1984

46. Rosenthall L, Burke DL: A radionuclide and radiographic diagnosis of sternocostoclavicular hyperostosis. Clin Nucl Med 11:322, 1986

47. Rosenthall L, Kaye M: Technetium-99m-pyrophosphate kinetics and imaging in metabolic bone disease. J Nucl Med 16:33, 1975

48. Sfakianakis GN, Haase GM, Ortiz VN: The value of bone scanning in the early recognition of deliberate child abuse. J Nucl Med 20:675, 1979

49. Silver L, Sarreck R: Bone scan in the hand-foot syndrome, Clin Nucl Med 9:710, 1984

50. Singh BN, Kesala A, Mehta SP, et al: Osteomalacia on bone scan simulating skeletal metastases. Clin Nucl Med 2:181, 1977

51. Singh BN, Spies SM, Mehta SP, et al: Unusual bone scan presentation in osteomalacia: Symmetrical uptake a suggestive sign. Clin Nucl Med 3:292, 1978

52. Sty JR, Babbit DR, Starshak RJ: Bone scintigraphy demonstrating Englemann's disease. Clin Nucl Med 3:69, 1978

53. Sy WM: Bone scan in primary hyperparathyroidism. J Nucl Med 15:1089, 1974

54. Terry DW, Isitman AT, Holmes RA: Radionuclide bone images in hypertrophic pulmonary osteoarthropathy. AJR 124:571, 1975

55. Tetalman M, Fordham E, Ali A, et al: Hypertrophic pulmonary osteoatrophy: An overview. J Nucl Med 20:602, 1979

56. Tien R, Barron BJ, Dhekne RD: Caffey's Disease: Nuclear medicine and radiologic correlation: A case of mistaken identity. Clin Nucl Med 13:583, 1988

57. Tondeur M, Ham HR: False-positive bone imaging. Clin Nucl Med 14:547, 1989

58. Tow DE, Garcia DA, Jansons D: Bone scan in dental diseases. J Nucl Med 19:845, 1978

59. Ueno K, Rikimaru S, Kawashima Y, et al: Bone imaging of sternocostoclavicular hyperostosis in palmoplantar pustulosis. Clin Nucl Med 11:420, 1986

60. Velchik MG, Heyman S, Makler PT, et al: Bone scintigraphy: Differentiating benign cortical irregularity of the distal femur from malignancy. J Nucl Med 25:72, 1984

61. Velchik MG, Makler PT, Alavi A: Osteomalacia: An imposter of osseous metastasis. Clin Nucl Med 10:783, 1985

62. Wagman E, Hsieh E, Schwinger A: A case of polyostotic fibrous dysplasia demonstrated by bone scan using 99m-Tc-stannous polyphosphate. Clin Nucl Med 1:215, 1976

63. Wahner HW, Kyle RA, Beabout JW: Scintigraphic evaluation of the skeleton in multiple myeloma. Mayo Clinic Proc 55:739, 1980

64. Wells RG, Sty JR: Bone scintigraphy cherubism. Clin Nucl Med 10:892, 1985

65. Whyte MP, Murphy WA, Siegel BA: 99m-Tc-pyrophosphate bone imaging in osteopoikilosis, osteopathia striata and melorheostosis. Radiology 127:439, 1978

66. Wiegmann T, Rosenthall L, Kaye M: Technetium-99m-pyrophosphate bone scans in hyperparathyroidism. J Nucl Med 18:231, 1977

67. Woolfenden JM, Pitt MJ, Durie BG, et al: Comparison of bone scintigraphy and radiography in multiple myeloma. Radiology 134:723, 1980

BONE IMAGING

Increased Uptake in an Extremity in an Adult

COMMON AND
    UNCOMMON: Disuse/paralysis
                        Infection
                        Paget's disease
                        Reflex sympathetic dystrophy
                        Sympathectomy
                        Vascular tumor in extremity

REFERENCES

1. Lin DS: Uniappendicular increased uptake in bone imaging. Semin Nucl Med XVIII:165, 1988
2. Prakash V, Kamel NJ, Lin MS, et al: Increased skeletal localization of ^{99m}Tc diphosphonate in paralyzed limbs. Clin Nucl Med 1:48, 1976

BONE IMAGING

Bilateral Lower Limb Osseous Uptake

COMMON: Arthritides (e.g., osteoarthritis, rheumatoid arthritis)
Fractures — posttraumatic
Hypertrophic pulmonary osteoarthropathy
Multiple metastases
Paget's disease
Postsurgical changes
Stress fractures

UNCOMMON: Aseptic necrosis
Fibrous dysplasia
Hyperparathyroidism
Lymphoma
Multiple exostoses — child
Multiple myeloma
Myelofibrosis
Osteomalacia
Osteomyelitis
Paralyzed limbs
Renal osteodystrophy

RARE: Acromegaly
Frostbite injury
Hyperthyroidism
Leprosy
Mastocytosis
Melorheostosis
Scurvy
Syphilis
Thrombophlebitis
Thyroid acropachy
Urine contamination

REFERENCES

1. De Luca S, McKusick KA, Winzelberg G, et al: Increased specificity of vertebral bone scans. J Nucl Med 20:674, 1979
2. Manoli RS, Sorn JS: Unilateral increased radioactivity in the lower extremities on routine Tc-99m-pyrophosphate bone imaging. Clin Nucl Med 3:374, 1978

3. Milton WJ, Datz FL: Thrombophlebitis: A potential cause for diffuse lower extremity uptake on bone imaging. Clin Nucl Med 11:26, 1986

4. Moreno AJ, Yedinak MA, Rahnema A, et al: Bone scintigraphy in latent congenital syphilis. Clin Nucl Med 10:824, 1985

5. Parker M, Cowan J: Symmetrical osteomyelitis of the lower extremities. Clin Nucl Med 4:303, 1979

6. Prakash V, Kamel NJ, Len MS, et al: Increased skeletal localization of Tc-99m-diphosphonate in paralyzed limbs. Clin Nucl Med 1:48, 1976

7. Spencer RP, Datu JA: Bilateral lower limb uptake of bone scanning agents. Semin Nucl Med 10:314, 1980

BONE IMAGING

Increased Lower Neck Uptake

COMMON: Calcified cricothyroid cartilage
           Metastases
           Normal
           Osteoarthritis
           Postsurgical

UNCOMMON: Fracture
           Osteomyelitis
           Poor tag

RARE   Metastatic calcification
       Other causes of solitary or multiple sites of uptake
         (See Gamuts)
       Paget's disease
       Rheumatoid arthritis
       Tumor (thyroid, neck, soft tissues)

REFERENCE

1. Lin DS: Increased uptake in lower neck on bone images. Semin Nucl Med
   XVIII:167, 1988

BONE IMAGING

Increased Uptake in the Patella — Unilateral and Bilateral

COMMON: Idiopathic
Chondromalacia
Osteoarthritis

UNCOMMON
AND RARE: Bursitis
Dorsal defect of the patella
Fracture
Hypertrophic pulmonary osteoarthropathy
Osteomyelitis
Paget's disease
Tumor — primary and metastatic

REFERENCES

1. Goergen TG, Resnick D, Greenway G, et al: Dorsal defect of the patella (DDP): A characteristic radiographic lesion. Radiology 130:333, 1979

2. Fogelman I, McKillop JH, Gray HW: The "hot patella" sign: Is it of any clinical significance? Concise communication. J Nucl Med 24:312, 1983

3. Kipper MS, Alazraki NP, Feiglin DH: The "hot" patella. Clin Nucl Med 7:28, 1982

4. Lin DS: "Hot" patella on bone images. Semin Nucl Med 16:218, 1986

5. Stoler B, Staple TW: Metastases to the patella. Radiology 93:853, 1969

BONE IMAGING

Linear Cortical Uptake

COMMON: Hypertrophic osteoarthropathy (primary and secondary)
Shin splints

UNCOMMON
AND RARE: Chronic venous stasis
Contiguous soft tissue tumor
Fluorosis
Leprosy
Paget's disease
Renal osteodystrophy
X-linked hypophosphatemia

REFERENCES

1. Ali A, Tetalman MR, Fordham EW, et al: Distribution of hypertrophic pulmonary osteoarthropathy. AJR 137:771, 1980
2. Datz FL: Erythema nodosum leprosum reaction of leprosy causing periostitis and the double-stripe sign on bone scan. Clin Nucl Med 12:212, 1987
3. DeVries N, Datz FL, Manaster BJ: Pachydermoperiostosis (primary hypertrophic osteoarthropathy): Radionuclide characterization. Skel Radiol 15:658, 1986
4. Kirshy DM, Dun EK, Sarkar SD, Strashun AM: Increased long-bone periosteal/cortical uptake in skeletal scintigraphy. Semin Nucl Med XXII:54, 1992

BONE IMAGING

Positive SPECT in Low Back Pain

COMMON: Any cause of solitary or multiple uptake
          Disk degeneration
          Facetal osteoarthritis

UNCOMMON: Schmorl's nodes
            Spondylolisthesis
            Spondylolysis

RARE: Hemangioma
        Pedicle fracture

REFERENCE

1. Ryan PJ, Evans PA, Gibson T, Fogelman I: Chronic low back pain: Comparison of bone SPECT with radiography and CT. Radiology 182:849, 1992

BONE IMAGING

Pediatric Patient with Acute Bone Pain — Positive Bone Scan

COMMON AND
UNCOMMON: Fractures (acute, toddlers, stress, child abuse)
Transient sinovitis
Septic arthritis
Cellulitis
Discitis
Legg-Calves-Perthes disease
Slipped femoral capital epiphysis

REFERENCES

1. Sty JR, Wells RG, Smith WB: Child with acute leg pain. Semin Nucl Med XVIII:137, 1988

BONE IMAGING

Whole Bone Uptake in a Pediatric Patient

COMMON:	Soft tissue pathology
	Cellulitis
	Lymphatic obstruction
	Venoocclusive disease
	Subperiosteal hematoma (child abuse)

UNCOMMON AND RARE:	Acute plastic bowing injury
	Arterial obstruction
	Osteomyelitis

REFERENCE

1. Glasier CM, Seibert JJ, Williamson SL: Gamut of increased whole bone activity in bone scintigraphy in children. Clin Nucl Med 17:192,1992

BONE IMAGING

Cold Defect

COMMON: Avascular necrosis (e.g., posttraumatic, sickle cell
disease, slipped capital femoral epiphysis, Legg-
Perthes disease)
Malignant bone tumors (e.g., multiple myeloma,
rarely osteogenic sarcoma)
Metastases (e.g., lung, breast)
Prosthesis or pacemaker

UNCOMMON: Barium in colon
Disuse atrophy
Electrical burn
Femoral heads — normal variant
Following radiation therapy
Jewelry, etc.
Lead shielding
Osteomyelitis (early)
Severe peripheral vascular disease

RARE: Attenuation from adipose tissue
Benign tumors (e.g., hemangioma, brown tumor of
hyperparathyroidism)
Bone cyst
Congenital absence of a pedicle
Congenital heart disease (absent sternum)
Faulty electronics
Following arthrography (transient)
Frostbite
Hemangioma
Incorrect photopeak
Parietal foramina
Parietal thinning
Pixel overflow artifact
Septic arthritis
Transient synovitis

REFERENCES

1. Antonmattei S, Tetalman MR, Lloyd TV: The multi scan appearance of eosinophilic granuloma. Clin Nucl Med 4:53, 1979

2. Bunker SR, Handmaker H, Torre DM, Schmidt WP: Pixel overflow artifacts in SPECT evaluation of skeleton. Radiology 174:229, 1990

3. Bushnell D, Shirazi P, Nhedkar N, et al: Ewing's sarcoma seen as a "cold" lesion on bone scans. Clin Nucl Med 8:172, 1983

4. Cheng TH, Holman BL: Radionuclide assessment of Gaucher's disease. J Nucl Med 19:1333, 1978

5. Danigelis JA, Fisher RL, Ozonoff MD, et al: 99m-Tc-polyphosphate bone imaging in Legg-Perthes disease. AJR 115:407, 1975

6. Embry RL, Delaplain CB: Scintigraphic pitfall in patient with steatopygia. Clin Nucl Med 17:824, 1992

7. Gelfand MJ, Ball WS, Oestreich AE, et al: Transient loss of femoral head Tc-99m diphosphonate uptake with prolonged maintenance of femoral head architecture. Clin Nucl Med 8:347, 1983

8. Gelfand MJ, Strife JL, Graham EJ, et al: Bone scintigraphy in slipped capital femoral epiphysis. Ciln Nucl Med 8:613, 1983

9. Gentili A, Miron SD, Adler LP: Review of some common artifacts in nuclear medicine. Clin Nucl Med 19:138, 1994

10. Goergen TG, Alazraki NP, Halpern SE, et al: "Cold" bone lesions: A newly recognized phenomenon of bone imaging. J Nucl Med 15:1120, 1974

11. Goergen TG, Halpern S, Alazraki N, et al: The "photon deficient" area: A new concept in bone scanning. J Nucl Med 15:495, 1974

12. Goris ML, Basso LV, Ectubanas E: Photopenic lesions in bone scintigraphy. Clin Nucl Med 5:299, 1980

13. Greyson ND, Kassel EE: Serial bone scan changes in recurrent bone infarction: J Nucl Med 17:184, 1976

14. Harcke HT: Bone imaging in infants and children: A review. J Nucl Med 19:324, 1978

15. Higgins WL: Symmetric photon deficiency in femoral heads of bone imaging: A normal variant. J Nucl Med 29:266, 1988

16. Karelitz JR, Richards JB: Pseudophotopenic defect due to barium in the colon. Clin Nucl Med 3:414, 1978

17. King MA, Weber DA, Casarett GW, et al: A study of irradiated bone. Part II. Changes in Tc-99m-pyrophosphate bone imaging. J Nucl Med 21:22, 1980

18. Kober B, Hermann HJ, Wetzel E: "Cold lesions" in bone scintigraphy. J Nucl Med 21:501, 1980

19. Levine SB, Haines JE, Larson SM, et al: Reduced skeletal localization of 99m-Tc-diphosphonate in the two cases of severe osteoporosis. Clin Nucl Med 2:318, 1977

20. Lieberman C, Hemingway DL: Photopenic defect due to penis prosthesis. Clin Nucl Med 4:481, 1979

21. Lisbona R, Rosenthall L: Assessment of bone viability by scintiscanning in frostbite injuries. J Trauma, 16:989, 1976

22. McKillop JH, Fogelman I, Boyle IT, et al: Bone scan appearance of a Paget's osteosarcoma: Failure to concentrate HEDP. J Nucl Med 18:1039, 1977

23. Makhija M, Bofill ER: Hemangioma, a rare cause of photopenic lesion on skeletal imaging. Clin Nucl Med 13:661, 1988

24. Makhija MC: Fibrosarcoma photopenic lesion on a bone scan. Clin Nucl Med 8:265, 1983

25. Mandell GAM, Harcke HT, Bowen JR, Sharkey CA: Transient photopenia of femoral head following arthrography. Clin Nucl Med 14:397, 1989

26. Prakash V: Image of Harrington Rods on a 99m-Tc-pyrophosphate scan. Clin Nucl Med 4:384, 1979

27. Rao BK, Lieberman LM: Parietal thinning: A cause for photopenia on bone scan. Clin Nucl Med 5:313, 1980

28. Russin LD, Staab EV: Unusual bone scan findings in acute osteomyelitis: Case report. J Nucl Med 17:617, 1976

29. Seo IS, Joo KG, Baeumler GR: Multiple manifestations of osteolytic lesions on bone imaging. J Nucl Med 21:896, 1980

30. Sorkin SJ, Horii SC, Passalaqua A, et al: Decreased activity on bone scan following therapeutic radiation: A source of possible error. Clin Nucl Med 3:67, 1978

31. Spencer RP: Pseudo-Legg-Perthes disease in metastatic neuroblastoma. Clin Med 4:82, 1979

32. Stadalnik RC: "Cold" spot bone imaging. Semin Nucl Med 9:2, 1979

33. Teates CD, Williamson BJR: "Hot and cold" bone lesion in acute osteomyelitis. AJR 129:517 1977

34. Thrall JH, Ghaed N, Geslien GE, et al: Pitfalls in the Tc-99m-polyphosphate skeletal imaging. AJR 121:739, 1974

35. Trackler RT, Miller KE, Sutherland PH, et al: Childhood pelvis osteomyelitis presenting as a "cold" lesion on bone scan: Case report. J Nucl Med 17:620, 1976

36. Vieras F: Radiation induced skeletal and soft tissue bone scan changes. Clin Nucl Med 2:93, 1977

37. Wahner HW, Kyle RA, Beabout JW: Scintigraphic evaluation of the skeleton in multiple myeloma. Mayo Clinic Proc 55:739, 1980

38. Williamson BJR, Sistrom CL: Femoral and acetabular photopenia associated with septic hip arthritis. Clin Nucl Med 16:52, 1991

39. Williamson BJR, Teates CD, Bray ST: Bone scanning in detecting soft tissue abnormalities. South Med J 73:853, 1980

40. Woolfenden JM, Pitt MJ, Durie BGM, et al: Bone scanning in multiple myeloma. J Nucl Med 20:647, 1979

41. Woolfenden JM, Pitt MJ, Durie BGM, et al: Comparison of bone scintigraphy and radiography in multiple myeloma. Radiology 134:723, 1980

BONE IMAGING

Cold Defect — Pediatric Patient

COMMON AND
UNCOMMON: Avascular necrosis (steroids, fracture)
Congenital absence of a pedicle
Congenital heart disease
Histiocytosis X
Infiltrative disorders (leukemia, Gaucher's)
Joint effusion
Legg-Perthes disease
Metastases (especially neuroblastoma)
Osteomyelitis
Parietal foramina
Primary tumor (osteosarcoma, Ewing's)
Radiation
Septic arthritis
Sickle cell anemia
Slipped capital femoral epiphysis
Transient synovitis

REFERENCES

1. Kloiber R, Pavlosky W, Portner O, et al: Bone scintigraphy of hip joint effusions in children. AJR 140:995, 1983

2. Mandell GA, Heyman S: Absent sternum on bone scan. Clin Nucl Med 8:327, 1983

3. Morrison SC, Adler LP: Photopenic areas on bone scanning associated with childhood leukemia. Clin Nucl Med 16:24, 1991

4. Smergel EM, Harcke H, Pizzutillo PD, Betz RR: Use of bone scintigraphy in management of slipped capital femoral epiphysis. Clin Nucl Med 12:349, 1987

5. Sty JR, Starshak RJ: Skull scintigraphy parietal foramina. Clin Nucl Med 8:87, 1983

6. Uren RF, Howman-Giles R: Cold hip sign on bone scan. Clin Nucl Med 16:553, 1991

7. Weingrad T, Heyman S, Alavi A: Cold lesions on bone scan in pediatric neoplasms. Clin Nucl Med 9:125, 1984

BONE IMAGING

Doughnut Sign — Osseous and Nonosseous

COMMON: Giant cell tumor
Metastatic carcinoma (e.g., follicular thyroid carcinoma, lung carcinoma)
Myocardial infarction
Primary tumor (Lung)

UNCOMMON: Amyloidosis (Cardiac)
Breast prosthesis
Coccidioidomycosis osteomyelitis
Craniotomy flap
Cystic ameloblastoma
Hematoma (in ovarian cyst, subperiosteal)
Hyperostosis frontalis
Meningioma
Mucocele
Multiple myeloma
Osteoporosis
Pregnancy

REFERENCES

1. Chun JH, Ackerman L, Subramanian K, et al: Doughnut sign on bone scintigraphy in angioblastic meningioma. Clin Nucl Med 10:48, 1985

2. Dhawan VM, Turner JW, Spencer RP: Osseous and nonosseous "doughnut" sign during bone scanning. Clin Nucl Med 5:423, 1980

3. Dionne D, Taillefer R, LeBlond R, et al: Osteoporosis circumscripta cranii: A cause for "doughnut" sign on cerebral and bone scans. Clin Nucl Med 8:377, 1983

4. Dumont M, Danais S, Taillefer R: "Doughnut" sign in avascular necrosis of the bone. Clin Nucl Med 9:44, 1984

5. Freeman ML, Van Drunnen M, Gergans G, et al: Accumulation of bone scanning agent in multiple myeloma. Clin Nucl Med 9:49, 1984

6. Front D, Hardoff R: Doughnut phenomenon in bone scintigraphy. Clin Nucl Med 3:82, 1978

7. Ghaeed N, Marsden RJ: Accumulation of ^{99m}Tc-diphosphonate in hepatic neoplasm. Radiology 126:192, 1978

8. Jayabalan V, Berry S: Accumulation of Tc-99m-pyrophosphate in breast prosthesis. Clin Nucl Med 2:452, 1977

9. Levine E, De Smet AA, Neff JR, et al: Scintigraphic evaluaton of giant cell tumor of bone. AJR 143:343, 1984

10. Mandell GA, Harcke HT: Subperiosteal hematoma: Another scintigraphic "doughnut." Clin Nucl Med 11:35, 1986

11. Mandell GA, Harcke HT: Pelvic doughnut — sign of incidental pregnancy on bone scintigraphy. Clin Nucl Med 12:116, 1987

12. McGinty G, Charron M: Bull's eye appearance of hyperostosis frontalis interna. Clin Nucl Med 17:602, 1992

13. Nocera R, Nusynowitz ML, Swischuk LE, et al: The "doughnut sign" on bone scintigraphy due to coccidioidomycosis. Clin Nucl Med 8:501, 1983

14. Parkey RW, Bonte FJ, Biya LM, et al (eds): Clinical Nuclear Cardiology. New York, Appleton-Century-Crofts, 1979

15. Shih W-J, DeLand FH, Domstad PA, et al: Ring-like uptake pattern of a skeletal imaging agent in a huge renal cell carcinoma. Clin Nucl Med 11:219, 1986

16. Shibuya H, Hanafusa K, Shagdarsuren M, et al: Use of CT and scintigraphy in diagnosing cystic ameloblastoma of jaw. Clin Nucl Med 19:15, 1994

17. Silberstein EB, Daly D: Mucocele of skull. Clin Nucl Med 13:135, 1988

18. Van Nostrand D, Madewell JE, McNiesh LM, et al: Radionuclide bone scanning in giant cell tumor. J Nucl Med 27:329, 1986

19. Veluvolu P, Collier BD, Isitman AT, et al: Scintigraphic skeletal "doughnut" sign due to giant cell tumor of the fibula. Clin Nucl Med 9:631, 1984

20. Wegener WA, Williams HT: Meningioma extending through skull — a palpable lesion with scintigraphic doughnut sign. Clin Nucl Med 15:441, 1990

BONE IMAGING

Beautiful Bone Scan

COMMON: Delayed imaging — in normal patient
Metastases (e.g., breast, lung, prostate, bladder, lymphoma)
Renal osteodystrophy

UNCOMMON: Hyperparathyroidism — secondary and rarely primary
Osteomalacia
Paget's disease

RARE: Aplastic anemia
Chronic familial hyperphosphatemia
Fibrous dysplasia
Forced diuresis
Hypervitaminosis D
Leukemia
Malnutrition
Myelofibrosis
Osteoporosis
Polychondritis
Scleroderma
Systemic lupus erythematosis
Systemic mastocytosis
Waldenström's macroglobulinemia

REFERENCES

1. Cheng TH, Holman BL: Increased skeletal: Renal uptake ratio — etiology and characteristics, Radiology 136:455, 1980
2. de Graaf P, Schicht IM, Pauwels EKJ, et al: Bone scintigraphy in renal osteodystrophy. J Nucl Med 19:1289, 1978
3. Epstein DA, Alter AA, Levin EJ, et al: Bone scintigraphy in myelofibrosis. Clin Nucl Med 1:51, 1976
4. Fogelman I, Greig WR, Bessent RG, et al: Skeletal uptake of Tc-99m-HEDP in primary hyperparathyroidism. J Nucl Med 18:1040, 1977
5. Fogelman I, McKillop JH, Bessent RG, et al: The role of bone scanning in osteomalacia. J Nucl Med 19:245, 1978
6. Fogelman I, McKillop JH, Cowden EA, et al: Bone scan findings in hypervitaminosis D: Case report. J Nucl Med 18:1205, 1977

7. Gupta SM, Gupta A, Spencer RP, et al: Bone and spleen lesions in systemic mastocytosis. Clin Nucl Med 8:34, 1983

8. Holmes RA: Tc-99m-pyrophosphate in demonstrating bone disease of parathyroid dysfunction. J Nucl Med 18:309, 1977

9. Iancu TC, Almagor G, Friedman E, et al: Chronic familial hyperphosphatemia. Radiology 129:669, 1978

10. Juma S, Lin DS, Kutka N: Diffuse bone metastases in a case of astrocytoma. Clin Nucl Med 10:353, 1985

11. Karimeddini MK, Spencer RP: Forced diuresis — a cause of absent renal uptake of bone imaging agent. Clin Nucl Med 12:407, 1987

12. Kim EE, DeLand FH: Myelofibrosis presenting as hypermetabolic bone disease by radionuclide imaging in a patient with asplenia. Clin Nucl Med 3:406, 1978

13. Lubat E, Kramer EL, Sanger JJ: "Supernormal" bone image in a case of Waldenström macroglobulinemia. Clin Nucl Med 11:279, 1986

14. Lunia SL, Heravi M, Goel V, et al: Pitfalls of absent or faint kidney sign on bone scan. J Nucl Med 21:894, 1980

15. Ohashi K, Smith HS, Jacobs MP: Superscan appearance in distal renal tubular acidosis. Clin Nucl Med 16:318, 1991

16. Schatzki SS, McIlmoyle G, Lowis SL, et al: Diffuse osteoblastic metastases from an intracranial glioma. AJR 128:321, 1977

17. Sy WM, Bonventre MV, Camera A: Bone scan in mastocytosis: Case report. J Nucl Med 17:699, 1976

18. Sy WM, Patel D, Faunce H: Significance of absent or faint kidney sign on bone scan. J Nucl Med 16:454, 1975

19. Van Leendert RJM, Flendrig JA: A patient with primary hyperparathyroidism and an abnormal bone scan. Clin Nucl Med 11:701, 1986

20. Witherspoon LR, Blonde L, Shuler SE, et al: Bone scan patterns of patients with diffuse metastatic carcinoma of the axial skeleton. J Nucl Med 17:253, 1976

BONE IMAGING

Unilateral Decreased Uptake in a Limb

COMMON AND
  UNCOMMON: Amputation
               Arterial insufficiency/occlusion
               Disuse
               Following radiation therapy
               Reflex sympathetic dystrophy

REFERENCES

1. Joyce RC, Conrad G, Shih WJ, Ryo UY: Arterial thrombosis and insufficiency causing diffusely decreased uptake by skeleton of a limb. Semin Nucl Med XXI:165, 1991
2. Slavin JD, Peracha HU, Spencer RP: Reduced accumulation of ^{99m}Tc MDP in the leg related to vascular occlusion. Clin Nucl Med 12:971, 1987

BONE IMAGING

Generalized Decreased Osseous Uptake

COMMON: Congestive heart failure (e.g., myocardial infarction,
cardiomyopathy)
Idiopathic
Poor radiopharmaceutical preparation —
dissociation of tag
Poor hydration

UNCOMMON: Contrast media after injection of bone agent
Elevated aluminum levels in generator
Elevated serum aluminum levels
Iron overload (e.g., hemosiderosis, iron
supplementation)
Osteoporosis

RARE: Advanced osteopetrosis
Advanced renal osteodystrophy
Medications (e.g., phospha-soda, EHDP)
Rhabdomyolysis
Thalassemia major

REFERENCES

1. Charkes ND: Mechanisms of skeletal tracer uptake. J Nucl Med 20:794, 1979

2. Costello P, Gramm HF, Steinberg D: Simultaneous occurrence of functional asplenia and splenic accumulation of diphosphonate in metastatic breast carcinoma. J Nucl Med 18:1237, 1977

3. Crawford JA, Gumerman LW: Alteration of body distribution of ^{99m}Tc-pyrophosphate by radiographic contrast material. Clin Nucl Med 3:305, 1978

4. de Graaf P, Schicht M, Pauwels EKJ, et al: Bone scintigraphy in renal osteodystrophy. J Nucl Med 19:1289, 1978

5. Hommeyer SH, Varney DM, Eary JF: Skeletal nonvisualization in bone scan secondary to intravenous etidronate therapy. J Nucl Med 33:748, 1992

6. Levine SB, Haines JE, Larson SM, et al: Reduced skeletal localization of ^{99m}Tc-diphosphonate in two cases of severe osteoporosis. Clin Nucl Med 2:318, 1977

7. McRae J, Hambright P, Valk P, et al: Chemistry of ^{99m}Tc tracers. II. In vitro conversion of tagged HEDP and pyrophosphate (bone seekers) into gluconate (renal agent). Effects of Ca and Fe (II) on in vivo distribution. J Nucl Med 17:208, 1976

8. Parker JA, Jones AG, Davis MA, et al: Reduced uptake of bone-seeking radiopharmaceuticals related to iron excess. Clin Nucl Med 1:267, 1976

9. Saha GB, Herzberg DL, Boyd CM: Unusual in vivo distribution of ^{99m}Tc-diphosphonate. Clin Nucl Med 2:303, 1977

10. Stadalnik RC: Etidronate sodium therapy — a cause of poor skeletal radiopharmaceutical uptake. Semin Nucl Med XXI:332, 1991

BONE IMAGING

Periarticular Uptake

COMMON: Infectious arthritis
Osteoarthritis
Prosthesis — first six months following implantation
Rheumatoid arthritis

UNCOMMON: Ankylosing spondylitis
Cruciate ligament tear
Disuse osteoporosis
Fracture or tumor proximal to joint
Gout
Hypertrophic pulmonary osteoarthropathy
Juvenile rheumatoid arthritis
Polymyaglia rheumatica
Prosthesis — infection
Prosthesis — loosening
Psoriasis
Reflex sympathetic dystrophy syndrome
Reiter's syndrome
Seronegative arthritis
Synovial osteochondromatosis

RARE: Arthritis of Crohn's disease
Arthritis of ulcerative colitis
Avascular necrosis
Calcium pyrophosphate deposition disease
Congenital lipodystrophy
Enthesopathy
Exercise between injection and imaging
Gaucher's disease
Hajdu-Cheney syndrome
Hemarthrosis
Hyperparathyroidism
Interleukin-2
Intraosseous ganglion
Lyme disease
Myelofibrosis
Osteomalacia
Osteopetrosis
Other metabolic bone diseases
Pachydermoperiostitis

Pelligrini-Stieda syndrome
Pigmented villonodular synovitis
Progressive systemic sclerosis
Prosthesis foreign body reaction
Pseudoarthrosis
Regional migratory osteoporosis
Systemic lupus erythematosis
Tumor
Tumoral calcinosis

REFERENCES

1. Bekerman C, Genant HK, Hoffer PB, et al: Radionuclide imaging of the bones and joints of the hand. Radiology 118:653, 1975

2. Bray ST, Partain CL, Teates CD, et al: The value of the bone scan in idiopathic regional migratory osteoporosis. J Nucl Med 20:1268, 1979

3. Brown ML, Thrall JH, Cooper RA, et al: Radiography and scintigraphy in tumoral calcinosis. Radiology 124:757, 1977

4. Desaulniers M, Fuks A, Hawkins D, et al: Radiotechnetium polyphosphate joint imaging. J Nucl Med 15:417, 1974

5. Epstein DA, Alter AA, Levin EJ: Bone scintigraphy in myelofibrosis. Clin Nucl Med 1:51, 1976

6. Freeman LM, Weissman HS (eds): Nuclear Medicine Annual. New York, Raven Press, 1980

7. Harcke HT: Bone imaging in infants and children: A review. J Nucl Med 19:324, 1978

8. Goldman AB, Braunstein P: Augmented radioactivity on bone scans of limbs bearing osteosarcomas. J Nucl Med 16:423, 1975

9. Hoffer PB, Genant HK: Radionuclide joint imaging. Semin Nucl Med 6:121, 1976

10. Holder LE, Mackinnon SE: Reflex sympathetic dystrophy in the hands: Clinical and scintigraphic criteria. Radiology 152:517, 1984

11. Jackson ML, Goldfarb CR, Ongseng F: The offensive wrist. Clin Nucl Med 11:130, 1985

12. Krishnamurthy GT, Brickman AS, Blahd WH: Technetium 99m-sn-pyrophosphate pharmacokinetus and bone image changes in parathyroid disease. J Nucl Med 18:236, 1977

13. Lentle BC, Russell AS, Percy JS, et al: Scintigraphic findings in ankylosing spondylitis. J Nucl Med 18:524, 1977

14. Lin MS, Fawcett HD, Goodwin DA: Bone scintigraphy demonstrating arthropathy of central joints in ankylosing spondylitis. Clin Nucl Med 5:364, 1980

15. Majd M, Frankel RS: Radionuclide imaging in skeletal inflammatory and ischemic disease in children. AJR 126:832, 1976

16. Makhija MC, Lopano AJ: Intraosseous ganglion bone imaging with Tc-99m MDP. Clin Nucl Med 8:54, 1984

17. Mishkin J, Makler PT, Velchik MG: Bone imaging appearance of Pelligrini-Stieda syndrome. Clin Nucl Med 11:291, 1986

18. Namey TC, Rosenthall L: Generalized periarticular uptake of ^{99m}Tc-pyrophosphate in progressive systemic sclerosis. Clin Nucl Med 2:26, 1977

19. Namey TC, Rosenthall L: Periarticular uptake of ^{99m}technetium-diphosphonate in psoriasis. Arthritis Rheum 19:607, 1976

20. Park HM, Lambertus J: Skeletal and reticuloendothelial imaging in osteopetrosis: Case report. J Nucl Med 18:1091, 1977

21. Reeder MM, Felson B: Gamuts in Radiology. Cincinnati, Audiovisual Radiology of Cincinnati, Inc., 1975

22. Rosenthall L, Hawkins D: Radionuclide joint imaging in the diagnosis of synovial disease. Semin Arthritis Rheum 7:49, 1977

23. Salimi Z, Restrepo G: Joint scintigraphy using ^{99m}Tc pyrophosphate in experimental hemarthrosis. J Nucl Med 27:246, 1986

24. Salimi Z, Vas W, Restrepo G: Joint scintigraphy using technetium-99m pyrophosphate in experimental hemarthrosis. J Nucl Med 27:246, 1986

25. Sandler MS, Heyman S, Watts H: Localization of ^{99m}Tc methylene diphosphonate within synovial fluid in osteosarcoma. AJR 143:349, 1984

26. Sewell JR, Black CM, Chapman AH, et al: Quantitative scintigraphy in diagnosis and management of plantar fasciitis (calcaneal periostitis): Concise communication. J Nucl Med 21:633, 1980

27. Shafa MH, Fernandez-Ulloa M, Rost RC, et al: Diagnosis of aseptic necrosis of the talus by bone scintigraphy: Case report. Clin Nucl Med 8:50, 1983

28. Shuler SE, Helve WW: Peripheral joint imaging in juvenile rheumatoid arthritis. South Med J 67:789, 1974

29. Velchik MG: Acroosteolysis in a patient with Hajdu-Cheney syndrome demonstrated by bone scintigraphy. Clin Nucl Med 9:659, 1984

30. Weissberg DL, Resnick D, Taylor A, et al: Rheumatoid arthritis and its variants: Analysis of scintiphotographic, radiographic, and clinical examinations. AJR 131:665, 1978

31. Whyte MP, Murphy WA, Siegal BA: ^{99m}Tc-pyrophosphate bone imaging in osteopoikilosis, osteopathia stricita, and melorheostosis. Radiology 127:439, 1978

32. Yip TCK, House S, Griffiths HJ: Scintigraphic findings in congenital lipodystrophy. Clin Nucl Med 14:28, 1988

33. Yon JW, Spicer KM, Gordon L: Synovial visualization during Tc-99m MDP bone scanning in septic arthritis of the knee. Clin Nucl Med 8:249, 1983

34. Yudd AP, Velchik MG: Pigmented villonodular synovitis of the hip. Clin Nucl Med 10:441, 1985

BONE IMAGING

Increased Uptake in the Sacroiliac Joints

COMMON: Ankylosing spondylitis
Osteoarthritis
Trauma

UNCOMMON: Metabolic bone disease
Psoriatic spondylitis
Reiter's syndrome
Sacroiliac pyarthrosis

RARE: Acute anterior uveitis
Crohn's disease
Juxtaarticular bone abnormalities
Systemic lupus erythematosus
Ulcerative colitis

REFERENCES

1. Barrachough D, Russell AS, Percy JS: Psoriatic spondylitis: A clinical radiological and scintiscan survey. J Rheumatol 4:282, 1977

2. Berghs H, Remans J, Drieskens L, et al: Diagnostic value of sacro-iliac joint scintigraphy with ^{99m}technetium-pyrophosphate in sacro-illiitis. Ann Rheum Dis 37:190, 1978

3. Davis P, Thomson AB, Lentle BC: Quantitative sacro-iliac scintigraphy in patients with Crohn's disease. Arthritis Rheum 21:234, 1978

4. Dequeker J, Goddeeris T, Walravens M, et al: Evaluation of sacro-illiitis: comparison of radiological and radionuclide techniques. Radiology 128:687, 1978

5. De Smet AA, Mahmood T, Robinson RG, et al: Elevated sacro-iliac joint uptake ratios in systemic lupus erythematosus. AJR 143:351, 1984

6. Lentle BC, Russell AS, Percy JS, et al: Scintigraphic findings in ankylosing spondylitis. J Nucl Med 18:524, 1977

7. Miller JH, Gates GF: Scintigraphy of sacro-iliac pyarthritis in children. JAMA 238:2701, 1977

8. Namey TC, McIntyre J, Buse M, et al: Nucleographic studies of axial spondarthritides. Arthritis Rheum 20:1058, 1977

9. Russell AS, Davis P, Percy JS, et al: the sacro-illiitis of acute Reiter's syndrome. J Rheumatol 4:293, 1977

10. Russell AS, Lentle BC, Percy JS, et al: Scintigraphy of sacro-iliac joints in acute anterior uveitis. Ann Int Med 85:606, 1976

11. Szanto E, Axelsson B, Lindvall N: Detection of sacro-illiitis. Scand J Rheumatology 6:129, 1977

BONE IMAGING

Polyarticular Involvement

COMMON: Ankylosing spondylitis
Gout
Osteoarthritis
Rheumatoid arthritis

UNCOMMON
AND RARE: Most other causes of periarticular uptake

REFERENCES

1. Beikerman C, Genant HK, Hoffer PB, et al: Radionuclide imaging of the bones and joints of the hand. Radiology 118:653, 1975

2. Desanlniers M, Fuks A, Hawkins D, et al: Radiotechnetium-polyphosphate joint imaging. J Nucl Med 15:417, 1974

3. Freeman LM, Weissmann HS (eds): Nuclear Medicine Annual 1980. New York, Raven Press, 1980

4. Hoffer PB, Genant HK: Radionuclide joint imaging. Semin Nucl Med 6:121, 1976

5. Lentle BC, Russell AS, Percy JS, et al: The scintigraphic investigation of sacro-iliac disease. J Nucl Med 18:529, 1977

6. Lin MS, Fawcett HD, Goodwin DA: Bone scintigraphy demonstrating arthropathy of central joints in ankylosing spondylitis. Clin Nucl Med 5:364, 1980

7. Reeder MM, Felson B: Gamuts in Radiology. Cincinnati, Audiovisual Radiology of Cincinnati, Inc., 1975

8. Rosenthall L, Hawkins D: Radionuclide joint imaging in the diagnosis of synovial disease. Semin Arthritis Rheum 7:49, 1977

9. Shuler SE, Helvie WW: Peripheral joint imaging in juvenile rheumatoid arthritis. South Med J 67:789, 1974

10. Weissberg DL, Resnick D, Taylor A, et al: Rheumatoid arthritis and its variants: Analysis of scintiphotographic, radiographic and clinical examinations. AJR 131:665, 1978

BONE IMAGING

Increased Arterial Blood Flow to the Hands

COMMON: Arthritis (septic, inflammatory)
Fracture
Kienbock's disease
Postsurgical
Posttrauma
Reflex sympathetic dystrophy
Technical (tourniquet effect, intraarterial injection)

UNCOMMON
AND RARE: AVM
Hemangioma
Osteoid osteoma
Synovitis
Tendinitis

REFERENCES

1. Desai A, Intenzo C: Tourniquet effect. J Nucl Med 25:697, 1984

2. Duong RB, Nishiyama H, Mantil JC, et al: Kienbock's disease: Scintigraphic demonstration in correlation with clinical, radiographic, and pathologic findings. Clin Nucl Med 7:418, 1982

3. Holder LE, Mackinnon SE: Reflex sympathetic dystrophy in hands: Clinical and scintigraphic criteria. Radiology 152:517, 1984

4. Lecklitner ML, Douglas KP: Abnormalities of hands during arterial phase of skeletal scintigraphy. Semin Nucl Med XVII:360, 1987

5. Maurer AH, Holder LE, Espinola DA, et al: Three-phase radionuclide scintigraphy of hand. Radiology 146:761, 1983

BONE IMAGING

Positive Three-Phase

COMMON: Metastatic tumor
Osteomyelitis
Paget's disease
Postsurgical
Primary bone tumor (osteoid osteoma,
   chondroblastoma, giant cell, Ewing's)
Reflex sympathetic dystrophy syndrome

UNCOMMON: Acute fracture
Arthritis
Avulsion injury
Bone graft
Cellulitis
Diabetic osteoarthropathy
Fibrous dysplasia
Heterotopic ossification
Plantar fasciitis
Sympathetic blockage
Tendinitis

RARE: Aseptic necrosis
Following radiation
Fracture malunion
Freiberg's disease
Intraosseous ganglion
Leukemia
Medial meniscus tear
Melorheostosis
Pellegrini-Stieda disease
Pigmented villonodular synovitis
Regional migratory osteoporosis
Sarcoidosis
Skeletal angiomatosis
Soft tissue tumors (MFH, hemangioma,
   adenosarcoma)
Spontaneous osteonecrosis
Traumatic myositis

REFERENCES

1. Bilchik T, Heyman S, Siegel A, Alavi A: Osteoid osteoma: Role of radionuclide bone imaging, conventional radiography and computed tomography in its management. J Nucl Med 33:269, 1992

2. Braeuning MP, Park HM: Three-phase ^{99m}Tc MDP scan findings of a soft tissue sarcoma. Clin Nucl Med 15:572, 1990

3. Davis DC, Syklawer R, Cole RL: Melorheostosis on three-phase bone scintigraphy. Clin Nucl Med 17:561, 1992

4. Delbeke D, Habibian MR: Noninflammatory entities and differential diagnosis of positive three-phase bone imaging. Clin Nucl Med 13:844, 1988

5. Ferris JV, Ziessman HA: ^{99m}Tc MDP imaging of acute radiation-induced inflammation. Clin Nucl Med 13:430, 1988

6. Ginsberg HN, Swayne LC: Three-phase bone scan in chronic myelogenous leukemia. Clin Nucl Med 12:823, 1987

7. Intenzo CM, Wapner KL, Park CH, Kim SM: Evaluation of plantar fasciitis by three-phase bone scintigraphy. Clin Nucl Med 16:325, 1991

8. Kahn D, Wilson MA: Bone scintigraphic findings in patellar tendinitis. J Nucl Med 28:1768, 1987

9. Kim SM, Desai AG, Krakovitz M, et al: Scintigraphic evaluation of regional migratory osteoporosis. Clin Nucl Med 14:36, 1988

10. Krasnow AZ, Isitman AT, Collier BD, et al: Flow study and SPECT imaging for diagnosis of giant cell tumor of bone. Clin Nucl Med 13:89, 1988

11. Krubsack AJ: Three-phase bone scan in muscular sarcoidosis. J Nucl Med 32:1829, 1991

12. Liu RS, Chou CS, Yeh SH: Three-phase bone scintigraphy in Pellegrini-Stieda disease. Clin Nucl Med 12:47, 1987

13. Makhija M, Stein I, Grossman R: Bone imaging in pigmented villonodular synovitis of the knee. Clin Nucl Med 17:340, 1992

14. Mandell GA, Harcke T, Sharkey C, Brooks K: Uterine blush in multiphase bone imaging. J Nucl Med 27:51, 1986

15. Maurer AH, Paczolt EA, Myers AR: Diagnosis of traumatic myositis of intrinsic muscles of hand by use of three-phase skeletal scintigraphy. Clin Nucl Med 15:535, 1990

16. Orzel JA, Rudd TG: Heterotopic bone formation: Clinical, laboratory, imaging correlation. J Nucl Med 26:125, 1985

17. Palestro CJ, Vega A, Kim CK, Goldsmith SJ: Paget's disease of the skull: Serendipity on gallium scintigraphy. Clin Nucl Med 15:574, 1990

18. Ramsay SC, Yeates MG, Ho LCY: Bone scanning in early assessment of nasal bone graft viability. J Nucl Med 32:33, 1991

19. Rockett JF: Demonstration of medial meniscus tear by three-phase bone imaging. Clin Nucl Med 16:47, 1991

20. Rockett JF: Three-phase radionuclide bone imaging in stress injury of anterior iliac crest. J Nucl Med 31:1554, 1990

21. Shih WJ, Magoun S, Purcell M, Domstad P: Malunion of a femoral fracture mimicking osteomyelitis in three-phase bone imaging. Clin Nucl Med 13:38, 1988

22. Smith FJ, Powe JE: Effect of sympathetic blockage on bone imaging. Clin Nucl Med 17:665, 1992

23. Sud AM, Wilson MW, Mountz JM: Unusual clinical presentation and scintigraphic pattern in myositis ossificans. Clin Nucl Med 17:198, 1992

24. Toxey J, Achong DM: Skeletal angiomatosis limited to hand: Radiographic and scintigraphic correlation. J Nucl Med 32:1912, 1991

25. Traflet R, Desai A, Park C: Spontaneous osteonecrosis of knee: Scintigraphic findings. Clin Nucl Med 12:525, 1987

26. Wardlaw JM, Best JJK: Triple-phase bone scan of an intraosseous ganglion. Clin Nucl Med 13:647, 1988

BONE IMAGING

Soft Tissue Uptake in Any Organ System

COMMON: Breast uptake — normal
Cartilage calcification (e.g., costal, thyroid, cricoid)
Cellulitis
Chronic renal failure
Electrical burn
Infarct — myocardial, cerebral, splenic
Injection site
Instrument contamination
Metastases
Muscle necrosis secondary to peripheral vascular
disease
Muscle trauma (e.g., crush injury)
Myositis ossificans
Pooling in calyces — normal
Previous technetium-99m-sulfur colloid scan
simulating uptake
Primary soft tissue tumor — benign
Primary soft tissue tumor — malignant
Radiopharmaceutical breakdown with free
technetium
Radiopharmaceutical colloid formation
Renal — normal
Urine contamination
Vascular calcification — especially femoral artery

UNCOMMON: Abscess
Adriamycin cardiotoxicity
Aneurysm
Any cause of metastatic calcification
Breast — benign disease (e.g., fibrocystic disease)
Breast — malignant
Calcific tendinitis
Cardiomyopathy
Cellulitis
Chemotherapy
Contrast media after bone dose injected
Contusion
Dermatomyositis
Following cardioversion
Hyperparathyroidism

Increased serum aluminum levels
Intestinal infarction — other causes
Intramuscular injections with local uptake (e.g., iron
    dextran, meperidine hydrochloride)
Iron dextran
Lactating breast
Lymph node visualization due to subcutaneous
    infiltration of bone agents
Lymphatic obstruction
Mitral stenosis
Myocardial contusion
Necrotizing enterocolitis
Nephrocalcinosis
Pediatrics — bowel uptake
Pediatrics — gallbladder uptake
Pericardial fluid
Pericarditis/myocarditis
Pleural fluid
Polymyositis
Renal artery stenosis
Renal obstruction
Rhabdomyolysis (e.g., alcoholism)
Soft tissue edema
Surgical wound or scar
Synovitis
Thrombophlebitis
Unstable angina
Valvular calcification

RARE: Alveolar microlithiasis
        Amyloidosis
        Aplastic anemia
        Benign Brenner tumor (ovary)
        Breast prosthesis
        Calcinosis universalis
        Chronic venous insufficiency
        Cyst (adrenal)
        Fetus
        Fibrothorax
        Filarial infestation
        Following liposuction
        Glucose-6-phosphate dehydrogenase deficiency
        Gout

Gynecomastia
Hemangioma
Hematoma
Hepatocellular disease
High dose bone scan
HIV-associated myositis
Hydroxyapatite orbital implants
Hyperhidrosis
Hypervitaminosis D
Inguinal hernia
Intraarterial injection
Klippel-Trenaunay syndrome
Liver necrosis
McArdle's syndrome
Milk-alkali syndrome
Mönckeberg's sclerosis
Neonatal subcutaneous fat necrosis
Neurofibromatosis
Osseous formation in the breast
Paraneoplastic syndrome
Paroxysmal nocturnal hemoglobinuria
Pellegrini-Stieda syndrome
Pseudogout
Radiographic contrast media extravasation
Renal stones
Sarcoidosis
Scurvy
Sickle cell disease
Sickle-thalassemia
Skin lesion of pseudoxanthoma elasticum
Subcutaneous nodules of rheumatoid arthritis
Surrounding a bone infarct
Synovial osteochondromatosis
Teratoma
Thalessemia major
Tietze's syndrome
Traumatic NG tube placement
Tumor lysis syndrome
Tumoral calcinosis
Uremic myopathy

REFERENCES

1. Abbud Y, Balanchandran S, Prince MJ, et al: Scintiscans of two siblings with tumoral calcinosis. Clin Nucl Med 4:117, 1979

2. Ajmani SK, Lerner SR, Pircher FJ: Bone scan artifact caused by hyperhidrosis: Case report. J Nucl Med 18:801, 1977

3. Aquino S, Villaneuva-Meyer J: Uptake of ^{99m}Tc MDP in soft tissues related to radiographic contrast media extravasation. Clin Nucl Med 17:974, 1992

4. Arbona GL, Antonmattci S, Tetalman MR, et al: Tc-99m-diphosphonate distribution in a patient with hypercalcemia and metastatic calcifications. Clin Nucl Med 5:422, 1980

5. Aston JK: Ovarian carcinoma detection during bone imaging. Clin Nucl Med 2:30, 1977

6. Baker J, Ali A, Groch MW, et al: Bone scanning in pregnant patients with breast carcinoma. Clin Nucl Med 12:519, 1987

7. Balanchandran S: Localization of ^{99m}Tc-Sn-pyrophosphate in liver metastasis from carcinoma of colon. Clin Nucl Med 1:165, 1976

8. Balanchandran S, Abbud Y, Prince MJ, et al: Tumoral calcinosis: Scintigraphic studies of an affected family. J Nucl Med 20:675, 1979

9. Batte WG, Yeh SDJ, Rosenblum MK, Larson SM: Intense muscle uptake of ^{67}Ga citrate and ^{99m}Tc MDP in patient with aplastic anemia. Clin Nucl Med 421, 1991

10. Baumert JE, Lantieri RL, Horning S, et al: Liver metastases of breast carcinoma detected on ^{99m}Tc-methylene diphosphate bone scan. AJR 134:389, 1980

11. Bekier A: Extraosseous accumulation of Tc-99m-pyrophosphate in soft tissue after radiation therapy. J Nucl Med 19:225, 1978

12. Blair RJ, Schroeder ET, McAfee JG, et al: Skeletal muscle uptake of bone seeking agents in both traumatic and nontraumatic rhabdomyolysis with acute renal failure. J Nucl Med 16:515, 1975

13. Bossuyt A, Verbeelen D: Accumulation of ^{99m}Tc-pyrophosphates in the skin lesions of pseudoaxanthoma elasticum. Clin Nucl Med 1:245, 1976

14. Bossuyt A, Verbeelen D, Jonckheer MH, et al: Usefulness of ^{99m}Tc-methylene diphosphonate scintigraphy in nephrocalcinosis. Clin Nucl Med 4:333, 1979

15. Braun SD, Lisbona R, Novales-Diaz JA, et al: Myocardial uptake of ^{99m}Tc-phosphate tracer in amyloidosis. Clin Nucl Med 4:244, 1979

16. Brill DR: Radionuclide imaging of nonneoplastic soft tissue disorders. Semin Nucl Med 11:277, 1981

17. Brown ML, Swee RG, Olson RJ, et al: Pulmonary uptake of ^{99m}Tc-diphosphonate in alveolar microlithiasis. AJR 131:703, 1978

18. Brown ML, Thrall JH, Cooper RA, et al: Radiography and scintigraphy in tumoral calcinosis. Radiology 124:757, 1977

19. Byun HH, Rodman SG, Chung KE: Soft tissue concentration of ^{99m}Tc-phosphates associated with injections of iron dextran complex. J Nucl Med 17:374, 1976

20. Campeau RJ, Gottlieb S, Kallos N: Aortic aneurysm detected by ^{99m}Tc-pyrophosphate imaging: Case report. J Nucl Med 18:272, 1977

21. Cannon JR, Long RF, Berens SV, et al: Metastatic abdominal implants of endometrial carcinoma demonstrated on ^{99m}Tc-methylene diphosphonate bone scan. Clin Nucl Med 3:310, 1978

22. Chaudhuri TK: Liver uptake of ^{99m}Tc-diphosphonate. Radiology 118:485, 1976

23. Chaudhuri TK, Chaudhuri TK, Go RT, et al: Uptake of [87m]Sr by liver metastasis from carcinoma of colon. J Nucl Med 14:293, 1973

24. Chaudhuri TK, Chaudhuri TK, Gulesserian HP, et al: Extraosseous noncalcified soft tissue uptake of ^{99m}Tc-polyphosphate. J Nucl Med 15:1054, 1974

25. Chhabria PK, Stankey RM, Pinsky ST: Extraskeletal uptake of [99m]Sn-pyrophosphate in hypercalcemia associated with carcinoma of the urinary bladder. Clin Nucl Med 2:87, 1977

26. Cole-Beuglet C, Kirk ME, Selouan R, et al: Bone within the breast. Report of a case with radiographic and nuclear medicine features. Radiology 119:643, 1976

27. Conway JJ, Weiss SC, Khentigan A, et al: Gallbladder and bowel localization of bone imaging radiopharmaceuticals. J Nucl Med 19:622, 1979

28. Costello P, Gramm HF, Steinberg D: Simultaneous occurrence of functional asplenia and splenic accumulation of diphosphonate in metastatic breast carcinoma. J Nucl Med 18:1237, 1977

29. Crawford JA, Gumerman LW: Alteration of body distribution of ^{99m}Tc-pyrophosphate by radiographic contrast material. Clin Nucl Med 3:305, 1978

30. Curry SL: Accumulation of ^{99m}Tc-methylene diphosphonate in an adenocarcinoma of the lung. Clin Nucl Med 4:170, 1970

31. de Graaf P, Pauwels EKJ, Schicht IM, et al: Scintigraphic detection of gastric calcification in dialysis patients. Diagn Imaging 48:171, 1979

32. de Graaf P, Schicht IM, Pauwels EKJ, et al: Detection of uremic pulmonary calcification with bone scintigraphy. J Nucl Med 19:723, 1978

33. Desai A, Eymontt M, Alavi A, et al: ^{99m}Tc-MDP uptake in nonosseous lesions. Radiology 135:181, 1980

34. Dhawan V, Sziklas JJ, Spencer RP, et al: Surgically related extravasation of urine detected on bone scan. Clin Nucl Med 2:411, 1977

35. Dhawan V, Turner JW, Spencer RP: Osseous and nonosseous "doughnut" sign during bone scanning. Clin Nucl Med 5:423, 1980

36. Dogan AS, Rezai K: Incidental lymph node visualization on bone scan due to subcutaneous infiltration of ^{99m}Tc MDP. Clin Nucl Med 18:208, 1993

37. Echevarria RA, Bonanno C, Davis DK: Uptake of ^{99m}Tc-pyrophosphate in liver necrosis. Clin Nucl Med 2:322, 1977

38. Ell PJ, Breitfellner G, Meixner M: Technetium-99m-HEDP concentration in calcified myoma. J Nucl Med 17:323, 1976

39. Ell PJ, Dixon JH, Abdullah AZ: Unusual spread of juxtacortical osteosarcoma. J Nucl Med 21:190, 1980

40. Epstein DA, Solar M, Levin EJ: Demonstration of long standing metastatic soft tissue calcification by ^{99m}Tc-diphosphonate. AJR 128:145, 1977

41. Euglenidis N, Locher JT: Tumor calcinosis imaged by bone scanning: Case report. J Nucl Med 18:34, 1977

42. Fig LM, Shapiro B, Shulkin BL: Uptake of ^{99m}Tc MDP in soft tissue calcific deposits due to tumor lysis syndrome. Clin Nucl Med 13:765, 1988

43. Fratkin MJ: Hepatic uptake of bone seeking radiopharmaceuticals. Clin Nucl Med 2:286, 1977

44. Front D, Hardoff R, Levy J, et al: Bone scintigraphy in scurvy. J Nucl Med 19:916, 1978

45. Front D, Hardoff R, Mashour N: Stomach artifact in bone scintigraphy. J Nucl Med 19:974, 1978

46. Fuller C, Leonard JC: Extraosseous localization of technetium-99m MDP in benign cystic teratoma. Clin Nucl Med 11:574, 1986

47. Garcia AC, Yeh SDJ, Benua RS: Accumulation of bone seeking radionuclides in liver metastasis from colon carcinoma. Clin Nucl Med 2:265, 1977

48. Gates GF: Ovarian carcinoma imaged by ^{99m}Tc-pyrophosphate: Case report. J Nucl Med 17:29, 1976

49. Gelfand MJ, Planitz MK: Uptake of ^{99m}Tc-diphosphonate in soft tissue in sickle cell anemia. Clin Nucl Med 2:355, 1977

50. Goldberg RP, Genant HK: Calcified bodies in popliteal cysts: A characteristic radiographic appearance. AJR 131:857, 1978

51. Gordon L, Schabel SI, Holland RD, et al: ^{99m}Tc-methylene diphosphonate accumulation in ascitic fluid due to neoplasm. Radiology 139:699, 1981

52. Goy W, Crowe WJ: Splenic accumulation of ^{99m}Tc-diphosphonate in a patient with sickle cell disease: Case report. J Nucl Med 17:108, 1976

53. Guest J, Park HM: Splenic uptake of ^{99m}Tc-diphosphonate in sickle cell disease. Clin Nucl Med 2:121, 1977

54. Guiberteau MJ, Potsaid MS, McKusick KA: Accumulation of ^{99m}Tc-diphosphonate in four patients with hepatic neoplasm: Case reports. J Nucl Med 17:1060, 1976

55. Hansen S, Stadalnik RC: Liver uptake of ^{99m}Tc-pyrophosphate. Semin Nucl Med 12:89, 1982

56. Harwood SJ: Splenic visualization using ^{99m}Tc-methylene diphosphonate in a patient with sickle cell disease. Clin Nucl Med 3:308, 1978

57. Heck LL: Extraosseous localization of phosphate bone agents. Semin Nucl Med 10:311, 1980

58. Holbert BL, Lamki LM, Holbert JM: Uptake of bone scanning agent in neurofibromatosis. Clin Nucl Med 12:66, 1987

59. Holmes RA, Mandi RS, Isitman AT: Tc-99m-labeled phosphates as an indicator of breast pathology. J Nucl Med 16:536, 1975

60. Howman-Giles R, Rahilly PM: Technetium-99m methylene diphosphonate accumulation in the diaphragm after severe ischemia. Clin Nucl Med 8:416, 1983

61. Howman-Giles RB, Gilday DL, Ash JM, et al: Splenic accumulation of Tc-99m-diphosphonate in thalassemia major. J Nucl Med 19:976, 1978

62. Howman-Giles R, McCauley D, Brown J: Multifocal pyomyositis: Diagnosis on technetium-99m MDP bone scan. Clin Nucl Med 9:149, 1984

63. Hunt J, Lewis S, Parkey R, et al: The use of technetium-99m-stannous pyrophosphate scintigraphy to identify muscle damage in acute electrical burns. J Trauma 19:409, 1979

64. Itoh K, Furudate M: Diffuse lung uptake on bone imaging in primary hyperparathyroidism before and after excision of parathyroid adenoma. Clin Nucl Med 4:382, 1979

65. Janowitz WR, Serafini AN: Intense myocardial uptake of ^{99m}Tc-diphosphonate in a uremic patient with secondary hyperparathyroidism and pericarditis: Case report. J Nucl Med 17:896, 1976

66. Jayabalan V, Berry S: Accumulation of ^{99m}Tc-pyrophosphate in breast prosthesis. Clin Nucl Med 2:452, 1977

67. Jayabalan V, DeWitt B: Gastric calcification detected in vivo by ^{99m}Tc-pyrophosphate imaging. Clin Nucl Med 3:27, 1978

68. Karanauskas S, Starshak RJ, Sty JR: Heterotopic ^{99m}Tc MDP uptake secondary to phlebitis. Clin Nucl Med 16:329, 1991

69. Kimmel RL, Sty JR: ^{99m}Tc-methylene diphosphonate renal images in a battered child. Clin Nucl Med 4:166, 1979

70. Kramer EL, Sanger JJ, Benjamin DD, et al: Detection of lacrimal gland infiltration on routine bone scintigraphy. Clin Nucl Med 8:546, 1983

71. Krasnow AZ, Collier BD, Isitman AT, et al: Diffuse muscle uptake of ^{99m}Tc MDP in patient with lung cancer. Clin Nucl Med 13:538, 1988

72. Landgarten S: Uptake of Tc-99m-pyrophosphate by the lactating breast. J Nucl Med 18:943, 1977

73. Lantieri RL, Lin MS, Martin W, et al: Increased renal accumulation of Tc-99m-MDP in renal artery stenosis. Clin Nucl Med 5:305, 1980

74. LeBel L, Carrier L, Chartrand R, Picard D: Hepatic hemangioma — unexpected bone scan finding. Clin Nucl Med 13:132, 1988

75. LeBovie J, Waxman AD, Siemsen JK: Localization of ^{99m}Tc-pyrophosphate in an islet cell tumor of the pancreas. Clin Nucl Med 3:289, 1978

76. Lee VW, Rubinow A, Pehrson J, et al: Amyloid goiter: Preoperative scintigraphic diagnosis using Tc-99m pyrophosphate. J Nucl Med 25:468, 1984

77. Lentle BC, Russell AS: Uptake of Tc-99m MDP in muscle anticipating clinical evidence of a carcinomatous myopathy. J Nucl Med 25:1320, 1984

78. Lentle BC, Scott JR, Noujaim AA, et al: Iatrogenic alterations in radionuclide biodistributions. Semin Nucl Med 9:131, 1979

79. Lessig HJ, Devenney JE: Localization of bone seeking agent within a desmoid tumor. Clin Nucl Med 4:164, 1979

80. Lieberman CM, Hemingway DL: Splenic visualization in a patient with glucose-6-phosphate dehydrogenase deficiency. Clin Nucl Med 4:405, 1979

81. Lunia S, Chandramouly BS, Chodos RB, et al: Uptake of ^{99m}Tc-methylene diphosphonate in squamous cell carcinoma of the penis. Clin Nucl Med 4:204, 1979

82. Lunia S, Chodos RB, Vedder DK: Localization of ^{99m}Tc-methylene diphosphonate in skin lesions of pseudoxanthoma elasticum. Clin Nucl Med 4:196, 1979

83. Lutrin CL, McDougall IR, Goris ML: Intense concentration of technetium 99m-pyrophosphate in the kidneys of children treated with chemotherapeutic drugs for malignant disease. Radiology 128:165, 1978

84. McCartney W, Nusynowitz ML: Reimann BEF, et al: ^{99m}Tc-diphosphonate uptake in neuroblastoma. AJR 126:1077, 1976

85. McLaughlin AF: Uptake of ^{99m}Tc-bone scanning agent by lungs with metastatic calcification. J Nucl Med 16:322, 1975

86. Manoli RS, Soin JS: Concentration of ^{99m}Tc-pyrophosphate in a benign leiomyoma of the uterus. Clin Nucl Med 2:60, 1977

87. Manoli RS, Soin JS: Unilateral increased radioactivity in the lower extremities on routine ^{99m}Tc-pyrophosphate bone imaging. Clin Nucl Med 3:374, 1978

88. Martin-Simmerman P, Cohen MD, Siddiqui A, et al: Calcification and uptake of Tc-99m diphosphonates in neuroblastomas: Concise communication. J Nucl Med 25:656, 1984

89. Numerow LM, Kloiber R, Mitchell RJ, et al: Hydroxyapatite orbital implants — Scanning with ^{99m}Tc MDP. Clin Nucl Med 19:9, 1994

90. Oren VO, Uszler JM: Liver metastases of oat cell carcinoma of lung detected on ^{99m}Tc-diphosphonate bone scan. Clin Nucl Med 3:355, 1978

91. Ortiz VN, Sfakianakis G, Haase GM, et al: The value of radionuclide scanning in early diagnosis of intestinal infarction. J Pediatr Surg 13:616, 1978

92. Orzel JA, Rudd TG: Heterotopic bone formation: Clinical, laboratory, and imaging correlation. J Nucl Med 26:125, 1985

93. Oster Z: Appearance of filarial infestations on a bone scan. J Nucl Med 17:425, 1976

94. Palestro CJ, Malat J, Collica CJ, et al: Incidental diagnosis of pregnancy on bone and gallium scintigraphy. J Nucl Med 27:370, 1986

95. Palmer-Lawrence JL, Mahan EF, Logic JR: Lateral inguinal hernia detected on routine bone scan. Clin Nucl Med 15:926, 1990

96. Park CH, Glassman LM, Thompson NL, et al: Reliability of renal imaging obtained incidentally in ^{99m}Tc-polyphosphate bone scanning. J Nucl Med 14:534, 1973

97. Parker JA, Jones AG, Davis MA, et al: Reduced uptake of bone seeking radiopharmaceuticals related to iron excess. Clin Nucl Med 1:267, 1976

98. Powers TA, Touya JJ: Tc-99m-pyrophosphate bone scan in calcinosis universalis. Clin Nucl Med 5:302, 1980

99. Prakash V, Lin MS, Perkash I: Detection of heterotopic calcification with ^{99m}Tc-pyrophosphate in spinal cord injury patients. Clin Nucl Med 3:167, 1978

100. Quaife MA, Boschult P, Baltaxe HA Jr, et al: Myocardial accumulation of labeled phosphate in malignant pericardial effusion. J Nucl Med 20:392, 1979

101. Ram Singh PS, Pujara S, Logic JR: ^{99m}Tc-pyrophosphate uptake in drug-induced gynecomastia. Clin Nucl Med 2:206, 1977

102. Renner JB, McCartney WH: Benign Brenner tumor of the ovary detected on Tc-99m methylene diphosphonate bone scan. Clin Nucl Med 9:643, 1984

103. Richards AG: Metastatic calcification detected through scanning with ^{99m}Tc-polyphosphate. J Nucl Med 15:1057, 1974

104. Richman LS, Gumerman LW, Levine G, et al: Localization of Tc-99m polyphosphate in soft tissue malignancies. AJR 124:577, 1975

105. Rosenfield N, Treves S: Osseous and extraosseous uptake of fluorine-18 and technetium-99m-polyphosphate in children with neuroblastoma. Radiology 111:127, 1974

106. Rosenthall L: ^{99m}Tc-methylene diphosphonate concentration in soft tissue malignant fibrous histiocytoma. Clin Nucl Med 3:58, 1978

107. Sagar VV, Meckelnburg RL, Chaikin HL: Bone scan in rhabdomyolysis. Clin Nucl Med 5:321, 1980

108. Sain A, Sham R, Silver L: Bone scan in sickle cell crisis. Clin Nucl Med 3:85, 1978

109. Samuels LD: Uptake of bone seeking radionuclides by malignant soft tissue tumors. J Nucl Med 19:674, 1979

110. Sarmiento AH, Alba J, Lanaro AE, et al: Evaluation of soft tissue calcifications in dermatomyositis with ^{99m}Tc-phosphate compounds: Case report. J Nucl Med 16:467, 1975

111. Sarreck R, Sham R, Alexander LL, et al: Increased ^{99m}Tc-pyrophosphate uptake with radiation pneumonitis. Clin Nucl Med 4:403, 1979

112. Schwegel DK, Lamki LM: Scintigraphic appearance of extraosseous uptake of ^{99m}Tc MDP following liposuction therapy. Clin Nucl Med 12:558, 1987

113. Scott JA, Palmer EL, Fischman AJ: HIV-associated myositis detected by radionuclide bone scanning. J Nucl Med 30:556, 1989

114. Serafini AN, Raskin MM, Zand LC, et al: Radionuclide breast scanning in carcinoma of the breast. J Nucl Med 15:1149, 1974

115. Sfakianakis GN, Damoulaki-Sfakianakis E, Bass JC, et al: Tc-99m-polyphosphate scanning in calcinosis universalis of dermatomyositis. J Nucl Med 16:568, 1975

116. Sfakianakis GN, Oritz VN, Haase GM, et al: Tc-99m-diphosphonate abdominal imaging in necrotizing enterocolitis. J Nucl Med 19:691, 1978

117. Sham R, Sain A, Silver L, et al: Localization of ^{99m}Tc-phosphate compounds in renal tumors. J Nucl Med 18:311, 1977

118. Shanley DJ, Buckner AB: Soft tissue uptake on bone scan in a patient with uremic myopathy. Clin Nucl Med 17:65, 1992

119. Siddiqui AR: Increased uptake of technetium-99m-labeled bone imaging agents in the kidney. Semin Nucl Med 12:101, 1982

120. Silberstein EB, Bove KE: Visualization of alcohol-induced rhabdomyolysis: A correlative radiotracer, histochemical, and electron microscopic study. J Nucl Med 20:127, 1979

121. Silverstein EB, Francis MD, Tofe AJ, et al: Distribution of ^{99m}Tc-Sn-diphosphonate and free ^{99m}Tc-pertechnetate in selected soft and hard tissues. J Nucl Med 16:58, 1975

122. Simpson AJ: Localization of ^{99m}Tc-pyrophosphate in an ischemic leg. Clin Nucl Med 2:400, 1977

123. Singh BN, Cisternino SJ, Kesala BA, et al: ^{99m}Tc-diphosphonate uptake in mucinous adenocarcinoma of the stomach. Clin Nucl Med 2:357, 1977

124. Singh BN, Ryerson TW, Kesala BA, et al: ^{99m}Tc-diphosphonate uptake in renal cell carcinoma. Clin Nucl Med 2:95, 1977

125. Snow RD, Lecklitner ML: Musculoskeletal findings in Klippel-Trenaunay syndrome. Clin Nucl Med 16:928, 1991

126. Spies SM, Swift TR, Brown M: Increased ^{99m}Tc-polyphosphate muscle uptake in a patient with polymyositis: Case report. J Nucl Med 16:1125, 1975

127. Starshak RJ, Hubbard AM, Sty Jr: Bone imaging: Adrenal cyst. Clin Nucl Med 8:448, 1983

128. Sty JR, Babbitt DP, Casper JT, et al: Technetium-99m-methylene diphosphonate imaging in neural crest tumors. Clin Nucl Med 4:12, 1979

129. Sty JR, Babbitt DP, Kun L: Atlas of ^{99m}Tc-methylene diphosphonate renal images in pediatric oncology. Clin Nucl Med 4:122, 1979

130. Sty JR, Babbitt DP, Sheth K: Abnormal Tc-99m-methylene diphosphonate accumulation in the kidneys of children with sickle cell disease. Clin Nucl Med 5:445, 1980

131. Swift TR, Brown M: Tc-99m-pyrophosphate muscle labeling in McArdle syndrome. J Nucl Med 19:295, 1978

132. Teates CD, Brower AC, Williamson BRJ: Osteosarcoma extraosseous metastases demonstrated on bone scans and radiographs. Clin Nucl Med 2:298, 1977

133. Teplick JG, Haskin ME, Alavi A: Calcified intraperitoneal metastases from ovarian carcinoma. AJR 127:1003, 1976

134. Thrall JH, Ghaed N, Geslien GE, et al: Pitfalls in Tc-99m-polyphosphate skeletal imaging. AJR 121:739, 1974

135. Tonami N, Sugihara M, Hisada K: Concentration of ^{99m}Tc-diphosphonate in calcified thyroid carcinoma. Clin Nucl Med 2:204, 1977

136. Truwit CL, Harshorne MF, Peters VJ: Subcutaneous ossification of legs examined by SPECT. Clin Nucl Med 13:423, 1988

137. Valdez VA, Jacobstein JB: Decreased bone uptake technetium-99m-polyphosphate in thalassemia. J Nucl Med 21:47, 1980

138. Van Antwerp JD, Hall JN, O'Mara RE: Soft tissue concentration of Tc-99m-phosphates associated with injections of iron dextran complex. J Nucl Med 18:855, 1977

139. Van Antwerp JD, O'Mara RE, Pitt MJ, et al: Technetium-99m-diphosphonate accumulation in amyloid. J Nucl Med 16:238, 1975

140. Vanek JA, Cook SA, Bukowski RM: Hepatic uptake of Tc-99m-labeled diphosphonate in amyloidosis: Case report. J Nucl Med 18:1086, 1977

141. Vieras F: Radiation-induced skeletal and soft tissue bone scan changes. Clin Nucl Med 2:93, 1977

142. Weissberg DL, Resnick D, Taylor A, et al: Rheumatoid arthritis and its variants: Analysis of scintiphotographic, radiographic, and clinical examinations. AJR 131:665, 1978

143. Williams JL, Capitanio MA, Harcke HT: Bone scanning in neonatal subcutaneous fat necrosis. J Nucl Med 19:861, 1978

144. Williamson BRJ, Teates CD, Bray ST: Bone scanning in detecting soft tissue abnormalities. South Med J 73:853, 1980

145. Winter PF: Splenic accumulation of ^{99m}Tc-diphosphonate. J Nucl Med 17:850, 1976

146. Winter PF, Perl LJ: Cold areas in bone scanning. J Nucl Med 17:755, 1976

147. Wistow BW, McAfee JG, Sagerman RH, et al: Renal uptake of ^{99m}Tc-methylene diphosphonate after radiation therapy. J Nucl Med 20:32, 1979

148. Wymer DC, Kies MS: Adrenal simulation by renal uptake of ^{99m}Tc-diphosphonate after radiotherapy. AJR 134:1256, 1980

149. Zimmer AM, Pavel DG: Experimental investigations of the possible cause of liver appearance during bone scanning. Radiology 126:813, 1978

150. Zuckier LS, Patel KA, Wexler JP, et al: Hot clot sign — a new finding in deep venous thrombosis on bone scintigraphy. Clin Nucl Med 15:790, 1990

BONE IMAGING

Diseases Causing Metastatic Calcification

COMMON: Cystic bone metastases
Hypervitaminosis D
Hyperparathyroidism (primary and secondary)
Primary bone tumors

UNCOMMON
AND RARE: Hypoparathyroidism
Iatrogenic (calcium infusion, phosphate, steroid
  therapy)
Leukemia
Lymphoma
Osteomalacia
Milk-alkali syndrome
Multiple myeloma
Sarcoidosis

REFERENCE

1. Davidson RM, Dhekne RD, Moore WH, Butler DB: Metastatic calcification in patient with malignant parathyroid carcinoma. Clin Nucl Med 15:692, 1990

BONE IMAGING

Organs Involved with Metastatic Calcification

COMMON: Kidney
Lung
Stomach

UNCOMMON: Blood vessels
Heart
Liver
Skeletal muscles
Thyroid

RARE: Cornea
Periarticular
Spleen

REFERENCE

1. Davidson RM, Dhekne RD, Moore WH, Butler DB: Metastatic calcification in patient with malignant parathyroid carcinoma. Clin Nucl Med 15:692, 1990

BONE IMAGING

Skin and Subcutaneous Tissue Uptake

COMMON   Cardioversion
Cellulitis
Electrical burns
Infiltrated injection
Spinal cord injury
Surgical wound or scar
Urine contamination
Vascular calcification — especially femoral artery

UNCOMMON: Contusion
Thrombophlebitis

RARE: Amyloidosis
Aneurysm
Calcinosis universalis
Chronic venous insufficiency
Extravasation of intravenous calcium
Extravasation of radiographic contrast
Fat necrosis
Filariasis
Following liposuction
Hemangioma
Hyperhidrosis
Injection sites
Lymph node
Lymphedema
Metastatic calcification of skin (calcinosis cutis)
Pseudoxanthoma elasticum
Radiation therapy
Subcutaneous heparin injection sites
Transcutaneous nitroglycerin
Tumor
Tumoral calcinosis

REFERENCES

1. Abbud Y, Balachandran S, Prince MJ, et al: Scintiscans of two siblings with tumoral calcinosis. Clin Nucl Med 4:117, 1979

2. Ajmani SK, Lerner SR, Pircher FJ: Bone scan artifact caused by hyperhidrosis: Case report. J Nucl Med 18:801, 1977

3. Balachandran S, Abbud Y, Prince MJ, et al: Tumoral calcinosis: Scintigraphic studies of an affected family. J Nucl Med 20:675, 1979

4. Balsam D, Goldfarb CR, Stringer B, et al: Bone scintigraphy for neonatal osteomyelitis: Simulation by extravasation of intravenous calcium. Radiology 135:185, 1980

5. Boxen I: Inadvertent lymphoscintigraphy? Clin Nucl Med 10:25, 1985

6. Brill DR: Radionuclide imaging of nonneoplastic soft tissue disorders. Semin Nucl Med 11:277, 1981

7. Brown ML, Thrall JH, Cooper RA, et al: Radiography and scintigraphy in tumoral calcinosis. Radiology 124:757, 1977

8. Chaudhuri TK, Chaudhuri TK, Go RT, et al: Uptake of [87m]Sr by liver metastasis from carcinoma of colon. J Nucl Med 14:293, 1973

9. Desai A, Eymontt M, Alavi A, et al: ^{99m}Tc-MDP uptake in nonosseous lesions. Radiology 135:181, 1980

10. Dhawan V, Sziklas JJ, Spencer RP, et al: Surgically related extravasation of urine detected on bone scan. Clin Nucl Med 8:505, 1983

11. Duong RB, Volarich DT, Fernandez-ulloa M, et al: Tc-99m MDP bone scan artifact. Clin Nucl Med 9:47, 1984

12. Euglendis N, Locher JT: Tumor calcinosis imaged by bone scanning: Case report. J Nucl Med 18:34, 1977

13. Heck LL: Extraosseous localization of phosphate bone agents. Semin Nucl Med 10:311, 1980

14. Hunt J, Lewis S, Parkey R, et al: The use of technetium-99m-stannous pyrophosphate scintigraphy to identify muscle damage in acute electrical burns. J Trauma 19:409, 1979

15. Larsen MJ, Adcock KA, Satterlee WG: Dermal uptake of technetium-99m MDP in calcinosis cutis. Clin Nucl Med 10:781, 1985

16. Lunia S, Chandramouly BS, Chodos RB, et al: Uptake of ^{99m}Tc-methylene diphosphonate in squamous cell carcinoma of the penis. Clin Nucl Med 4:204, 1979

17. Lunia S, Chodos RB, Vedder DK: Localization of ^{99m}Tc-methylene diphosphonate in skin lesions of pseudoxanthoma elasticum. Clin Nucl Med 4:196, 1979

18. Oster Z: Appearance of filarial infestations on a bone scan. J Nucl Med 17:425, 1976

19. Powers TA, Touya JJ: Tc-99m-pyrophosphate bone scan in calcinosis universalis. Clin Nucl Med 5:302, 1980

20. Prakash V, Lin MS, Perkash I: Detection of heterotopic calcification with ^{99m}Tc-pyrophosphate in spinal cord injury patients. Clin Nucl Med 3:167, 1978

21. Pugh BR, Buja LM, Parkey RW, et al: Cardioversion and "false-positive" technetium-99m stannous pyrophosphate myocardial scintigrams. Circulation 54:399, 1976

22. Sarmiento AH, Alba J, Lanaro AE, et al: Evaluation of soft tissue calcifications in dermatomyositis with ^{99m}Tc-phosphate compounds: Case report. J Nucl Med 16:467, 1975

23. Sfakianakis GN, Damoulaki-Sfakianakis E, Bass JC, et al: Tc-99m-polyphosphate scanning in calcinosis universalis of dermatomyositis. J Nucl Med 16:568, 1975

24. Shih W-J, DeLand FH, Domstad PA, et al: Unusual persistence of Tc-99m MDP uptake in the incisional scar after thoracotomy. Clin Nucl Med 9:596, 1984

25. Silberstein EB, DeLong S: Femoral artery calcification: Detection by bone scintigraphy. Clin Nucl Med 10:738, 1985

26. Thrall JH, Ghaed N, Geslien GE, et al: Pitfalls in Tc-99m-polyphosphate skeletal imaging. AJR 121:739, 1974

27. Van Antwerp JD, O'Mara RE, Pitt MJ, et al: Technetium-99m-diphosphonate accumulation in amyloid. J Nucl Med 16:238, 1975

28. Vieras F: Radiation induced skeletal and soft tissue bone scan changes. Clin Nucl Med 2:93, 1977

29. Vieras F: Serendipitous lymph node visualization during bone imaging. Clin Nucl Med 11:434, 1986

30. Wallner RJ, Dadparvar S, Croll MN, et al: Demonstration on an infected popliteal (Baker's) cyst with three-phase skeletal scintigraphy. Clin Nucl Med 10:153, 1985

31. William JL, Capitanio MA, Harcke HT: Bone scanning in neonatal subcutaneous fat necrosis. J Nucl Med 19:861, 1978

32. Williams HT, Sorsdahl OA: SPECT imaging of intense bone tracer uptake by extensive extraosseous hemangioma. Clin Nucl Med 18:358, 1993

BONE IMAGING

Skeletal Muscle and Periarticular Uptake

COMMON: Cardioversion
Electrical burns
Muscle trauma
Myositis ossificans
Peripheral vascular disease with ischemia
Rhabdomyolysis (e.g., alcoholism)

UNCOMMON: Calcific tendinitis
Dermatomyositis
Iron dextran injection
Muscular dystrophy
Polymyositis
Synovitis

RARE: Amyloidosis
Aplastic anemia
Chemoperfusion
Exertion
Frostbite
Gouty tophi
HIV-associated myositis
Klippel-Trenaunay syndrome
McArdle syndrome
Overexertion
Paraneoplastic syndrome
Pellegrini-Stieda disease
Postrevascularization
Pyomyositis
Radiotherapy
Sickle cell disease
Subcutaneous nodules of rheumatoid arthritis
Synovial osteochondromatosis
Tumor lysis syndrome
Uremic myopathy

REFERENCES

1. Alarion-Segovia D, Lazo C, Sejpulveda J, et al: Uptake of ^{99m}Tc-labeled phosphate by gouty tophi. J Rheumatol 1:314, 1974

2. Bekier A: Extraosseous accumulation of Tc-99m-pyrophosphate in soft tissue after radiation therapy. J Nucl Med 19:225, 1978

3. Blair RJ, Schroeder ET, McAfee JG, et al: Skeletal muscle uptake of bone seeking agents in both traumatic and nontraumatic rhabdomyolysis with acute renal failure. J Nucl Med 16:515, 1975

4. Brill DR: Radionuclide imaging of nonneoplastic soft tissue disorders. Semin Nucl Med 11:277, 1981

5. Byun HH, Rodman SG, Chung KE: Soft tissue concentration of ^{99m}Tc-phosphates associated with injections of iron dextran complex. J Nucl Med 17:374, 1976

6. Chaudhuri TK, Chaudhuri TK, Gulesserian HP, et al: Extraosseous noncalcified soft tissue uptake of ^{99m}Tc-polyphosphate. J Nucl Med 15:1054, 1974

7. Datz FL: Uptake of technetium-99m MDP in synovial osteochrondromatosis: Another cause of nonosseous activity on bone scan. Clin Nucl Med 367, 1984

8. Datz FL, Lewis SE, Conrad MR, et al: Pyomyositis diagnosed by radionuclide imaging and ultrasonography. South Med J 73:649, 1980

9. Ell PJ, Dixon JH, Abdullah AZ: Unusual spread of juxtacortical osteosarcoma. J Nucl Med 21:190, 1980

10. Epstein DA, Solar M, Levin EJ: Demonstration of long standing metastatic soft tissue calcification by ^{99m}Tc-diphosphonate. AJR 128:145, 1977

11. Floyd JL, Prather JL: ^{99m}Tc-EHDP uptake in ischemic muscle. Clin Nucl Med 2:281, 1977

12. Front D, Hardoff R, Levy J, et al: Bone scintigraphy in scurvy. J Nucl Med 19:916, 1978

13. Gelfand MJ, Planitz MK: Uptake of ^{99m}Tc-diphosphonate in soft tissue in sickle cell anemia. Clin Nucl Med 2:355, 1977

14. Goldberg RP, Genant HK: Calcified bodies in popliteal cysts: A characteristic radiographic appearance. AJR 131:857, 1978

15. Heck LL: Extraosseous localization of phosphate bone agents. Semin Nucl Med 10:311, 1980

16. Hunt J, Lewis S, Parkey R, et al: The use of technetium-99m-stannous pyrophosphate scintigraphy to identify muscle damage in acute electrical burns. J Trauma 19:409, 1979

17. Lee JY: Positive bone scan after strenuous physical therapy. Clin Nucl Med 8:229, 1983

18. Lentle BC, Percy JR, Regal WM, et al: Localization of Tc-99m-pyrophosphate in muscle after exercise. J Nucl Med 19:223, 1978

19. Lentle BC, Scott JR, Noujaim AA, et al: Iatrogenic alterations in radionuclide biodistributions. Semin Nucl Med 9:131, 1979

20. Prakash V, Lin MS, Perkash I: Detection of heterotopic calcification with ^{99m}Tc-pyrophosphate in spinal cord injury patients. Clin Nucl Med 3:167, 1978

21. Sagar VV, Meckelnburg RL, Chaikin HL: Bone scan in rhabdomyolysis. Clin Nucl Med 5:321, 1980

22. Sarmiento AH, Alba J, Lanaro AE, et al: Evaluation of soft tissue calcifications in dermatomyositis with ^{99m}Tc-phosphate compounds: Case Report. J Nucl Med 16:467, 1975

23. Sfakianakis GN, Damoulaki-Sfakianakis E, Bass JC, et al: Tc-99m-polyphosphate scanning in calcinosis universalis of dermatomyositis. J Nucl Med 16:568, 1975

24. Silverstein EB, Bove KE: Visualization of alcohol-induced rhabdomyolysis: A correlative radiotracer, histochemical, and electron-microscopic study. J Nucl Med 20:127, 1979

25. Simpson AJ: Localization of ^{99m}Tc-pyrophosphate in an ischemic leg. Clin Nucl Med 2:400, 1977

26. Spies SM, Swift TR, Brown M: Increased ^{99m}Tc-polyphosphate muscle uptake in a patient with polymyositis: Case Report. J Nucl Med 16:1125, 1975

27. Swift TR, Brown M: Tc-99m-pyrophosphate muscle labeling in McArdle syndrome. J Nucl Med 19:295, 1978

28. Valk P: Muscle localization of Tc-99m MDP after exertion. Clin Nucl Med 9:493, 1984

29. Van Antwerp JD, Hall JN, O'Mara RE: Soft tissue concentration of Tc-99m-phosphates associated with injections of iron dextran complex. J Nucl Med 18:855, 1977

30. Van Antwerp JD, O'Mara RE, Pitt MF, et al: Technetium-99m-diphosphonate accumulation in amyloid. J Nucl Med 16:238, 1975

31. Vieras F: Radiation induced skeletal and soft tissue bone scan changes. Clin Nucl Med 2:93, 1977

32. Weissberg DL, Resnick D, Taylor A, et al: Rheumatoid arthritis and its variants: Analysis of scintiphotographic, radiographic, and clinical examinations. AJR 131:665, 1978

33. Williamson BRJ, Teates CD, Bray ST: Bone scanning in detecting soft tissue abnormalities. South Med J 73: 853, 1980

BONE IMAGING

Increased Genitourinary Uptake

COMMON: Idiopathic
Normal
Pooling in calyces
Urinary tract obstruction

UNCOMMON: Chemotherapy
Metastatic calcification (e.g., hyperparathyroidism,
   transitional cell carcinoma, malignant melanoma)
Nephrocalcinosis
Radiation therapy

RARE: Acute pyelonephritis
Acute tubular necrosis
Antibiotics
Benign Brenner tumor of ovary
Contusion
Di Guglielmo's erythroleukemia
Fetus
Following radiographic contrast
Hematoma
Hydrocele
Iron overload
Metastases (e.g., lung carcinoma)
Multiple myeloma
Orchitis
Paroxysmal nocturnal hemoglobinuria
Phimosis
Primary renal tumors (e.g., renal cell carcinoma)
Radiation
Renal artery stenosis
Renal vein thrombosis
Scrotal lymphedema
Sickle cell anemia
Thalassemia major
Urinoma
Uterine leiomyoma
Wolman's disease

REFERENCES

1. Arbona GL, Antonmattei S, Tetalman MR, et al: Tc-99m-diphosphonate distribution in a patient with hypercalcemia and metastatic calcifications. Clin Nucl Med 5:422, 1980

2. Bossuyt A, Verbeelen D, Jonckheer MH, et al: Usefulness of ^{99m}Tc-methylene diphosphonate scintigraphy in nephrocalcinosis. Clin Nucl Med 4:333, 1979

3. Brill DR: Radionuclide imaging of nonneoplastic soft tissue disorders. Semin Nucl Med 11:277, 1981

4. Crawford JA, Gumerman LW: Alteration of body distribution of ^{99m}Tc-pyrophosphate by radiographic contrast material. Clin Nucl Med 3:305, 1978

5. Ell PJ, Breitfellner G, Meixner M: Technetiumn-99m-HEDP concentration in calcified myoma. J Nucl Med 17:323, 1976

6. Garty I, Tanzman M, Reiner S: Accumulation of technetium-99m MDP in distended ureter: A potential error in diagnosing osteoblastic bone activity. Clin Nucl Med 9:667, 1984

7. Heck LL: Extraosseous localization of phosphate bone agents. Semin Nucl Med 3:305, 1978

8. Lamki LM, Wyatt JK: Renal Vein thrombosis as a cause of excess renal accumulation on bone seeking agents. Clin Nucl Med 8:267, 1983

9. Lantieri RL, Lin MS, Martin W, et al: Increased renal accumulation of Tc-99m-MDP in renal artery stenosis. Clin Nucl Med 3:305, 1978

10. Lavelle KJ, Park HM, Moseman AM, et al: Renal hyperconcentration of ^{99m}Tc-HEDP in experimental acute tubular necrosis. Radiology 131:491, 1979

11. Lentle BC, Scott JR, Noujaim AA, et al: Iatrogenic alterations in radionuclide biodistributions. Semin Nucl Med 9:131, 1979

12. Lutrin CL, McDougall IR, Goris ML: Intense concentration of technetium-99m-pyrophosphate in the kidneys of children treated with chemotherapeutic drugs for malignant disease. Radiology 128:165, 1978

13. McCartney W, Nusynowitz ML, Reimann BEF, et al: ^{99m}Tc-diphosphonate uptake in neuroblastoma. AJR 126:1077, 1976

14. Manoli RS, Soin JS: Concentration of ^{99m}Tc-pyrophosphate in a benign leiomyoma of the uterus. Clin Nucl Med 2:60, 1977

15. Palestro C, Fineman D, Goldsmith SJ: Acute radiation nephritis — Its evolution on sequential bone imaging. Clin Nucl Med 13:789, 1988

16. Palestro CJ, Solomon RW, Kim CK, et al: Uterine leiomyomata — Discrepancy between scintigraphic and radiographic images. Clin Nucl Med 15:930, 1990

17. Park CH, Glassman LM, Thompson NL, et al: Reliability of renal imaging obtained incidentally in ^{99m}Tc-polyphosphate bone scanning. J Nucl Med 14:534, 1973

18. Parker JA, Jones AG, Davis MA, et al: Reduced uptake of bone seeking radiopharmaceuticals related to iron excess. Clin Nucl Med 1:267, 1976

19. Rao BR, Hodgens DW: Soft-tissue uptake of Tc-99m MDP in secondary scrotal lymphedema (letter to the editor). J Nucl Med 24:275, 1983

20. Sham R, Sain A, Silver L, et al: Localization of ^{99m}Tc-phosphate compounds in renal tumors. J Nucl Med 18:311, 1977

21. Siddiqui AR: Increased uptake of technetium-99m-labeled bone imaging agents in the kidney. Semin Nucl Med 12:101, 1982

22. Singh BN, Ryerson TW, Kesala BA, et al: ^{99m}Tc-diphosphonate uptake in renal cell carcinoma. Clin Nucl Med 2:95, 1977

23. Slavin JD, Skarzinski JJ, Spencer RP: Bone scans: Incidental detection of urinary tract etiology of abdominopelvic pain. Clin Nucl Med 9:667, 1984

24. Sty JR, Babbitt DP, Casper JT, et al: Technetium-99m-methylene diphosphonate imaging in neural crest tumors. Clin Nucl Med 4:12, 1979

25. Sty JR, Babbitt DP, Kun L: Atlas of ^{99m}Tc-methylene diphosphonate renal images in pediatric oncology. Clin Nucl Med 4:122, 1979

26. Sty JR, Babbitt DP, Sheth K: Abnormal Tc-99m-methylene diphosphonate accumulation in the kidneys of children with sickle cell disease. Clin Nucl Med 5:445, 1980

27. Sty JR, Starshak RJ: Scintigraphy in Wolman's disease. Clin Nucl Med 3:397, 1978

28. Swayne LC: Bone scan detection of renal vein thrombosis secondary to hypernephroma. Clin Nucl Med 11:133, 1986

29. Ward T, McClees E, Fajman W, et al: Hydrocele visualization on bone scan. Clin Nucl Med 9:360, 1984

30. Wilansky DL, Sidenberg L, Silverberg L: Renal and hepatic scintigraphy in paroxysmal nocturnal hemoglobinuria (PNH). Clin Nucl Med 10:369, 1985

31. Wistow BW, McAfee JG, Sagerman RH, et al: Renal uptake of ^{99m}Tc-methylene diphosphonate after radiation therapy. J Nucl Med 20:32, 1979

32. Wymer DC, Kies MS: Adrenal simulation by renal uptake of ^{99m}Tc-diphosphonate after radiotherapy. AJR 134:1256, 1980

BONE UPTAKE

Increased Renal Uptake — Focal

COMMON: Normal
Pooling in calyces
Urinary tract obstruction

UNCOMMON
AND RARE: Contusion
Hematoma
Metastatic calcification
Radiation
Tumor (renal cell carcinoma, metastases, etc.)

REFERENCES

1. Brill DR: Radionuclide imaging of nonneoplastic soft tissue disorders. Semin Nucl Med 11:277, 1981
2. Kimmel RL, Sty JR: ^{99m}Tc-methylene diphosphonate renal images in a battered child. Clin Nucl Med 4:166, 1979
3. Park CH, Glassman LM, Thompson NL, et al. Reliability of renal imaging obtained incidentally in ^{99m}Tc-polyphosphate bone scanning. J Nucl Med 14:534, 1973
4. Salimi Z, Vas W, Tang-Barton P, et al: Increased renal parenchymal accumulation of Tc-99m HDP in kidney contusion. Clin Nucl Med 9:574, 1984
5. Siddiqui AR: Increased uptake of technetium-99m-labeled bone imaging agents in the kidney. Semin Nucl Med 12:101, 1982
6. Singh BN, Ryerson TW, Kesala BA, et al: ^{99m}Tc-diphosphonate uptake in renal cell carcinoma. Clin Nucl Med 2:95, 1977
7. Sty JR, Babbitt DP, Kun L: Atlas of ^{99m}Tc-methylene diphosphonate renal images in pediatric oncology. Clin Nucl Med 4:122, 1979
8. Titelbaum DS, Fowble BF, Powe JE, Martinez FJ: Renal uptake of ^{99m}Tc methylene diphosphonate following therapeutic radiation for vertebral metastases. J Nucl Med 30:1113, 1989
9. Wymer DC, Kies MS: Adrenal simulation by renal uptake of ^{99m}Tc-diphosphonate after radiotherapy. AJR 134:1256, 1980

BONE IMAGING

Increased Renal Uptake — Diffuse

COMMON: Idiopathic
Urinary tract obstruction

UNCOMMON: Chemotherapy
Metastatic calcification

RARE: Acute pyelonephritis
Acute tubular necrosis
Antibiotics
Following radiographic contrast
Hepatorenal syndrome
Iron overload
Medullary sponge kidney
Multiple myeloma
Paroxysmal nocturnal hemoglobinuria
Radiation
Renal artery stenosis
Renal vein thrombosis
Sickle cell anemia
Thalassemia major

REFERENCES

1. Arbona GL, Antonmattei S, Tetalman MR, et al: Tc-99m-diphosphonate distribution in a patient with hypercalcemia and metastatic calcifications. Clin Nucl Med 5:422, 1980

2. Bernard MS, Hayward M, Hayward C, Mundy L: Evaluation of intense renal parenchymal activity (hot kidneys) on bone scintigraphy. Clin Nucl Med 15:154, 1990

3. Brill DR: Radionuclide imaging of nonneoplastic soft tissue disorders. Semin Nucl Med 11:277, 1981

4. Crawford JA, Gumerman LW: Alteration of body distribution of ^{99m}Tc-pyrophosphate by radiographic contrast material. Clin Nucl Med 3:305, 1978

5. Juweid M, Richards CH, Heyman S: Unilateral medullary sponge kidney detected on bone scan. Clin Nucl Med 18:73, 1993

6. Lamki LM, Wyatt JK: Renal vein thrombosis as a cause of excess renal accumulation of bone seeking agents. Clin Nucl Med 8:267, 1983

7. Lantieri RL, Lin MS, Martin W, et al: Increased renal accumulation of Tc-99m-MDP in renal artery stenosis. Clin Nucl Med 5:305, 1980

8. Lavelle KJ, Park HM, Moseman AM, et al: Renal hyperconcentration of ^{99m}Tc-HEDP in experimental acute tubular necrosis. Radiology 131:491, 1979

9. Lentle BC, Scott JR, Noujaim AA, et al: Iatrogenic alterations in radionuclide biodistributions. Semin Nucl Med 9:131, 1979

10. Lutrin CL, McDougall IR, Goris ML: Intense concentration of technetium-99m-pyrophosphate in the kidneys of children treated with chemotherapeutic drugs for malignant disease. Radiology 128:165, 1978

11. Parker JA, Jones AG, Davis MA, et al: Reduced uptake of bone seeking radiopharmaceuticals related to iron excess. Clin Nucl Med 1:267, 1976

12. Sheth KJ, Sty JR, Johnson F, et al: Myoglobinuria with acute renal failure and hot kidneys seen on bone imaging. Clin Nucl Med 8:498, 1984

13. Siddiqui AR: Increased uptake of technetium-99m-labeled bone imaging agents in the kidney. Semin Nucl Med 12:101, 1982

14. Sty JR, Babbitt DP, Kun L: Atlas of ^{99m}Tc-methylene diphosphonate renal images in pediatric oncology. Clin Nucl Med 4:122, 1979

15. Sty JR, Babbitt DP, Sheth K: Abnormal Tc-99m-methylene diphosphonate accumulation in the kidneys of children with sickle cell disease. Clin Nucl Med 5:445, 1980

16. Watanabe N, Shimizu M, Kageyama M, et al: Diffuse increased renal uptake on bone scintigraphy in acute tubular necrosis. Clin Nucl Med 19:19, 1994

17. Yang KTA, Lin KE, Wu SS, Wang DJ: Uptake of ^{99m}Tc MDP by renal cortex in patient with advanced hepatic disease and oliguria. Clin Nucl Med 17:143, 1992

BONE IMAGING

Increased Activity in Pelvic Soft Tissues

COMMON: Bladder diverticulum
Normal genitalia
Urinary diversion
Urine contamination

UNCOMMON: Pelvic kidney (transplant, ptosis, etc.)
Tampon-simulating uptake
Ureteral obstruction

RARE: Abscess
Aneurysm
Ascites
Extrophy of bladder
Fetus
Hydrocele
Hyperhidrosis
Inguinal hernia
Intestinal infarction
Orchitis
Peritoneal metastases
Phimosis
Scrotal lymphedema
Surgical scar
Tumor (ovarian carcinoma, embryonal cell
carcinoma, squamous cell carcinoma penis,
teratoma, cyst)
Ureteral/bladder rupture
Ureterocele
Uterine gliomyoma
Vascular calcification
Vesicovaginal fistula

REFERENCES

1. Ajmani SK, Lerner SR, Pirchen FJ: Bone scan artifact caused by hyperhidrosis. J Nucl Med 18:801, 1977
2. Cannon JR, Long RF, Berens SV, et al: Metastatic abdominal implants of endometrial carcinoma demonstrated on ^{99m}Tc methylene diphosphonate bone scan. Clin Nucl Med 3:310, 1978

3. Ell PH, Breitfellner G, Meixner M: [99m]Tc HEDP concentration in calcified myoma. J Nucl Med 17:323, 1976

4. Glassman AB, Selby JB: Another bone imaging agent false-positive: Phimosis. Clin Nucl Med 5:34, 1980

5. Goldfarb CR, Ongseng F, Kuhn M, Metzger T: Nonskeletal accumulation of bone-seeking agents: Pelvis. Semin Nucl Med XVIII:159, 1988

6. Heck LL: Extraosseous localization of phosphate bone agents. Semin Nucl Med 3:305, 1978

7. Lunia S, Chandrainouly BS, Chodos R, et al: Uptake of ^{99m}Tc methylene diphosphonate in squamous cell carcinoma of the penis. Clin Nucl Med 5:204, 1979

8. Mandell GA, Pzzica A, Zegel H, et al: Radionuclide diagnosis of hematoma of an ovarian cyst. J Nucl Med 22:930, 1981

9. Manoli RS, Soin JS: Concentration of ^{99m}Tc pyrophosphate in benign leiomyoma of uterus. Clin Nucl Med 2:60, 1977

10. Moinuudin M, Rockett JF: Ureteral rupture and bone scintigraphy. J Urol 120:365, 1978

11. Rao BR, Hodgens DW: Soft tissue uptake of ^{99m}Tc MDP in secondary scrotal lymphedema. J Nucl Med 24:275, 1983

12. Rao BK, Weir JG, Lieberman LM: Exstrophy of the bladder: Diagnosis on bone scan. Clin Nucl Med 6:552, 1981

13. Ward T, McClees E, Fajman W, et al: Hydrocele visualization on bone scan. Clin Nucl Med 9:360, 1984

BONE IMAGING

Liver Uptake — Focal or Diffuse

COMMON: Hepatic metastases (primarily colon, also breast, lung, esophagus, melanoma)
Overlying soft tissue activity simulating liver uptake
Prior technetium-99m-sulfur colloid scan simulating uptake
Radiopharmaceutical preparation causing colloid formation
Radiopharmaceutical preparation — elevated aluminum level in generator eluate

UNCOMMON: Diffuse hepatic necrosis
Elevated serum aluminum level
Injection of contrast media after bone agent injection
Metastatic calcification
Repeated iron dextran injections

RARE: Amyloidosis
Cavernous hemangioma
Primary liver tumor (e.g., cholangiocarcinoma, hepatoma, infantile hemangioendothelioma)
Thalassemia major

REFERENCES

1. Balachandran S: Localization of ^{99m}Tc-Sn-pyrophosphate in liver metastasis from carcinoma of colon. Clin Nucl Med 1:165, 1976

2. Baumert JE, Lantieri RL, Horning S, et al: Liver metastases of breast carcinoma detected on ^{99m}Tc-methylene. AJR 134:389, 1980

3. Brill DR: Radionuclide imaging of nonneoplastic soft tissue disorders. Semin Nucl Med 11:277, 1981

4. Burke T, Fukumoto D, Cohen A, et al: Hepatoma accumulation of Tc-99m hydroxymethylene diphosphonate. Clin Nucl Med 8:275, 1983

5. Burkhalter JL, Morano JU, Patel BR: Accumulation of technetium-99m MDP in a cavernous hemangioma of the liver. Clin Nucl Med 11:498, 1986

6. Chaudhuri TK: Liver uptake of ^{99m}Tc-diphosphonate. Radiology 118:485, 1976

7. Chaudhuri TK, Chaudhuri TK, Go RT, et al: Uptake of ^{87m}Sr by liver metastasis from carcinoma of colon. J Nucl Med 14:293, 1973

8. Crawford JA, Gumerman LW: Alteration of body distribution of ^{99m}Tc-pyrophosphate by radiographic contrast material. Clin Nucl Med 3:305, 1978

9. Desai AG, Schaffer B, Park CH: Accumulation of bone-scanning agents in hepatoma. Radiology 149:292, 1983

10. Eagel BA, Stier SA, Wakem C: Nonosseous bone scan abnormalities in multiple myeloma associated with hypercalcemia. Clin Nucl Med 14:869, 1988

11. Echevarria RA, Bonanno C, Davis DK: Uptake of ^{99m}Tc-pyrophosphate in liver necrosis. Clin Nucl Med 2:322, 1977

12. Ferraro EM, Alfelor FR, Lee M, Poon TT: Hepatic amyloidosis in IV drug abuser detected by bone scintigraphy. Clin Nucl Med 12:274, 1987

13. Fratkin MJ: Hepatic uptake of bone seeking radiopharmaceuticals. Clin Nucl Med 2:286, 1977

14. Garcia AC, Yeh SDJ, Benua RS: Accumulation of bone seeking radionuclides in liver metastasis from colon carcinoma. Clin Nucl Med 2:265, 1977

15. Growcock G, Lecklitner ML: Metastatic ovarian cystoadenocarcinoma during bone scintigraphy. Clin Nucl Med 8:274, 1983

16. Guiberteau MJ, Potsaid MS, McKusick KA: Accumulation of ^{99m}Tc-diphosphonate in four patients with hepatic neoplasm: Case reports. J Nucl Med 17:1060, 1976

17. Hakim S, Joo KG, Baeumler GR: Visualization of acute hepatic necrosis with a bone imaging agent. Clin Nucl Med 10:697, 1985

18. Hansen S, Stadalnik RC: Liver uptake of ^{99m}Tc-pyrophosphate. Semin Nucl Med 12:89, 1982

19. Hiltz A, Iles SE: Abnormal distribution of ^{99m}Tc iminodiphosphonate due to iron dextran therapy. Clin Nucl Med 15:818, 1990

20. Lentle BC, Scott JR, Noujaim AA, et al: Iatrogenic alterations in radionuclide biodistributions. Semin Nucl Med 9:131, 1979

21. Levy HM, Smith R: Hepatic uptake of technetium-99m diphosphonate in thalassemia major. Clin Nucl Med 11:110, 1986

22. Oren VO, Uszler JM: Liver metastases of oat cell carcinoma of lung detected on ^{99m}Tc-diphosphonate bone scan. Clin Nucl Med 3:355, 1978

23. Shih WJ, Coupal J: Diffuse and intense ^{99m}Tc HMDP localization in liver due to hypoxia secondary to respiratory failure. Clin Nucl Med 19:116, 1994

24. Shih W-J, Domstad PA, Lieber A, et al: Localization of [99M]Tc-HMDP in hepatic metastases from colonic carcinoma. AJR 146:333, 1986

25. Vanek JA, Cook SA, Bukowski RM: Hepatic uptake of Tc-99m-labeled diphosphonate in amyloidosis: Case report. J Nucl Med 18:1086, 1977

26. Zimmer AM, Pavel DG: Experimental investigations of the possible cause of liver appearance during bone scanning. Radiology 126:813, 1978

BONE IMAGING

Liver Uptake — Focal

COMMON: Hepatic metastases
Breast carcinoma
Colon carcinoma
Lung carcinoma

UNCOMMON: Hepatic metastases
Esophageal carcinoma
Lymphoma
Malignant melanoma
Osteosarcoma
Ovarian carcinoma
Prostate carcinoma

RARE: Angiosarcoma
Cavernous hemangioma
Cholangiocarcinoma
Hepatoblastoma
Hepatoma
Primary malignant liver tumor

REFERENCES

1. Balachandran S: Localization of ^{99m}Tc-Sn-pyrophosphate in liver metastasis from carcinoma of colon. Clin Nucl Med 1:165, 1976

2. Baumert JE, Lantieri RL, Horning S, et al: Liver metastases of breast carcinoma detected on ^{99m}Tc methylene. Am J Roentgenol 134:389, 1980

3. Brill DR: Radionuclide imaging of nonneoplastic soft tissue disorders. Semin Nucl Med 11:277, 1981.

4. Burkhalter JL, Morano JU, Patel Br: Accumulation of ^{99m}Tc MDP in a cavernous hemangioma of the liver. Clin Nucl Med 11:498, 1986

5. Chaudhuri TK, Chaudhuri TK, Go RT, et al: Uptake of ^{87m}Sr by liver metastasis from carcinoma of colon. J Nucl Med 14:293, 1973

6. Desai AG, Schaffer B, Park CH: Accumulation of bone scanning agents in hepatoma. Radiology 149:292, 1983

7. Garcia AC, Yeh SDJ, Benua RS: Accumulation of bone seeking radionuclides in liver metastasis from colon carcinoma. Clin Nucl Med 2:265, 1977

8. Growcock G, Lecklitner ML: Metastatic ovarian cystoadenocarcinoma during bone scintigraphy. Clin Nucl Med 8:274, 1983

9. Guiberteau MJ, Potsaid MS, McKusick KA: Accumulation of [99mTc] diphosphonate in four patients with hepatic neoplasm. J Nucl Med 17:1060, 1976

10. Ibis E, Krasnow AZ, Isitman AT, et al: Liver uptake of [99mTc]-labeled phosphate compounds: An updated gamut, 1992. Semin Nucl Med XXII:202, 1992

11. Oren VO, Uszler JM: Liver metastases of oat cell carcinoma of lung detected on [99mTc] diphosphonate bone scan. Clin Nucl Med 3:355, 1978

12. Shih WJ, Domstad PA, Lieber A, et al: Localization of [99mTc] HMDP in hepatic metastases from colonic carcinoma. Am J Roentgenol 146:333, 1986

BONE IMAGING

Liver Uptake — Diffuse

COMMON: Prior ^{99m}Tc sulfur colloid scan simulating uptake
Radiopharmaceutical preparation — elevated
aluminium level in generator eluate
Radiopharmaceutical preparation causing colloid
formation

UNCOMMON: Diffuse hepatic necrosis
Elevated serum aluminium level
Injection of contrast media after bone agent
injection
Metastatic calcification
Repeated iron dextrose injections

RARE: Amyloidosis
Thalassemia major

REFERENCES

1. Chaudhuri TK: Liver uptake of ^{99m}Tc diphosphonate. Radiology 118:485, 1976

2. Crawford JA, Gumerman LW: Alteration of body distribution of ^{99m}Tc pyrophosphate by radiographic contrast material. Clin Nucl Med 3:305, 1978

3. Echevarria RA, Bonanno C, Davis DK: Uptake of ^{99m}Tc pyrophosphate in liver necrosis. Clin Nucl Med 2:322, 1977

4. Fratkin MJ: Hepatic uptake of bone seeking radiopharmaceuticals. Clin Nucl Med 2:286, 1977

5. Hakim S, Joo KG, Baeumler GR: Visualization of acute hepatic necrosis with a bone imaging agent. Clin Nucl Med 10:697, 1985

6. Hansen S, Stadalnik RC: Liver uptake of ^{99m}Tc pyrophosphate. Semin Nucl Med 2:89, 1982

7. Lentle BC, Scott JR, Noujaim AA, et al: Iatrogenic alterations in radionuclide biodistributions. Semin Nucl Med 9:131, 1979

8. Levy HM, Smith R, Hepatic uptake of ^{99m}Tc diphosphonate in thalassemia major. Clin Nucl Med 11:110, 1986

9. Vanek JA, Cook SA, Bukowski RM: Hepatic uptake of ^{99m}Tc labeled diphosphonate in amyloidosis. J Nucl Med 18:1086, 1977

10. Zimmer AM, Pavel DG: Experimental investigations of possible cause of liver appearance during bone scanning. Radiology 126:813, 1978

BONE IMAGING

Splenic Uptake

COMMON: Hemosiderosis
            Sickle cell disease

UNCOMMON: Metastatic disease to spleen (e.g., breast, Hodgkin's
              disease)
            Sickle-thalassemia
            Thalassemia major

RARE: Angiosarcoma
            Aplastic anemia
            Autoimmune hemolytic anemia
            Glucose-6-dehydrogenase deficiency
            Iohexol injection
            Leukemia
            Lymphoma
            Splenic artery calcification
            Splenic hemangioma
            Subcapsular hematoma

REFERENCES

1. Brill DR: Radionuclide imaging of nonneoplastic soft tissue disorders. Semin Nucl Med 11:277, 1981

2. Charron M, Rosenthall L: Visualization of spleen with radiophosphate in severe combined immunodeficiency disease. Clin Nucl Med 13:339, 1988

3. Cooper SG, Strauss EB, Levine AH: Detection of noncalcified splenic hemangioma by radionuclide bone scan. J Nucl Med 30:1111, 1989

4. Costello P, Gramm HF, Steinberg D: Simultaneous occurrence of functional asplenia and splenic accumulation of diphosphonate in metastatic breast carcinoma. J Nucl Med 18:1237, 1977

5. Dravid VS, Heyman S: Splenic uptake on bone scan in autoimmune hemolytic anemia. Clin Nucl Med 15:584, 1990

6. Franceschi D, Nagel JS, Holman BL: Splenic accumulation of ^{99m}Tc methylene diphosphonate in transfusion-dependent patient with chronic myelogenous leukemia. J Nucl Med 31:1552, 1990

7. Goy W, Crowe WJ: Splenic accumulation of ^{99m}Tc-diphosphonate in a patient with sickle cell disease. Case report. J Nucl Med 17:108, 1976

8. Guest J, Park HM: Splenic uptake of ^{99m}Tc-diphosphonate in sickle cell disease. Clin Nucl Med 2:121, 1977

9. Harwood SJ: Splenic visualization using ^{99m}Tc-methylene diphosphonate in a patient with sickle cell disease. Clin Nucl Med 3:308, 1978

10. Howman-Giles RB, Gilday DL, Ash JM, et al: Splenic accumulation of Tc-99m-diphosphonate in thalassemia major. J Nucl Med 19:976, 1978

11. Lieberman CM, Hemingway DL: Splenic visualization in a patient with glucose-6-phosphate dehydrogenase deficiency. Clin Nucl Med 4:405, 1979

12. Negrin JA, Sziklas JJ, Spencer RP, et al: Resolving splenic uptake of ^{99m}Tc MDP in aplastic anemia. Clin Nucl Med 16:944, 1991

13. Poulton TB, Rauchenstein JN, Murphy WD: Diffuse liver and splenic activity with ^{99m}Tc MDP associated with iohexol injection. 17:864, 1992

14. Sain A, Sham R, Silver L: Bone scan in sickle cell crisis. Clin Nucl Med 3:85, 1978

15. Shukla LW, Lin DS, Kutka N: Splenic uptake in bone imaging. Semin Nucl Med XVIII:71, 1988

16. Spencer RP, Sziklas JJ, Zubi SM: Disassociation of splenic accumulation of ^{99m}Tc MDP and radiocolloid. Clin Nucl Med 16:747, 1991

17. Vanek JA, Cook SA, Bukowski RM: Hepatic uptake of Tc-99m-labeled diphosphonate in amyloidosis: Case report. J Nucl Med 18:1086, 1977

18. Winter PF: Splenic accumulation of ^{99m}Tc-diphosphonate. J Nucl Med 17:850, 1976

BONE IMAGING

Pulmonary Uptake

COMMON: Any cause of metastatic calcification
Fibrothorax
Metastases (e.g., osteogenic sarcoma)
Pleural fluid
Primary lung tumors (e.g., lung carcinoma,
osteogenic sarcoma)
Radiation therapy

UNCOMMON
AND RARE: Alveolar microlithiasis
Idiopathic pulmonary ossification
Infection
Liver transplantation
Mitral stenosis
Radiopharmaceutical preparation
Sarcoidosis

REFERENCES

1. Arbona GL, Antonmattei S, Tetalman MR, et al: Tc-99m-diphosphonate distribution in a patient with hypercalcemia and metastatic calcifications. Clin Nucl Med 5:422, 1980

2. Babbel RW, Jackson DE, Conte FA: ^{99m}Tc MDP accumulation in nonmalignant pleural effusion. Clin Nucl Med 13:298, 1988

3. Batte WG, Teh SDJ, Larson SM: Diffuse lung uptake of ^{99m}Tc MDP associated with pneumocystis carinii pneumonia in patient with neuroblastoma. Clin Nucl Med 16:321, 1991

4. Brill DR: Radionuclide imaging of nonneoplastic soft tissue disorders. Semin Nucl Med 11:277, 1981

5. Brown ML, Swee RG, Olson RJ, et al: Pulmonary uptake of ^{99m}Tc-diphosphonate in alveolar microlithiasis. AJR 131:703, 1978

6. Curry SL: Accumulation of ^{99m}Tc-methylene diphosphonate in an adenocarcinoma of the lung. Clin Nucl Med 4:170, 1970

7. de Graaf P, Schicht IM, Pauwels EKJ, et al: Detection of uremic pulmonary calcification with bone scintigraphy. J Nucl Med 19:723, 1978

8. DuCret RP, Boudreau RJ, Miller SJ, et al: Skeletal imaging after pleurodesis. Clin Nucl Med 12:896, 1987

9. Felson B, Schwarz J, Lukin RR, et al: Idiopathic pulmonary ossification. Radiology 153:303, 1984

10. Goldstein HA, Gefter WB: Detection of unsuspected malignant pleural effusion by bone scan. Clin Nucl Med 9:556, 1984

11. Heck LL: Extraosseous localization of phosphate bone agents. Semin Nucl Med 10:311, 1980

12. Itoh K, Furudate M: Diffuse lung uptake on bone imaging in primary hyperparathyroidism before and after excision of parathyroid adenoma. Clin Nucl Med 4:382, 1979

13. Levy HA, Park CH: Unilateral thoracic soft tissue accumulation of bone agent in lung cancer. J Nucl Med 28:1275, 1987

14. McLaughlin AF: Uptake of ^{99m}Tc-bone scanning agent by lungs with metastatic calcification. J Nucl Med 16:322, 1975

15. Peterson M: Radionuclide detection of primary pulmonary osteogenic sarcoma. J Nucl Med 31:1110, 1990

16. Raisis IP, Park CH, Yang SL, Maddrey W: Lung uptake of ^{99m}Tc phosphate compounds after liver transplantation. Clin Nucl Med 15:188, 1990

17. Ravin CE, Hoyt TS, DeBlanc H: Concentration of 99m-technetium-polyphosphate in fibrothorax following pneumonectomy. Radiology 122:405, 1977

18. Richards AG: Metastatic calcification detected through scanning with ^{99m}Tc-polyphosphate. J Nucl Med 15:1057, 1974

19. Sarreck R, Sham R, Alexander LL, et al: Increased ^{99m}Tc-pyrophosphate uptake with radiation pneumonitis. Clin Nucl Med 4:403, 1979

20. Shigeno C, Fukunaga M, Morito R, et al: Bone scintigraphy in pulmonary alveolar microlithiasis. Clin Nucl Med 7:103, 1982

21. Silberstein EB, Vasavada PJ, Hawkins H: Idiopathic pulmonary ossification with focal pulmonary uptake of technetium-99m HMDP bone scanning agent. Clin Nucl Med 10:436, 1983

22. Tatum JL, Burke TS, Hirsch JI, et al: Artifactual focal accumulation of Tc-99m bone imaging tracer in the chest: Technical note (bone imaging artifact). Clin Nucl Med 10:16, 1985

23. Teates CD, Brower AC, Williamson BRJ: Osteosarcoma extraosseous metastases demonstrated on bone scans and radiographs. Clin Nucl Med 2:298, 1977

BONE IMAGING

Gastrointestinal Uptake

COMMON: Free pertechnetate

UNCOMMON: Choleithiasis/cholecystitis
Excretion by liver in pediatric patients
Metastatic calcification
Necrotizing enterocolitis
Other causes of intestinal infarction
Surgical diversion of urine

RARE: Milk-alkali syndrome
Pediatric patients
Tumor
Vesicoenteric fistula

REFERENCES

1. Ackerman L, Elam E, Bushnell D, et al: Bowel visualization in bone scintigraphy. Semin Nucl Med XVII:81, 1987

2. Brill DR: Radionuclide imaging of nonneoplastic soft tissue disorders. Semin Nucl Med 11:277, 1981

3. Conway JJ, Weiss SC, Khentigan A, et al: Gallbladder and bowel localization of bone imaging radiopharmaceuticals. J Nucl Med 19:622, 1979

4. Corstens F, Kerremans A, Claessens R: Resolution of massive technetium-99m methylene diphosphonate uptake in the stomach in vitamin D intoxication. J Nucl Med 27:219, 1986

5. de Graaf P, Pauwels EKJ, Schicht IM, et al: Scintigraphic detection of gastric calcification in dialysis patients. Diagn Imaging 48:171, 1979

6. Delcourt E, Baudoux M, Neve P: Tc-99m-MDP bone scanning detection of gastric calcification. Clin Nucl Med 5:546, 1980

7. Front D, Hardoff R, Mashour N: Stomach artifact in bone scintigraphy. J Nucl Med 19:974, 1978

8. Goldstein R, Ryo UY, Pinsky SM: Metastatic calcification of the stomach imaged on a bone scan. Clin Nucl Med 9:591, 1984

9. Heck LL: Extraosseous localization of phosphate bone agents. Semin Nucl Med 10:311, 1980

10. Jayabalan V, DeWitt B: Gastric calcification detected in vivo by ^{99m}Tc-pyrophosphate imaging. Clin Nucl Med 3:27, 1978

11. Lentle BC, Scott JR, Noujaim AA, et al: Iatrogenic alterations in radionuclide biodistributions. Semin Nucl Med 9:131, 1979

12. McLean RG: Carcinoma of the stomach with osseous and extraosseous metastases: Visualization of primary and secondary sites with Tc-99m medronate. Clin Nucl Med 10:199, 1985

13. Makhija M, Brodie M: Vesicocolonic fistula. Clin Nucl Med 10:604, 1983

14. Ortiz VN, Sfakianakis GN, Haase GM, et al: The value of radionuclide scanning in early diagnosis of intestinal infarction. J Pediatr Surg 13:616, 1978

15. Reitz MD, Vasinrapee P, Mishkin FS: Myocardial, pulmonary, and gastric uptake of technetium-99m MDP in a patient with multiple myeloma and hypercalcemia. Clin Nucl Med 11:730, 1986

16. Sfakianakis GN, Ortiz VN, Haase GM, et al: Tc-99m-diphosphonate abdominal imaging in necrotizing enterocolitis. J Nucl Med 19:691, 1978

17. Singh BN, Cisternino SJ, Kesala BA, et al: ^{99m}Tc-diphosphonate uptake in mucinous adenocarcinoma of the stomach. Clin Nucl Med 2:357, 1977

BONE IMAGING

Breast Uptake

COMMON: Breast carcinoma
Chronic cystic mastitis
Mastoplasia
Normal
Postmastectomy

UNCOMMON: Gynecomastia
Lactation

RARE: Amyloidosis
Bone formation in the breast
Breast prosthesis
Fat necrosis
Hematoma
Other tumors
Primary osteogenic sarcoma of the breast
Superimposed pulmonary uptake

REFERENCES

1. Brill DR: Radionuclide imaging of nonneoplastic soft tissue disorders. Semin Nucl Med 11:277, 1981

2. Burnett KR, Lyons KP, Brown WT: Uptake of osteotropic radionuclides in the breast. Semin Nucl Med 14:48, 1984

3. Cole-Beuglet C, Kirk ME, Selouan R, et al: Bone within the breast. Report of a case with radiographic and nuclear medicine features. Radiology 119:643, 1976

4. Holmes RA, Mandi RS, Isitman AT: Tc-99m-labeled phosphates as an indicator of breast pathology. J Nucl Med 16:536, 1975

5. Jayabalan V, Berry S: Accumulation of ^{99m}Tc-pyrophosphate in breast prosthesis. Clin Nucl Med 2:452, 1977

6. Landgarten S: Uptake of Tc-99m-pyrophosphate by the lactating breast. J Nucl Med 18:943, 1977

7. Lumsden AB: Demonstration of a primary bone tumor of the breast by technetium-99m diphosphonate bone imaging. Clin Nucl Med 11:362, 1986

8. McLellan GL, Stewart JH, Balachandran S: Localization of Tc-99m-MDP in amyloidosis of the breast. Clin Nucl Med 6:579, 1981

9. O'Connell ME, Sutton H: Excretion of radioactivity in breast milk following ^{99m}Tc-(sn)-polyphosphate. Br J Radiol 49:377, 1976

10. Ram Singh PS, Pujara S, Logic JR: ^{99m}Tc-pyrophosphate uptake in drug induced gynecomastia. Clin Nucl Med 2:206, 1977

11. Serafini AN, Raskin MM, Zand LC, et al: Radionuclide breast scanning in carcinoma of the breast. J Nucl Med 15:1149, 1974

12. Schmitt GH, Holmes RA, Isitman AT, et al: A proposed mechanism for ^{99m}Tc-labeled polyphosphate and diphosphonate uptake by human breast tissue. Radiology 112:733, 1974

BONE IMAGING

Thyroid Uptake

COMMON: Free pertechnetate
               Normal (lower neck uptake)

UNCOMMON
AND RARE: Amyloidosis
               Hyperthyroidism
               Multinodular goiter

REFERENCE

1. Peterdy E: The diagnosis of thyroid disease on bone scans. Clin Nucl Med 10:177, 1985

BONE IMAGING

Extraosseous Uptake in a Pediatric Patient

COMMON AND
UNCOMMON: Calcium gluconate infusion
Dystrophic calcification (e.g., calcinosis universalis,
  fat necrosis, hematoma, disk, postsurgical)
Infarction (e.g., cerebral, myocardial, splenic)
Intramuscular injection sites
Malignant effusion
Postradiation
Tumor (e.g., hamartoma, neuroblastoma, metastatic
  osteosarcoma)

REFERENCES

1. Sty JR, Starshak RJ, Oechler HW: Extraosseous uptake of Tc-99m-MDP in congenital fibromatosis. Clin Nucl Med 6:123, 1981
2. Wells RG, Sty JR: Comparative imaging: Disk calcification in childhood. Clin
   Nucl Med 10:821, 1985

BONE IMAGING

Extraosseous Chest Uptake in a Pediatric Patient

COMMON AND
UNCOMMON: Cardiac injury
Infarction
Pericarditis
Toxicity
Trauma
Hyperparathyroidism
Idiopathic pulmonary calcification
Myositis
Postsurgical
Tumor
Mesenchymoma
Metastasis (esp. osteogenic sarcoma)
Neuroblastoma
Plasma cell granuloma
Teratoma

REFERENCE

1. Wells RG, Sty JR: Estraosseous bone-tracer uptake: Plasma cell granuloma. Clin Nucl Med 11:527, 1986

BONE IMAGING

Diffusely Increased Thoracoabdominal (Lower Thorax and/or Upper Abdomen) Uptake

COMMON: Metastases
Metastatic calcification
Pleural effusion
Radiopharmaceutical problem
Recent liver-spleen scan
Sickle-thalassemia and functional asplenia

UNCOMMON: G-6-PD deficiency
Hepatic necrosis
Subcapsular hematoma of spleen

RARE: Amyloidosis
Wolman's disease (adrenal)

REFERENCES

1. Shih W-J, Coupal JJ, Domstad PA, et al: Diffuse thoracoabdominal radioactivity seen in bone imaging. Clin Nucl Med 11:254, 1986
2. Shih W-J, Domstad PA, Deland FH: Diffuse radioactivity in the thoracoabdominal region seen in bone scintigraphy. Semin Nucl Med 16:211, 1986

BONE IMAGING

Cup Defect in Bladder

COMMON: Postprostatectomy

UNCOMMON
AND RARE: Contamination
Diverticulae (bladder)
Metastasis
Urinary tract fistula

REFERENCE

1. Slavin JD, Mathews J, Spencer RP: Infrabladder "cup defect" following prostatectomy: Recognition on bone scintigram. J Nucl Med 26:149, 1985

BONE IMAGING

Dual-photon Absorptiometry of Spine — Misleading Results

COMMON AND
UNCOMMON: Aortic calcifications
Compression fracture
Hypertrophic degenerative joint disease
Intrinsic bone disease (metastases, Paget's disease)
Metallic orthopedic devices (Harrington rods, etc.)
Postsurgical (laminectomy, bone grafting)
Radiographic contrast (GI, CNS)
Scoliosis and other congenital spine deformities

REFERENCES

1. VonMoll LK, Shulkin BL: Dual-photon absorptiometry — importance of clinical correlation. Clin Nucl Med 13:175, 1988
2. Wahner HW: Assessment of metabolic bone disease: Review of new nuclear medicine procedures. Mayo Clin Proc 60:827, 1985

4

Pulmonary

LUNG IMAGING

Perfusion Defect

COMMON: Acute pulmonary thromboembolism
Atelectasis — postoperative
Bronchitis acute/chronic
Bronchogenic carcinoma
Bullae, cysts
Emphysema
Pleural effusion
Pneumonia
Previous pulmonary thromboembolism

UNCOMMON: Air embolism
Asthma
Atelectasis — foreign body
Bronchiectasis
Cardiomegaly
Collagen vascular disease
Congestive heart failure
Fat embolism
Fibrosing mediastinitis (histoplasmosis)
Fibrothorax
Intravenous drug abuse
Jewelry
Lobectomy, pneumonectomy

Lymphangitic carcinomatosis
Mitral valve disease
Mucous plug syndrome
Obesity
Pacemaker
Primary pulmonary hypertension
Pulmonary hypertension
Sarcoidosis
Scapular defect — normal
Sickle cell anemia
Tuberculosis

RARE: Agenesis of the lung
Aortic aneurysm
Congenital absence of left pericardium
Congenital cystic adenomatoid malformation
Congenital lobar emphysema
Dirofilaria immitis
Elevated diaphragm
Endobronchial adenoma
Following surgical correction of congenital heart
   disease
Hemangioendotheliomatosis
Injection in a pulmonary catheter
Interstitial lobar emphysema
Intrathoracic kidney
Intrathoracic stomach
Lung transplantation-obliterative bronchiolitis
Metastases
Pneumothorax
Prominent clavicles and upper ribs
Pulmonary arteriovenous fistula
Pulmonary arteriovenous malformation
Pulmonary artery agenesis or stenosis
Pulmonary artery sarcoma
Pulmonary contusion
Pulmonary venoocclusive disease
Sequestration
Substernal goiter
Sywer-James syndrome
Takayasu's arteritis
Tortuous aorta
Traumatic pulmonary artery pseudoaneurysm
Tumor microembolism

REFERENCES

1. Alderson PO, Secker-Walker RH, Forrest JV: Detection of obstructive pulmonary disease: Relative sensitivity of ventilation-perfusion studies and chest radiography. Radiology 112:643, 1974.

2. Alderson PO, Secker-Walker RH, Strominger DB, et al: Quantitative assessment of regional ventilation and perfusion in children with cystic fibrosis. Radiology 111:151, 1974

3. Balon HR, Meier DA: Large substernal goiter as cause of pulmonary perfusion defect. Clin Nucl Med 15:806, 1990

4. Bedont RA, Datz FL: Lung scan perfusion defects limited to matching pleural effusions: Low probability of pulmonary embolism. AJR 145:1155, 1985

5. Bray ST, Johnstone WH, Dee PM, et al: The "mucous plug syndrome": A pulmonary embolism mimic. Clin Nucl Med 9:513, 1984

6. Bryant LR, Spencer FC, Greenlaw RH, et al: Postoperative changes in regional pulmonary blood flow. J Thorac Cardiovasc Surg 53:64, 1967

7. Carrol RG, Albin M, Waterman P, et al: Lung scan patterns in fifty cases of proven pulmonary air embolism. J Nucl Med 18:606, 1977

8. Crane R, Rudd TG, Dail D: Tumor microembolism: Pulmonary perfusion pattern. J Nucl Med 25:877, 1984

9. Dillon WP, Taylor AT, Mineau DE, et al: Traumatic pulmonary artery pseudoaneurysm simulating pulmonary embolism. AJR 139:818, 1982

10. Friedman SA, Schub HM, Smith EH: Perfusion defects in the aging lung. Am Heart J 79:160, 1970

11. Gilday DL, James EA Jr: Lung scan patterns in pulmonary embolism versus those in congestive heart failure and emphysema. AJR Radium Ther Nuc Med 115:739, 1972

12. Green N, Swanson L, Kenn W: Lymphangitis carcinomatosis, lung scan abnormalities. J Nucl Med 17:258, 1976

13. Hallisey MJ, Caride VJ: Single perfusion defect secondary to intrathoracic kidney. Clin Nucl Med 15:268, 1990

14. Halvorsen RA, DeCret RP, Kuni CC, et al: Obliterative bronchiolitis following lung transplantation diagnostic utility of aerosol ventilation lung scanning and high-resolution CT. Clin Nucl Med 16:256, 1991

15. Harding JA, Velchik MG: Pulmonary scintigraphy in a patient with multiple pulmonary arteriovenous malformations and pulmonary embolism. J Nucl Med 26:151, 1985

16. Houzard C, Andre M, Guilhen S, et al: Perfusion lung scan in patients operated for transposition of great arteries. Clin Nucl Med 14:268, 1989

17. Jones ET, Rao RB: Abnormal perfusion scan due to intrathoracic stomach and colon. J Nucl Med 24:543, 1983

18. Kim CK, Heyman S: Ventilation/perfusion mismatch caused by positive pressure ventilatory support. J Nucl Med 30:1268, 1989

19. Lee VW, Dedick P, Shapiro JH: The diagnosis of pneumothorax by radionuclide lung scan. Clin Nucl Med 9:13, 1984

20. Lee HK, Skarzynski J: Attenuation defects caused by prominent clavicles and first ribs in perfusion lung imaging. Clin Nucl Med 13:545, 1988

21. Lisbona R, Hakim TS, Dean GW, et al: Regional pulmonary perfusion following human heart-lung transplantation. J Nucl Med 30:1297, 1989

22. Lopez-Majano V, Kieffer RF, Marine DN, et al: Pulmonary resection in bullous disease. Am Rev Respir Dis 99:554, 1969

23. Lopez-Majano V, Wagner HN, Tow DE, et al: Radioisotope scanning of the lungs in pulmonary tuberculosis. JAMA 194:1053, 1965

24. Lull RJ, Tatum JL, Sugerman HJ, et al: Radionuclide evaluation of lung trauma. Semin Nucl Med 13:223, 1983

25. McIntyre KM, Sasahara AA: Correlation of pulmonary photoscan and angiogram as measures of the severity of pulmonary embolic involvement. J Nucl Med 12:732, 1971

26. Milstein D, Nusynowitz ML, Lull RJ: Radionuclide diagnosis in chest disease resulting from trauma. Semin Nucl Med 4:339, 1974

27. Mishkin FS, Wagner HN: Regional abnormalities in pulmonary arterial blood flow during acute asthmatic attacks. Radiology 88:142, 1967

28. Moncada R, Baker O, Kenny J, et al: Reversible unilateral pulmonary hypoperfusion secondary to acute check-valve obstruction of a main bronchus. Radiology 106:361, 1973

29. Moreno AJ, Weismann I, Billingsley JL, et al: Angiographic and scintigraphic findings in fibrosing mediastinitis. Clin Nucl Med 8:167, 1983

30. Nielsen PE, Kirchner PT, Gerger RH: Oblique views in lung perfusion scanning: Clinical utility and limitations. J Nucl Med 18:967, 1977

31. Padilla L, Orzel JA, Kreins CM: Congenital lobar emphysema: Segmental lobar involvement demonstrated on ventilation and perfusion imaging (letter to the editor). J Nucl Med 26:1343, 1985

32. Palestro C, Fineman D, Goldsmith SJ: Pulmonary scintigraphy in surgically corrected congenital heart disease. Clin Nucl Med 12:967, 1987

33. Park H-M, Ducret RP, Brindley DC: Pulmonary imaging in fat embolism syndrome. Clin Nucl Med 11:521, 1986

34. Pendarvis BC, Swischuk LE: Lung scanning in the assessment of respiratory disease in children. AJR Radium Ther Nucl Med 107:313, 1969

35. Reinig JW, Simmons JT, Bielroy L: Multiple lung perfusion defects in a patient with Takayasu's arteritis. Clin Nucl Med 10:893, 1985

36. Robinson AE, Goodrich JK, Spock A: Inhalation and perfusion radionuclide studies of pediatric chest diseases. Radiology 93:1123, 1969

37. Rocha AF, Harbert JC (eds): Textbook of Nuclear Medicine: Clinical Applications. Philadelphia, Lea and Febiger, 1979

38. Seaton D: Regional lung function in asbestos workers. Thorax 32:40, 1977

39. Secker-Walker RH, Goodwin J: Quantitative aspects of lung scanning. Proc R Soc Med 64:344, 1971

40. Senyk J, Arborelius M Jr, Lilja B: Respiratory function in esophageal hiatus hernia. II. Regional lung function. Respiration 32:103, 1975

41. Singh A, Holmes RA, Witten DM: Rapid resolution of perfusion/ventilatory abnormalities in pulmonary air embolism. Clin Nucl Med 10:327, 1985

42. Sharzynski JJ, Slavin JD, Spencer RP, et al: "Matching" ventilation/perfusion images in fat embolization. Clin Nucl Med 11:40, 1986

43. Soin JS, McKusck MA, Wagner HN Jr: Regional lung function abnormalities in narcotic addicts. JAMA 224:1717, 1973

44. Suga K, Kuramitsu T, Yoshimuzu T, et al: Scintigraphic analysis of hemodynamics in patient with single large pulmonary arteriovenous fistula. Clin Nucl Med 17:110, 1992

45. Tow DE, Wagner HN Jr: Effect of pleural fluid on the appearance of the lung scan. J Nucl Med 11:138, 1970

46. Umehara I, Shibuya H, Nakagawa T, Numano F: Comprehensive analysis of perfusion scintigraphy in Takayasu's arteritis. Clin Nucl Med 16:252, 1991

47. Wagner HN Jr, Lopez-Majano V, Tow DE, et al: Radioisotope scanning of the lungs in early diagnosis of bronchogenic carcinoma. Lancet 1:344, 1965

LUNG IMAGING

Unilateral Decreased Perfusion

COMMON: Bronchogenic carcinoma

UNCOMMON: Congenital heart disease following shunt (e.g.,
tetralogy of Fallot with Blalock-Taussig shunts)
Following pneumonectomy
Pulmonary embolism
Severe pleural or parenchymal disease (e.g.,
emphysema with pneumonia, tuberculosis)
Swyer-James syndrome

RARE: Aortic aneurysm
Bronchial adenoma
Broncholithiasis
Bullae (giant)
Fibrosing mediastinitis (e.g., histoplasmosis)
Foreign body obstructing main bronchus
Injection in a pulmonary artery catheter
Malposition of endotracheal tube
Mucous plug syndrome
Postatelectatic
Pulmonary artery hypoplasia or agenesis
Pulmonary vein atresia
Pulmonary venoocclusive disease
Sarcoid
Takayasu's arteritis
Tumor embolization

REFERENCES

1. Apan RL, Saenz R, Siemsen JR: Bloodless lung due to bronchial obstruction.
J Nucl Med 13:561, 1972

2. Brachman M, Tanasescw D, Ramanna L, et al: False positive lung imaging:
Inadvertent injection into a pulmonary artery catheter. Clin Nucl Med 4:415,
1979

3. Calderon M, Burdine JA. Pulmonary venoocclusive disease. J Nucl Med 15:455,
1974

4. Charnsangavej C: Occlusion of the right pulmonary artery by acute dissecting
aortic aneurysm. AJR 132:274, 1979

5. Chaudhuri TK, Chaudhuri TK, Schapiro RL, et al: Abnormal lung perfusion in a patient with bronchial adenoma. Chest 62:110, 1972

6. Chung CJ, Grossnickle M, Rosenthal P, et al: Postatelectatic ventilation perfusion mismatch simulating a pulmonary embolus. J Nucl Med 31:1397, 1990

7. Cowan RJ, Short DB, Maynard CD: Nonperfusion of one lung secondary to improperly positioned endotrachael tube. JAMA 227:1165, 1974

8. Garty I, Koren A, Moguilner G, et al: Nearly total absence of pulmonary perfusion with corresponding technetium-99m MDP and gallium-67 uptake in a patient with mediastinal neuroblastoma. Clin Nucl Med 10:579, 1985

9. Held BT, Siegelman SS: Pulmonary infarction secondary to bronchogenic carcinoma. AJR 120:145, 1974

10. Isawa T, Taplin GV: Unilateral pulmonary artery agenesis, stenosis, and hypoplasia. Radiology 99:605, 1971

11. Lloyd TV: Decreased lung perfusion due to broncholithiasis. Clin Nucl Med 4:523, 1979

12. Lloyd TV, Johnson JC: Pulmonary artery occlusion following fibrosing mediastinitis due to histoplasmosis. Clin Nucl Med 4:35, 1979

13. Makler PT, Malmud LS, Charkes ND: Diminished perfusion to an entire lung due to mucus plug. Clin Nucl Med 2:160, 1977

14. Olsson HE, Spitzer RM, Erston WF: Primary and secondary pulmonary artery neoplasia mimicking acute pulmonary embolism. Radiology 118:49, 1976

15. Puyau FA, Meckstroth GR: Evaluation of pulmonary perfusion patterns in children with tetralogy of Fallot. AJR 122:119, 1974

16. Rosen RJ, Goodman LR: Occult bronchogenic carcinoma masquerading as recurrent pulmonary embolism. AJR 132:133, 1979

17. Stanley DC, Cho S, Tisnado J, et al: Pulmonary arteriography in patients with hilar or mediastinal masses and lung scans suggesting pulmonary embolism. South Med J 74:960, 1981

18. Stjernholm MR, Landis GA, Marcus FI, et al: Perfusion and ventilation radioisotope lung scans in stenosis of the pulmonary arteries and their branches. Am Heart J 78:37, 1969

19. Thomas HM: Regulation of regional pulmonary blood flow in bronchial occlusion. Clin Nucl Med 2:173, 1977

20. Thomason CB, Rama Rao B: Lung imaging — unilateral absence or near absence of pulmonary perfusion on lung scanning. Semin Nucl Med 13:388, 1983

21. Tomsick TA, Holder LE: Unilateral absent perfusion of the lung. JAMA 234:89, 1975

22. White RI, James E, Wagner HN: The significance of unilateral absence of pulmonary artery perfusion by lung scanning. AJR 111:501, 1971

23. Zeiger LS, Moss EG: Ventilation and perfusion imaging Swyer-James syndrome. Clin Nucl Med 2:103, 1977

LUNG IMAGING

Mottled Perfusion Scan

COMMON AND
UNCOMMON: Congestive heart failure
             Collagen vascular disease
             Emboli
               Air
               Amniotic fluid
               Fat
               Oil
               Tumor
             Hemangioendotheliomatosis
             Intravenous drug abuse
             Insufficient number of particles
             Metastases
             Pneumonia
             Primary pulmonary hypertension
             Tuberculosis

REFERENCES

1. Lisbona R, Kreisman H, Novales-Diaz J, et al: Perfusion lung scanning: Differentiation of primary from thromboembolic pulmonary hypertension. AJR 144:27, 1985
2. Williams AG, Mettler FA, Christie JH, et al: Fat embolism syndrome. Clin Nucl Med 11:495, 1986

LUNG IMAGING

Extrapulmonary Activity

COMMON: Delayed imaging after particle breakdown ^{99m}Tc
dissociation
Radiopharmaceutical problem

UNCOMMON: Acute respiratory distress syndrome
Cardiac shunt — right-to-left
Pulmonary arteriovenous malformation
Superior vena cava obstruction

REFERENCES

1. Gale B, Chen C, Chun KJ, et al: Systemic to pulmonary venous shunting in superior vena cava obstruction — Unusual myocardial and thyroid visualization. Clin Nucl Med 15:246, 1990

2. Hellin DH, Ferrer AC, Alberti JFF: Extrapulmonary uptake in spleen during lung perfusion with ^{99m}Tc MAA. Clin Nucl Med 17:899, 1992

3. Hiltz A, Iles S: Abnormal ^{99m}Tc MAA accumulation. Clin Nucl Med 13:727, 1988

4. Maldonado A, Domper M, Garcia MJ, et al: Respiratory distress syndrome — suggestive pattern of shunt effect detected by means of macroparticles. Clin Nucl Med 18:19, 1993

5. Mills BJA, Krasnow AZ, Collier BD, et al: Extrapulmonary activity during perfusion lung imaging with ^{99m}Tc MAA. Clin Nucl Med 15:128, 1990

6. Trent C, Tupler RH, Wildenhain P, Turbiner EH: Macrovascular pulmonary arteriovenous malformations demonstrated by radionuclide method. Clin Nucl Med 18:231, 1993

7. Trombley BA, Marcus CS, Koci T: Unexpected demonstration of superior vena caval obstruction in third trimester lung imaging. Clin Nucl Med 13:407, 1988

LUNG IMAGING

Hot Spots

COMMON: Atelectasis
Faulty injection technique
Normal lung adjacent to pulmonary embolism
COPD

UNCOMMON: Thrombophlebitis

RARE: Congestive heart failure
Focal pulmonary edema secondary to pulmonary
embolism
Pneumonia

REFERENCES

1. Goldberg E, Liebermann C: "Hot spots" in lung scans. J Nucl Med 18:499, 1977

2. Lutzher LG, Perez LA: Radioactive embolization from upper-extremity thrombophlebitis. J Nucl Med 16:241, 1975

3. Meignan M, Palmer EL, Waltman AC, Strauss HW: Zones of increased perfusion (hot spots) on perfusion lung scans: Correlation with pulmonary arteriograms. Radiology 173:47, 1989

4. Natara B, Ugo F, Igor B: Pulmonary microemboli. J Nucl Med 19:1183, 1978

5. Preston DF, Greenlaw RH: "Hot spots" on lung scans. J Nucl Med 11:422, 1970

6. Tiu S, Liu D, Kramer EL, et al: Focal pulmonary edema: Correlation with perfusion lung scan. Clin Nucl Med 10:583, 1985

LUNG IMAGING

Liver Visualization on Perfusion Scan

COMMON: Inferior or superior vena cava obstruction

UNCOMMON
AND RARE: Right-to-left shunt (cardiac or pulmonary)
Radiopharmaceutical problem

REFERENCES

1. Edeburn GF, Kozlowski JF, Tumeh SS: Appearance of lung scan in venae cavae occlusion. AJR 145:273, 1985
2. Marcus CS, Parker LS, Rose JG, et al: Uptake of Tc-99m MAA by the liver during a thromboscintigram/lung scan. J Nucl Med 24:36, 1983
3. Siu K-S, Coel MN: Hepatic visualization after radionuclide venogram. Clin Nucl Med 9:358, 1984
4. Vea HW, Cerqueira MD: Hepatic localization of Tc-99m MAA in inferior vena cava obstruction. Clin Nucl Med 10:772, 1985
5. Weaver GR, Johnson JA, Sandler MP: Inferior vena cava obstruction with hot quadrate lobe on technetium-99m MAA scintivenography. Clin Nucl Med 11:731, 1986
6. Wraight EP: Re: Uptake of Tc-99m MAA by the liver during a lung scan (letter to the editor). J Nucl Med 24:747, 1983

LUNG IMAGING

Focal Retention of Xenon

COMMON: Bronchial asthma
Chronic bronchitis
Emphysema
Smoke inhalation

UNCOMMON: Bronchiectasis
Cystic fibrosis
Foreign body obstruction of a bronchus
Mucous plug syndrome
Tuberculosis
Tumor (e.g., carcinoma, adenoma)

RARE: Air embolism
Alpha-1-antitrypsin deficiency
Bronchopleural fistula
Congestive heart failure
Congenital lobar emphysema
Hiatal hernia
Idiopathic pulmonary fibrosis
Near drowning
Nonthermal inhalational injury
Pneumoconiosis (e.g., asbestosis)
Pneumonia
Pulmonary embolus
Radiation fibrosis
Swyer-James syndrome
Xenon accumulation in the liver
Xenon in the gastric fundus

REFERENCES

1. Agee RN, Long M, Hunt JL, et al: Use of Xenon-133 in early diagnosis of inhalational injury. J Trauma 16:218, 1976

2. Alderson PO, Doppman JL, Diamond SS, et al: Ventilation-perfusion lung imaging and selective pulmonary angiography in dogs with experimental pulmonary embolism. J Nucl Med 19:164, 1978

3. Boode WA, Gullickson C: Xenon ventilation studies: Potential use in infants. J Nucl Med 21:294, 1980

4. Hartshorne MF, Brown JM, Cawthon MA, et al: Profound xenon-133 trapping in left main bronchus: Obstruction by necrotic tumor. Clin Nucl Med 11:525, 1986

5. Lee HK, Granada M: Swyer-James syndrome: Diagnostic application of combined radionuclide ventilation and perfusion scanning. Clin Nucl Med 2:100, 1977

6. Leonidus JC, Moylan FM, Kahn PC, et al: Ventilation-perfusion scans in neonatal regional pulmonary emphysema complicating ventilatory assistance. AJR 131:243, 1978

7. Marx WJ, Courtney JV, MacMahon H, et al: Xenon in the gastric fundus: Potential pitfall in ventilation scan interpretation. AJR 132:676, 1979

8. Ramos M, Baumann HR, Muhberger F: Perfusion and ventilation imaging in pulmonary tuberculosis. Clin Nucl Med 3:233, 1978

9. Rocha AF, Harbert JC (eds): Textbook of Nuclear Medicine: Clinical Applications. Philadelphia, Lea and Febiger, 1979

10. Rocha AF, Harbert JC (eds): Textbook of Nuclear Medicine: Clinical Applications, Philadelphia, Lea and Febiger, 1986

11. Secker-Walker RH, Toban MM, Ho JE: Patterns of regional ventilation in patients with cardiomegaly or left heart failure. J Nucl Med 22:212, 1981

12. Zeigler LS, Moss EG: Ventilation and perfusion imaging in Swyer-James syndrome. Clin Nucl Med 2:103, 1977

13. Zelefsky MN, Freeman LM, Stern H: A simple approach to the diagnosis of bronchopleural fistula. Radiology 124:843, 1977

LUNG IMAGING

Xenon Retention in the Liver

COMMON: Alcoholic liver disease
Diabetes mellitus
Obesity

UNCOMMON
AND RARE: Hepatitis
Hepatotoxic drugs
Hyperlipidemias
Intravenous hyperalimentation

REFERENCES

1. Ahmad MA, Witztum KF, Fletcher JW, et al: Xenon-133 accumulation in hepatic steatosis. J Nucl Med 18:881, 1977

2. Baker MK, Schauwecker DS, Wenker JC, et al: Nuclear medicine evaluation of focal fatty infiltration of the liver. Clin Nucl Med 11:503, 1986

3. Beanco JA, Shafer RB: Implications of liver activity associated with ^{133}Xe ventilation lung scans. Clin Nucl Med 3:176, 1978

4. Carey JE, Purdy JM, Moses DC: Localization of ^{133}Xe in liver during ventilation studies. J Nucl Med 15:1179, 1974

5. Patel S, Sandler CM, Ranschkolb E: [133]Xe uptake in focal hepatic fat accumulation: CT correlation. AJR 138:541, 1982

LUNG IMAGING

Xenon Uptake in Skeleton

COMMON AND
UNCOMMON: Steroid therapy (increased fat in marrow)

REFERENCES:

1. Gordon L, Spicer KM, Yon JW Jr: Bone marrow uptake of xenon-133. Clin Nucl Med 10:891, 1985
2. Kramer EL, Tiu S, Sanger JJ, et al: Radioxenon retention in the skeleton on a routine ventilation study. Clin Nucl Med 8:299, 1983

LUNG IMAGING

Ventilation-Perfusion Mismatch

COMMON: Acute pulmonary thromboembolism
Bronchogenic carcinoma
Previous pulmonary embolism
Previous radiation therapy

UNCOMMON: Air embolism
Collagen vascular disease
Emphysema
Fat embolism
Fibrosing mediastinitis (histoplasmosis)
Intravenous drug abuse
Lymphangitic carcinomatosis
Mitral valve heart disease
Pneumonia
Pulmonary hypertension
Sarcoidosis
Sickle cell disease
Tuberculosis

RARE: Aortic aneurysm
Bronchopleural fistula
Dog heart worms (*Dirofilaria immitis*)
Hemangioendotheliomatosis
Hiatal hernia
Idiopathic pulmonary fibrosis
Immunologic pulmonary edema
Intrathoracic stomach
Malposition of intravenous catheter
Metastases
Pectus excavatum
Positive pressure ventilation/atelectasis
Pulmonary arteriovenous malformation
Pulmonary artery agenesis or stenosis
Pulmonary contusion
Pulmonary sarcoma
Pulmonary venoocclusive disease
Septic emboli
Surgical correction of congenital heart disease
Swallowed aerosol and paralyzed diaphragm

Systemic arterial supply
Traumatic pulmonary artery pseudoaneurysm
Tumor emboli
Wedging of Swan-Ganz catheter

REFERENCES

1. Agrons GA, Maslack MM, Parry CE, Latour MGN: Multiple coarctations of pulmonary artery: Scintigraphic appearance. Clin Nucl Med 15:19, 1990

2. Bateman NT, Crogt DN: False positive lung scans and radiotherapy. Br Med J 1:807, 1976

3. Calderon M, Burdine JA: Pulmonary venoocclusive disease. J Nucl Med 15:455, 1974

4. Campeau RJ, Faust JM, Ahmad S: Unusual ventilation perfusion scintigram in case of immunologic pulmonary edema clinically simulating pulmonary embolism. Clin Nucl Med 12:874, 1987

5. Dillon WP, Taylor AT, Mineau DE, et al: Traumatic pulmonary pseudoaneurism simulating pulmonary embolus. AJR 139:818, 1982

6. Dowdle SC, Human DG, Mann MD: Pulmonary ventilation and perfusion abnormalities and ventilation perfusion imbalance in children with pulmonary atresia or extreme tetralogy of Fallot. J Nucl Med 31:1276, 1990

7. Eary JF, Fisher MC, Cerqueira MD: Idiopathic pulmonary fibrosis: Another cause of ventilation/perfusion mismatch. Clin Nucl Med 11:369, 1986

8. Goodgold HM, Duffrin HJ: Ventilation/perfusion mismatch caused by emphysematous bullae. Clin Nucl Med 14:475, 1989

9. Green N, Swanson L, Kern W, et al: Lymphangitic carcinomatosis: Lung scan abnormalities. J Nucl Med 17:258, 1976

10. Griffith S, Hutchinson MA, Scott JW: False-positive V/Q study secondary to a central venous catheter in the pleural space. Clin Nucl Med 9:463, 1984

11. Housman JF, Fajman WA: False-positive V/Q imaging in pulmonary contusion. Clin Nucl Med 14:577, 1989

12. Isawa T, Taplin GV: Unilateral pulmonary artery agenesis, stenosis, and hypoplasia. Radiology 99:605, 1971

13. Kao CH, Liao SQ, Wang SJ, Yeh SH: Pulmonary scintigraphic findings in children with pectus excavatum by comparison of chest radiograph indices. Clin Nucl Med 17:874, 1992

14. Kim EE, DeLand FH: V/Q mismatch without pulmonary embolism in children with histoplasmosis. Clin Nucl Med 3:328, 1978

15. Kolla I, Holt D, Taylor A: Abnormal ventilation perfusion scan due to swallowed DTPA aerosol and a paralyzed hemidiaphragm. Clin Nucl Med 13:842, 1988

16. Li DK, Seltzer SE, McNeil BJ: V/Q mismatches unassociated with pulmonary embolism: Case report and review of the literature. J Nucl Med 19:1131, 1978

17. McNeil BJ: A diagnostic strategy using ventilation-perfusion studies in patients suspect for pulmonary embolism. J Nucl Med 17:613, 1976

18. Mehta T, Achong DM, Oates E: Septic pulmonary emboli from pulmonic valvular endocarditis demonstrated by serial ventilation perfusion lung imaging. Clin Nucl Med 18:11, 1993

19. Moser KM, Guisan M, Cuomo A, et al: Differentiation of pulmonary vascular from parenchymal diseases by ventilation-perfusion scintiphotography. Ann Intern Med 75:597, 1971

20. Myerson PJ, Myerson DA, Katz R, et al: Gallium imaging in pulmonary artery sarcoma mimicking pulmonary embolism: Case report. J Nucl Med 17:893, 1976

21. Narabayashi I, Otsuka N: Pulmonary ventilation and perfusion studies in lung cancer. Clin Nucl Med 9:97, 1984

22. Roswig DM, Sziklas JJ, Rosenberg RJ, et al: Bronchopleural fistula demonstrated by pulmonary scintigraphy: A "pseudo" ventilation/perfusion mismatch. Clin Nucl Med 9:240, 1984

23. Secker-Walker RH, Alderson PO, Wilhelm J, et al: Ventilation-perfusion scanning in carcinoma of the bronchus. Chest 65:660, 1974

24. Sidiqui AR, Wellman HN, Klatte EC, et al: Wedged Swan-Ganz catheter causing ventilation-perfusion mismatch: Case report and review of the literature. Clin Nucl Med 8:597, 1983

25. Siegal BA (ed): Nuclear Radiology Syllabus. Second Series. Chicago, American College of Radiology, 1978

26. Simon H: Ventilation-perfusion mismatch lung scan without pulmonary emboli. Clin Nucl Med 2:124, 1977

27. Soin JS, McKusick KA, Wagner HN Jr: Regional lung function abnormalities in narcotic addicts. JAMA 224:1717, 1973

28. Surprenant EL, Spellberg RD: Regional pulmonary function in supine patients with mitral valve disease. Radiology 117:99, 1975

29. Sy WM, Nissen AW: Radionuclide studies in hemangioendotheliomatosis: Case report. J Nucl Med 16:915, 1975

30. Szeklas JJ, Rosenberg R, Spencer RP: Ventilation-perfusion mismatch due to systemic arterial supply. Clin Nucl Med 4:231, 1979

31. Tiu S, Friedman DM, Klein B, Doyle EF: Lung scan in cardiac patient with Glenn anastomosis. Clin Nucl Med 12:567, 1987

32. Vieras F, Bradley EW, Alderson PO, et al: Regional pulmonary function after irradiation of the canine lung: Radionuclide evaluation. Radiology 147:839, 1983

33. Williams O, Lyall J, Vernon M, et al: Ventilation-perfusion lung scanning for pulmonary emboli. Br Med J 1:600, 1974

34. Wood MJ: Ventilation-perfusion mismatch: Lung imaging. Clin Nucl Med 8:181, 1983

35. Yussen PS, LaManna MM: Pulmonary scintigraphy in talc granulomatosis. Clin Nucl Med 12:949, 1987

LUNG IMAGING

Reverse Ventilation-Perfusion Mismatch

COMMON AND
UNCOMMON: Atelectasis in patient on positive pressure
mechanical ventilation
Chronic obstructive pulmonary disease
Lung cancer
Lung transplantation
Metabolic alkalosis
Pleural effusion
Pneumonia
Pulmonary hypertension

REFERENCES

1. Carvalho P, Lavender JP: Incidence and etiology of ventilation perfusion reverse mismatch defect. Clin Nucl Med 14:571, 1989

2. Goodwin CA, Epstein DH: Lung perfusion scanning: The case of "reverse mismatch." Clin Nucl Med 9:519, 1986

3. Kuni CC, Ducret RP, Nakhleh RE, Boudreau RJ: Reverse mismatch between perfusion and aerosol ventilation in transplanted lungs. Clin Nucl Med 18:313, 1993

4. Palmaz JC, Barnett CA, Reich SB, et al: Reverse ventilation-perfusion mismatch. Clin Nucl Med 9:6, 1984

5. Slavin JD, Mathews J, Spencer RP: Pulmonary ventilation/perfusion and reverse mismatches in an infant. Clin Nucl Med 10:708, 1985

6. Sostman HD, Neumann RD, Gottschalk A, et al: Perfusion of nonventilated lung: Failure of hypoxic vasoconstriction. AJR 141:151, 1983

7. Watanabe N, Hirano T, Inoue T, et al: Transient unilateral reverse ventilation perfusion mismatch in patient with lung cancer. Clin Nucl Med 17:705, 1992

LUNG IMAGING

Diffuse Gallium Uptake

COMMON: Adult respiratory distress syndrome
Bacterial pneumonia
Drug reaction (e.g., busulfan, cyclophosphamide,
amiodarone)
Early imaging — 24 hours
Following lymphangiography
Malignant process (e.g., lymphoma, lung, breast,
colon, other carcinomas)
Pneumoconiosis (e.g., silicosis, asbestosis)
Pneumocystitis carinii
Tuberculosis

UNCOMMON: Drug addicts — talc granulomatosis
Idiopathic pulmonary fibrosis
Radiation therapy
Sarcoidosis
Uremic pneumonitis

RARE: Acute leukemia
Bronchiectasis
Bronchiolitis obliterans
Cytomegalovirus
Empyema
Eosinophilic pneumonia
Hamman-Rich syndrome
Histiocytosis X
Lymphomatoid granulomatosis
Malignant pleural effusion
Mesothelioma
Metastatic calcification
Multiple myeloma with pulmonary dissemination
Normal or lactating breasts
Pulmonary alveolar proteinosis
Septic microemboli
Systemic lupus erythematosus
Wegener's granulomatosis

REFERENCES

1. Begin R, Bisson G, Lambert R, et al: Gallium-67 uptake in the lung of asbestos exposed sheep: Early association with enhanced macrophage-derived fibronectin accumulation. J Nucl Med 27:538, 1986

2. Bekerman C, Hoffer PB, Bitran JD, et al: Gallium-67-citrate imaging studies of the lung. Semin Nucl Med 10:286, 1980

3. Crystal RG, Gadek JE, Ferrans VJ, et al: Interstitial lung disease: Current concepts of pathogenesis, staging and therapy. Am J Med 70:524, 1981

4. Gupta SM, Sziklas JJ, Spencer RP, et al: Significance of diffuse pulmonary uptake in radiogallium scans: Concise communication. J Nucl Med 21:328, 1980

5. Hardoff R, Bursztein-DeMytteraere S: ⁶⁷Ga lung uptake in patients with adult respiratory distress syndrome — association with lung infection and patients' prognosis. Clin Nucl Med 17:853, 1992

6. Heshihi A, Schatz SI, McKusick KP, et al: Gallium-67-citrate scanning in patients with pulmonary sarcoidosis. AJR 122:744, 1974

7. Imbriano LJ, Mandel PR, Cordaro AF: Use of gallium scanning in predicting resolution of Legionnaires' pneumonia. Clin Nucl Med 8:19, 1983

8. Johnson DG, Johnson SM, Harris CC, et al: Ga-67 uptake in the lung in sarcoidosis. Radiology 150:551, 1984

9. Kim EE: Diffuse pulmonary gallium concentration. Semin Nucl Med 10:108, 1980

10. Kinoshita F, Ushio T, Maekawa A, et al: Scintiscanning of pulmonary diseases with Ga-67-citrate. J Nucl Med 15:227, 1974

11. Kubo A, Takagi Y, Ando Y, et al: Analysis of diffuse gallium lung uptake. J Nucl Med 20:674, 1979

12. Lecklitner ML, Johnson DR, Hughes JJ: ⁶⁷Ga and pulmonary complications of amoidarone. Clin Nucl Med 13:826, 1988

13. Lentle BC, Castor WR, Khaliz A, et al: The effect of contrast lymphangiography on localization of Ga-67-citrate. J Nucl Med 16:374, 1975

14. Levenson SM, Warren RD, Richman SD, et al: Abnormal pulmonary gallium accumulation in *P. carinii* pneumonia. Radiology 119:395, 1976

15. MacMahon H, Bekerman C: The diagnostic significance of gallium lung uptake in patients with normal chest radiographs. Radiology 127:189, 1978

16. Makhija MC, Davis G: Gallium-67 imaging in pulmonary eosinophilic granuloma. Clin Nucl Med 9:139, 1984

17. Manning DM, Strimlan CV, Turbiner EH: Early detection of busulfan lung: Report of a case. Clin Nucl Med 5:412, 1980

18. Morais J, Carrier L, Gariepy G, et al: ⁶⁷Ga pulmonary uptake in eosinophilic pneumonia. Clin Nucl Med 13:41, 1988

19. Richman SD, Levenson SM, Bunn PA, et al: Ga-67 accumulation associated bleomycin toxicity. Cancer 36:1966, 1975

20. Siemsen JK, Sargent EN, Grebe SF, et al: Pulmonary concentration of Ga-67 in pneumoconiosis. AJR 120:815, 1974

21. Simen T, Hoffer PB: The nonspecificity of diffuse pulmonary uptake of Ga-67 on 24-hour images. Radiology 135:445, 1980

22. Sullivan WT, Orzel JA, Reed KD, et al: Abnormal lung and liver uptake of gallium-67 and technetium-99m MDP in hypercalcemia of lymphoma and metastatic pulmonary calcification. Clin Nucl Med 11:545, 1986

23. Tien R, Moore WH, Glasser LM, et al: Thoracic gallium uptake in patients with lymphomatoid granulomatosis. Clin Nucl Med 13:886, 1988

24. Turbiner EH, Yeh SD, Rosen PP, et al: Abnormal gallium scintigraphy in *Pneumocystitis carinii* with a normal chest radiograph. Radiology 127:437, 1978

25. van Rooij WJ, van der Meer SC, van Royen EA, et al: Pulmonary gallium-67 uptake in amiodarone pneumonitis. J Nucl Med 25:211, 1984

26. Yeh SDJ, White DA, Stover-Pepe DE, et al: Abnormal gallium scintigraphy in pulmonary alveolar proteinosis (PAP). Clin Nucl Med 12:294, 1987

LUNG IMAGING

Diffuse Pulmonary Uptake of Gallium in a Pediatric Patient

COMMON: Bacterial pneumonia (including tuberculosis)
Bronchitis
Drug toxicity
Leukemia
Histiocytosis X
Pneumocystis carinii
Radiation

UNCOMMON
AND RARE: Collagen vascular disease
Idiopathic pulmonary fibrosis
Septic emboli

REFERENCE

1. Kapala GB, Chusid MJ, Sty JR: Ga-67 chest imaging: Chronic granulomatous disease. Clin Nucl Med 8:632, 1983

LUNG IMAGING

Gallium Uptake with a Normal Chest Radiograph

COMMON: *Pneumocystis carinii* infection
Subradiographic interstitial inflammatory reaction
Subradiographic malignant process (e.g., lymphoma,
carcinoma)

UNCOMMON
AND RARE: Drug addicts
Drug toxicity (bleomycin, amiodarone)
Following lymphangiography
Miliary tuberculosis
Mycobacterium avium in acquired immunodeficiency
syndrome
Pneumoconiosis
Radiation pneumonitis
Sarcoidosis
Sjögren's syndrome
SLE

REFERENCES

1. Barron TF, Birnbaum NS, Shane LB, et al: *Pneumocystis carinii* pneumonia studied by gallium-67 scanning. Radiology 154:791, 1985

2. Bekerman C, Hoffer PB, Bitran JD, et al: Gallium-67 citrate imaging studies of the lung. Semin Nucl Med 10:286, 1980

3. Collins RD Jr, Ball GV, Logic JR: Gallium-67 scanning in Sjögren's syndrome: Concise communication. J Nucl Med 25:299, 1984

4. Grieff M, Lisbona R: Detection of military tuberculosis by ⁶⁷Ga scintigraphy. Clin Nucl Med 16:910, 1991

5. Gupta SM, Syiklas JJ, Spencer RP, et al: Significance of diffuse pulmonary uptake in radiogallium scans: Concise communication. J Nucl Med 21:328, 1980

6. Lentle BC, Castor WR, Khaliz A, et al: The effect of contrast lymphangiography on localization of Ga-67-citrate. J Nucl Med 16:374, 1975

7. Levenson SM, Warren RD, Richman SD, et al: Abnormal pulmonary gallium accumulation in P. *carinii* pneumonia. Radiology 119:395, 1976

8. MacMahon H, Bekerman C: The diagnostic significance of gallium lung uptake in patients with normal chest radiographs. Radiology 127:189, 1978

9. Malhotra CM, Erickson AD, Feinsilver SH, et al: Ga-67 studies in a patient with acquired immunodeficiency syndrome and disseminated mycobacterial infection. Clin Nucl Med 10:96, 1985

10. Manning DM, Strimlan V, Turbiner EH: Early detection of busulfan lung: Report of a case. Clin Nucl Med 5:412, 1980

11. Moses SC, Baker SR, Seldin ME: Diffuse pulmonary gallium accumulation with a normal chest radiogram in a homosexual man with *Pneumocystis carinii* pneumonia: A case report. Clin Nucl Med 8:608, 1987

12. Moinuddin M, Rockett J: Gallium scintigraphy in the detection of amiodarone lung toxicity. AJR 147:607, 1986

13. Simon TR, Hoffer PB: The nonspecificity of diffuse pulmonary uptake of Ga-67 on 24-hour images. Radiology 135:445, 1980

14. Turbiner EH, Yeh SO, Rosen PP, et al: Abnormal gallium scintigraphy in *Pneumocystis carinii* with a normal chest radiograph. Radiology 127:427, 1978

LUNG IMAGING

Positive Chest X-Ray without Gallium Uptake

COMMON: Fibrosis
Non-Ga-67-avid primary or metastatic tumor

UNCOMMON
AND RARE: Hematoma
Leukopenia
Pulmonary infarct
Steroids

REFERENCE

1. Tiu S, Kramer EL, Sanger JJ, et al: Discordance between chest x-ray and gallium scan. Semin Nucl Med 14:149, 1984

LUNG IMAGING

Symmetrical Focal Gallium Uptake in Chest

COMMON: Aspiration pneumonia
Breast (physiologic)
Bronchiectasis
Idiopathic pulmonary fibrosis
Pneumoconiosis
Scleroderma

UNCOMMON
AND RARE: Alveolar proteinosis
Bilateral subdiaphragmatic abscess
Cystic fibrosis
Collagen vascular disease
Desquamitive interstitial pneumonitis
Lipoid pneumonia
Rheumatoid arthritis

REFERENCE

1. Wu S-Y, Brown T, Lyons KP: Symmetrical focal chest uptake in gallium-67 scintigraphy. Semin Nucl Med 14:146, 1984

LUNG IMAGING

Focal Indium Leukocyte Uptake

COMMON: Pneumonia

UNCOMMON
AND RARE: Adult respiratory distress syndrome
Aspiration
Atelectasis
Bleeding
Congestive heart failure
Empyema
Idiopathic
Nonseptic pulmonary embolism

REFERENCES

1. Cook PS, Datz FL, Disbro MA, et al: Pulmonary uptake in indium-111 leuko-cyte imaging: Clinical significance in patients with suspected occult infections. Radiology 150:557, 1984
2. Segall GM, McDougall IR: Diagnostic value of lung uptake of indium-111 oxine-labeled white blood cells. AJR 147:601, 1986

LUNG IMAGING

Diffuse Indium Leukocyte Uptake

COMMON: Adult respiratory distress syndrome
Congestive heart failure
Idiopathic

UNCOMMON
AND RARE: Aspiration
Atelectasis
Cardiopulmonary resuscitation
Diffuse metastases
Drug-induced pneumonitis
Hemodialysis
Increased numbers of immature leukocytes
Pneumonia
Radiation therapy

REFERENCES

1. Cook PS, Datz FL, Disbro MA, et al: Pulmonary uptake in indium-111 leukocyte imaging: Clinical significance in patients with suspected occult infections. Radiology 150:557, 1984

2. Palestro CJ, Padilla ML, Swyer AJ, Goldsmith SJ: Diffuse pulmonary uptake of ^{111}In-labeled leukocytes in drug-induced pneumonitis. J Nucl Med 33:1175, 1992

3. Segall GM, McDougall IR: Diagnostic value of lung uptake of indium-111 oxine-labeled white blood cells. AJR 147:601, 1986

5

Gastrointestinal

MECKEL'S DIVERTICULUM

Increased Uptake

COMMON: Meckel's diverticulum
Normal activity in the gastrointestinal tract
Normal activity in upper and lower urinary tract

UNCOMMON: Barrett's esophagus
Ectopic gastric mucosa in small bowel proper with
ulceration
Extrarenal pelvis
Hemangioma
Intussusception
Peptic intestinal ulceration
Retained gastric antrum
Uterine activity

RARE: Abdominal aortic aneurysm
Abscess
Appendiceal stump
Appendicitis
Angioblastic transformation of the intestine
Arteriovenous malformation
Carcinoid tumor
Carcinoma of colon and small bowel
Diverticulitis

Ectopic kidney
Gastric mucosal proliferation
Gastrointestinal duplication
Inflammatory bowel disease
Intestinal leiomyoma
Intestinal leiomyosarcoma
Intestinal lymphosarcoma
Intestinal neurinoma
Intrathoracic gastrogenic cyst
Medications which irritate the gastrointestinal tract
Neurinoma of jejunum
Nonrotation of bowel
Obstructive uropathy
Peutz-Jeghers syndrome
Prior barium enema
Prior endoscopic exam
Regional enteritis
Retained feces
Sacral meningomyelocele
Small bowel obstruction other than intussusception
Uterine fibroid
Vesicoureteral reflux

REFERENCES

1. Berquist TH, Nolan NG, Stephens DH, et al: Radioisotope scintigraphy in diagnosis of Barrett's esophagus. AJR 123:401, 1975

2. Berquist TH, Nolan NG, Stephens DH, et al: Specificity of ^{99m}Tc-pertechnetate in scintigraphic diagnosis of Meckel's diverticulum: Review of 100 cases. J Nucl Med 17:465, 1976

3. Bhatnagar A, Sawroop K, Pant CS, Chakravarty K: Radionuclide diagnosis of dual abdominal pathology. Clin Nucl Med 19:72, 1994

4. Burt TB, Knochel JQ, Datz FL, et al: Uterine activity: A potential cause of false-positive Meckel's scans. J Nucl Med 22:886, 1981

5. Colbert PM: Problems with radioisotope scan for Meckel's diverticulum. N Engl J Med 291:530, 1974

6. Conway JJ: Radionuclide diagnosis of Meckel's diverticulum. Gastrointest Radiol 5:209, 1980

7. Dunn EK, Farman J, Teitcher J, Smith T: Ileal leiomyosarcoma and leiomyoma — false-positive scintiscans for Meckel's diverticulum. Clin Nucl Med 12:440, 1987

8. Duszynski DO, Anthone R: Jejunal intussusception demonstrated by Tc^{99m} pertechnetate and abdominal scanning. AJR 109:729, 1970

9. Duszynski DO, Jewett TC, Allen JE: Tc^{99m}-Na pertechnetate scanning of the abdomen with particular reference to small bowel pathology. AJR 113:258, 1971

10. Fisher DR, Preston DF, Robinson RG, et al: Barrett's esophagus complicating lye ingestion: Demonstration by pertechnetate scintigraphy. Clin Nucl Med 8:550, 1983

11. Gardner RC, Kantrowitz PA, Chandler HL: Detection of cecal adenocarcinoma by Tc-99m pertechnetate scintigram. Clin Nucl Med 9:577, 1984

12. Gelfand MJ, Silberstein EB, Cox J: Radionuclide imaging of Meckel's diverticulum in children. Clin Nucl Med 3:4, 1978

13. Goel V: Meckel's diverticulum. Semin Nucl Med 12:97, 1982

14. Gordon F, Ramirez-DeGollado J, Munoz R, et al: Diagnosis of Barrett's esophagus with radioisotopes. AJR 121:716, 1974

15. Hertzog MS, Chacko AK, Pitts CM: Leiomyoma of terminal ileum producing a false-positive Meckel's scan. J Nucl Med 26:1278, 1985

16. Kwai AH, Tumeh SS: Early visualization of diverticulitis by ^{99m}Tc pertechnetate imaging. Clin Nucl Med 13:373, 1988

17. Lentle BC, Scott GW: A "false-positive" abdominal scan for Meckel's diverticulum. Br J Radiol 48:59, 1975

18. Mandell GA, Harcke HT, Sharkey C, Cooley L: Postprandial blush in multiphase bone scanning. J Nucl Med 28:1550, 1987

19. Mark R, Young L, Ferguson C, et al: Diagnosis of intrathoracic gastrogenic cyst using ^{99m}Tc-pertechnetate. Radiology 109:137, 1973

20. Maxwell ME, Baggenstoss B: False-positive Meckel's diverticulum scan of nonpathologic origin. J Nucl Med Technol 1:16, 1973

21. Mehall CJ, Klein RM, Muz J, Davis LP: Intestinal neoplasm mimicking a Meckel's diverticulum on scintigraphic imaging. Clin Nucl Med 16:233, 1991

22. Mukherji S, Harbert J, Lee T: Calyceal pertechnetate as a false-positive focus of ectopic gastric mucosa. Clin Nucl Med 10:570, 1985

23. No JE, Gleason WA, Thompson JS: The expanding spectrum of disease demonstrable by Tc-99m-pertechnetate abdominal imaging. J Nucl Med 19:691, 1978

24. Polga JP, Sargent J, Dickinson P: Positive intestinal scan caused by carcinoid tumor. J Nucl Med 15:365, 1974

25. Rodgers BM, Youssef S: "False-positive" scan for Meckel's diverticulum. J Pediatr 87:239, 1975

26. Rosenthall L, Henry JN, Murphy DA, et al: Radiopertechnetate imaging of the Meckel's diverticulum. Radiology 105:371, 1972

27. Schussheim A, Moskowitz GW, Levy LM: Radionuclide diagnosis of bleeding Meckel's diverticulum in children. Am J Gastroenterol 68:25, 1977

28. Schwesinger WH, Croom RD, Habibian MR: Diagnosis of an enteric duplication with pertechnetate-^{99m}Tc scanning. Ann Surg 181:428, 1975

29. Sciarretta G, Malaguti P, Turba E, et al: Retained gastric antrum syndrome diagnosed by ^{99m}Tc-pertechnetate scintiphotography in man: Hormonal and radioisotopic study of two cases. J Nucl Med 19:377, 1978

30. Sfakianakis GN, Conway JJ: Detection of ectopic gastric mucosa in Meckel's diverticulum and in other aberrations by scintigraphy. I. Pathophysiology and ten-year clinical experience. J Nucl Med 22:647, 1981

31. Sfakianakis GN, Conway JJ: Detection of ectopic gastric mucosa in Meckel's diverticulum and in other aberrations by scintigraphy. II. Indications and methods — a ten-year experience. J Nucl Med 22:732, 1981

32. Siddiqui A, Ryo UY, Pinsky SM: Arteriovenous malformation simulating Meckel's diverticulum on ^{99m}Tc-pertechnetate abdominal scintigraphy. Radiology 122:173, 1977

33. Sty JR, Boedecker RA, Thorp SM: Abdominal imaging in ulcerative colitis. Clin Nucl Med 4:427, 1979

34. Tauscher JW, Bryant DR, Gruenther RC: False-positive scan for Meckel's diverticulum. J Pediatr 92:1022, 1978

35. Yudd AP, Makler PT, Noel AW, et al: Nonrotation of bowel: Possible pitfalls in Meckel's scanning. Clin Nucl Med 10:377, 1985

MECKEL'S DIVERTICULUM

False-Negative

COMMON: Downstream wash of pertechnetate by active
bleeding or excessive secretions and motility
Meckel's diverticulum which does not contain
gastric mucosa

UNCOMMON: Small size of gastric mucosa in the Meckel's
diverticulum
Suboptimal technique

RARE: Autonecrosis of Meckel's diverticulum
Barium shielding of uptake
Drugs blocking uptake (e.g., perchlorate)
Obscuration by bladder activity
Obscuration by normal gastrointestinal activity

REFERENCES

1. Duszynski DO, Jewett TC, Allen JE: Tc^{99m}-Na pertechnetate scanning of the abdomen with particular reference to small bowel pathology. AJR 113:258, 1971

2. Goel V: Meckel's diverticulum. Semin Nucl Med 12:97, 1982

3. Sfakianakis GN, Conway JJ: Detection of ectopic gastric mucosa in Meckel's diverticulum and in other aberrations by scintigraphy. I. Pathophysiology and ten-year clinical experience. J Nucl Med 22:647, 1981

4. Sfakianakis GN, Conway JJ: Detection of ectopic gastric mucosa in Meckel's diverticulum and in other aberrations by scintigraphy. II. Indications and methods — ten-year experience. J Nucl Med 22:732,1981

5. Siegel BA, Alazraki NP, Alderson PO, et al (eds): Nuclear Radiology Syllabus, Second Series. Chicago, Waverly Press, 1978

GASTROINTESTINAL BLEEDING STUDIES

False-Positive Tc-99m Red Blood Cell Bleeding Study

COMMON: Bladder
Free pertechnetate in gastrointestinal tract
Kidney
Penis

UNCOMMON: Hepatic hemangioma
Varices

RARE: Abscess
Acute cholecystitis
Aneurysm
Angiodysplasia
Angiomyolipoma (tuberous sclerosis)
Arterial graft
Arteriovenous malformation
Cutaneous hemangioma
Fistula
Factitious bleeding
Gallbladder
Gastritis (without hemorrhage)
Gluteal hematoma
Hepatoma
Horseshoe kidney
Infantile hemangioendothelioma
Left ovarian vein
Leiomyosarcoma
Other tumor
Pelvic or ectopic kidney
Uterus

REFERENCES

1. Bakkers JTN, Crobach LFSJ, Pauwels EKJ: Factitious gastrointestinal bleeding (letter to the editor). J Nucl Med 26:666, 1985
2. Brill DR: Gallbladder visualization during technetium-99m-labeled red cell scintigraphy for gastrointestinal bleeding. J Nucl Med 26:1408, 1985
3. Camele RA, Bansal SK, Turbiner EH: Red blood cell gastrointestinal bleeding scintigraphy: Appearance of the left ovarian vein. Clin Nucl Med 9:275, 1984

4. Datz FL, Bilotta WR: Horseshoe kidney simulating acute gastrointestinal hemorrhage on ^{99m}Tc-labeled red blood cell imaging. Clin Nucl Med 13:123, 1988

5. Engel MA, Marks DS, Sandler MA, et al: Differentiation of focal intrahepatic lesions with ^{99m}Tc-red blood cell imaging. Radiology 146:777, 1983

6. Front D, Israel O, Groshar D, et al: Technetium-99m-labeled red blood cell imaging. Semin Nucl Med 14:226, 1984

7. Hollerman JJ, Bernstein MA, Froelich JW, et al: Detection of hemangiomas using whole-body imaging with technetium-99m labeled RBCs. Clin Nucl Med 11:716, 1986

8. Intenzo C, Desai A, Park C: False-positive gastrointestinal bleeding study due to a pelvic kidney. Clin Nucl Med 9:523, 1984

9. Lecklitner ML, Hughes JJ: Pitfalls of gastrointestinal bleeding studies with ^{99m}Tc-labeled RBCs. Semin Nucl Med 16:151, 1986

10. Moinuddin M, Allison JR, Montgomery JH, et al: Scintigraphic diagnosis of hepatic hemangioma: Its role in the management of hepatic mass lesions. AJR 145:223, 1985

11. Mountz JM, Ripley SD, Gross MD, et al: The appearance of a large mesenteric varix on a technetium-99m red blood cell gastrointestinal bleeding study. Clin Nucl Med 11:229, 1986

12. Noel AW, Heyman S: Scintigraphic findings in infantile hemangioendothelioma. Clin Nucl Med 11:413, 1986

13. Noel AW, Makler PT, Velchik MG, et al: Visualization of arterial grafts on a gastrointestinal bleeding scan. Clin Nucl Med 10:19, 1985

14. Orellana P, Olea E, Lillo R, et al: Gastroduodenal artery aneurysm detected by radionuclide studies. Clin Nucl Med 8:540, 1983

15. Oskin JE, Alexander JM, Bekerman C, et al: Alterations of dynamics in arterial mesenteric circulation secondary to atherosclerosis — a new pitfall of GI bleeding studies with ^{99m}Tc-tagged RBCs. Clin Nucl Med 15:524, 1990

16. Polga JP, Zubi SM, Spencer RP, et al: Gastrointestinal blood pool imaging in tuberous sclerosis. Clin Nucl Med 10:437, 1985

17. Rabinowitz SA, McKusick KA, Strauss HW: ^{99m}Tc red blood cell scintigraphy in evaluating focal liver lesions. AJR 143:63, 1984

18. Rachlin S, Sarkar SD, McCarthy CS, et al: Detection of acute cholecystitis on ^{99m}Tc: RBC scintiscans for hemangioma. Clin Nucl Med 19:163, 1994

20. Suzuki Y, Ootaki M: Abdominal scanning with Tc-99m red blood cells: False-positive study due to ectopic kidney. Clin Nucl Med 9:616, 1984

21. Wilton GP, Wahl RL, Juni JE, et al: Detection of gastritis by ^{99m}Tc-labeled red-blood-cell scintigraphy. AJR 143:759, 1984

GASTROINTESTINAL BLEEDING STUDIES

False-Positive Tc-99m Sulfur Colloid Study

COMMON: Bladder
Penis

UNCOMMON: Accessory or ectopic spleen
Asymmetric marrow uptake
Infarction
Myelofibrosis
Status postradiation therapy
Tumor
Transplanted kidney in rejection or acute tubular
necrosis

RARE: Aneurysm
Arterial graft
Bone chips
Kidney (normal)
Leiomyoma (ileal, uterine)
Metastasis
Paget's disease
Pancreatic pseudocyst
Varices

REFERENCES

1. Gilbert LA, Silberstein EB, Rauf GC, et al: Anorectal bleeding vs penile activity: A potential diagnostic problem. Clin Nucl Med 9:205, 1984

2. Goergen TG: Serendipity in scintigraphic gastrointestinal bleeding studies. Clin Nucl Med 8:396, 1983

3. Lecklitner ML: Pitfalls of gastrointestinal bleeding studies with ^{99m}Tc sulfur-colloid. Semin Nucl Med 16:155, 1986

4. Moreno AJ, Byrd BF, Berger DE, et al: Abdominal varices mimicking an acute gastrointestinal hemorrhage during technetium-99m red blood cell scintigraphy. Clin Nucl Med 10:248, 1985

5. Rowe DM, Schauwecker DS, Park H-M: Focal bone marrow activity: A false-positive on a sulfur colloid bleeding study. Clin Nucl Med 10:295, 1985

6. Veluvolu P, Isithman AT, Collier BD, et al: False-positive ^{99m}Tc sulfur colloid GI bleeding study due to Paget's disease. Clin Nucl Med 13:465, 1988

LABELED RED CELL IMAGING

Perfusion-Blood Pool Mismatch of Liver Lesion

COMMON: Cavernous hemangioma

UNCOMMON
AND RARE: Hepatic angiosarcoma
Hepatocellular carcinoma

REFERENCES

1. Ginsberg F, Slavin JD, Spencer RP: Hepatic angiosarcoma: Mimicking angioma on three-phase ^{99m}Tc red blood cell scintigraphy. J Nucl Med 27:1861, 1986

2. Groshar D, Ben-Haim S, Gips S, et al: Spectrum of scintigraphic appearance of liver hemangiomas. Clin Nucl Med 17:294, 1992

3. Kudo M, Ikekubo K, Yamamoto K, et al: Distinction between hemangioma of liver and hepatocellular carcinoma: Value of labeled RBC SPECT scan. Am J Roentgenol 152:977, 1989

4. Rabinowitz SA, McKusick KA, Strauss HW: ^{99m}Tc red blood cell scintigraphy in evaluating focal liver lesions. Am J Roentgenol 143:63, 1984

5. Tumeh SS, Benson C, Nagel JS, et al: Cavernous hemangioma of liver: Detection with single-photon emission computed tomography. Radiology 164:353, 1987

LABELED RED CELL IMAGING

Photopenic Lesion in Liver

COMMON AND
UNCOMMON: Abscess
Cyst
Hepatoma
Metastases

REFERENCES

1. Intenzo C, Kim S, Madsen M, et al: Planar and SPECT ^{99m}Tc RBC imaging in hepatic cavernous hemangioma and other hepatic lesions. Clin Nucl Med 13:3327, 1988

2. Rabinowitz SA, McKusick KA, Strauss HW: ^{99m}Tc red blood cell scintigraphy in evaluating focal liver lesions. Radiology 143:63, 1984

3. Shih WJ, Purcell M: Photopenic appearance of hepatic lesion(s) on ^{99m}Tc red blood cell imaging. Semin Nucl Med XXII:58,1992

4. Swayne LC, Diehl WL, Brown TD, et al: False-positive hepatic blood pool scintigraphy in metastatic colon carcinoma. Clin Nucl Med 16:630, 1991

LABELED RED CELL STUDY

Gallbladder Visualization

COMMON AND
UNCOMMON: Anemia
Intravenous radiographic contrast
Multiple transfusions
Renal failure

REFERENCES

1. Abello R, Haynie TP, Kim EE: Pitfalls of a ^{99m}Tc RBC bleeding study due to gallbladder and ileal-loop visualization. Gastrointest Radiol 16:32, 1991
2. Brill DR: Gallbladder visualization during ^{99m}Tc labeled red blood cell scintigraphy for GI bleeding. J Nucl Med 26:1408, 1985
3. Caslowitz P, Achong DM: Early gallbladder visualization during ^{99m}Tc RBC scintigraphy. Clin Nucl Med 17:365, 1992
4. Kotlyarov EV, Mattay VS, Reba RC: Gallbladder visualization during ^{99m}Tc RBC blood pool imaging. Clin Nucl Med 13:515, 1988
5. Wood MJ, Hennigan DB: Radionuclide tagged red blood cells in the gallbladder. Clin Nucl Med 9:289, 1984

BILIARY IMAGING

Delayed Visualization of the Gallbladder

COMMON: Chronic cholecystitis

UNCOMMON
AND RARE: Acalculous cholecystitis
Appendicitis
Carcinoma
Dubin-Johnson syndrome
Hepatocellular disease
Pancreatitis
Phrygian cap
Severe intercurrent disease
Total parenteral nutrition

REFERENCES

1. Bar-Meir S, Baron J, Seligson U, et al: ^{99m}Tc-HIDA cholescintigraphy in Dubin-Johnson and Rotor syndromes. Radiology 142:743, 1982

2. Drane WE, Nelp WB, Rudd TG: The need for routine delayed radionuclide hepatobiliary imaging in patients with intercurrent disease. Radiology 146:763, 1986

3. Edlund G, Kempi V, Linden W, et al: Transient non-visualization of the gallbladder by Tc-99m-HIDA cholescintigraphy in acute pancreatitis: Concise communication. J Nucl Med 23:117, 1982

4. Freeman LM, Frank MS, Sugarman LA, et al: Evaluation of biliary tract disorders with technetium-99m-HIDA cholescintigraphy. Tex Med 75:39, 1979

5. Freitas JE: Cholescintigraphy in acute and chronic cholecystitis. Semin Nucl Med 12:18, 1982

6. Miller JH, Sinatra FR, Thomas DW: Biliary excretion disorders in infants: Evaluation using 99mTc-PIPIDA. AJR 135:47, 1980

7. Rosenthall L: Cholescintigraphy in the presence of jaundice using Tc-IDA. Semin Nucl Med 12:53, 1982

8. Smergel EM, Haurere AH: Phrygian cap simulating mass lesion in hepatobiliary scintigraphy. Clin Nucl Med 9:131, 1984

9. Weissman HS, Frank MS, Bernstein LH, et al: Rapid and accurate diagnosis of acute cholecystitis with ^{99m}Tc-HIDA cholescintigraphy. AJR 132:523, 1979

BILIARY IMAGING

Nonvisualization of the Gallbladder

COMMON: Acute cholecystitis

UNCOMMON: Acute pancreatitis
Chronic cholecystitis
Complete common duct obstruction
Nonfasting normals
Postcholecystectomy
Prolonged fasting
Severe hepatocellular disease

RARE: Abscess adjacent to gallbladder
Agenesis of the gallbladder
AIDS cholangitis
Alcoholism
Asphyxiation
Choledochal cyst
Congenital absence of gallbladder
Dubin-Johnson syndrome
Gallbladder carcinoma
Hemobilia
Hyperalimentation
Intrahepatic gallbladder
Intrahepatic lithiasis
Kawasaki's syndrome
Rotor's syndrome
Severe intercurrent disease

REFERENCES

1. Ali A, Turner DA, Fordham EW: Re: Tc-99m IDA cholescintigraphy in acute pancreatitis. J Nucl Med 24:748, 1983
2. Bar-Meir S, Baron J, Seligson U, et al: ^{99m}Tc-HIDA cholescintigraphy in Dubin-Johnson and Rotor syndromes. Radiology 142:743, 1982
3. Brunetti JX, VanHeertum RL, Kempf JS, et al: ^{99m}Tc DISIDA hepatobiliary scintigraphy in AIDS cholangitis. Clin Nucl Med 19:36, 1994
4. Colletti PM, Ralls PW, Seigel ME, et al: Cholescintigraphy in gallbladder carcinoma. Clin Nucl Med 11:270, 1986

5. Dickinson CZ, Powers TA, Sandler MP, et al: Congenital absence of the gall-bladder: Another cause of false-positive hepatobiliary image. J Nucl Med 25:70, 1984

6. Dumont M, Danais S: Intrahepatic gallbladder simulating choledochal cyst on DISIDA scintigraphy. Clin Nucl Med 9:657, 1986

7. Edlund G, Kempi V, Linden W, et al: Transient nonvisualization of the gall-bladder by Tc-99m-HIDA cholescintigraphy in acute pancreatitis: Concise communication. J Nucl Med 23:117, 1982

8. Freeman LM, Frank MS, Sugarman LA, et al: Evaluation of biliary tract disorders with technetium-99m-HIDA cholescintigraphy. Tex Med 75:39, 1979

9. Freitas JE: Cholescintigraphy in acute and chronic cholecystitis. Semin Nucl Med 12:18, 1982

10. Harwood S, Zusmer N, Robbins R, et al: The detection of a choledochal cyst by combined grey-scale ultrasound and ^{131}I-Rose Bengal scintigraphy. Clin Nucl Med 1:113, 1976

11. Jackson DE, Floyd JL, Levesque PH: Hemobilia associated with hepatic artery aneurysms: Scintigraphic detection with technetium-99m-labeled red blood cells. J Nucl Med 27:491, 1986

12. Lecklitner ML, Growcock G: Hepatobiliary scintigraphy: Nonvisualization of activity in the area of the gallbladder associated with intestinal activity. Semin Nucl Med 14:264, 1984

13. Miller JH, Sinatra FR, Thomas DW: Biliary excretion disorders in infants: Evaluation using ^{99m}Tc-PIPIDA. AJR 135:47, 1980

14. Nagle CE, Freitas J, Dworkin HJ: Cholescintigraphy in cholecystic cancer. Clin Nucl Med 8:220, 1983

15. Oshiumi Y, Nakayama C, Morita K, et al: Serial scintigraphy of choledochal cysts using ^{131}I-Rose Bengal and ^{131}I-bromsulphalein. AJR 128:769, 1977

16. Pauwels S, Steels M, Piret L, et al: Clinical evaluation of Tc-99m-diethyl IDA in hepatobiliary disorders. J Nucl Med 19:783, 1978

17. Rosenthall L: Cholescintigraphy in the presence of jaundice using Tc-IDA. Semin Nucl Med 12:53, 1982

18. Shuman WP, Gibbs P, Rudd RG, et al: PIPIDA scintigraphy for cholecystitis: False positives in alcoholism and total parenteral nutrition. AJR 138:1, 1982

19. Sujov P, Herschkowitz S, Jerushalmi J: Transient nonvisualization of gallbladder in asphyxiated neonate. Clin Nucl Med 15:50, 1990

20. Swayne LC: Acute acalculous cholecystitis: Sensitivity in detection using technetium-99m iminodiacetic acid cholescintigraphy. Radiology 160:33, 1986

21. Swayne LC, Kolc J: Erythromycin hepatoxicity: A rare cause of a false-positive technetium-99m DISIDA study. Clin Nucl Med 11:10, 1986

22. Velchik MG, Makler PT, Alavi A: Gallbladder carcinoma: Another cause of the distended photon-deficient gallbladder in cholescintigraphy. Clin Nucl Med 9:137, 1984

23. Warshauer DM, Sulzer JL: Agenesis of gallbladder — rare cause for false-positive hepatobiliary image. Clin Nucl Med 13:468, 1988

24. Weiss PE, Lanzafame RJ, Hinshaw JR: Abscess adjacent to gallbladder: A new cause of false-positive DISIDA scan. Clin Nucl Med 10:615, 1985

25. Weissman HS, Frank MS, Bernstein LH, et al: Rapid and accurate diagnosis of acute cholecystitis with ^{99m}Tc-HIDA cholescintigraphy. AJR 132:523, 1979

26. Weissman HS, Gliedman ML, Wilk PJ, et al: Evaluation of the postoperative patient with ^{99m}Tc-IDA cholescintigraphy. Semin Nucl Med 12:27, 1982

27. Weissman HS, Rosenblatt R, Sugarman LA, et al: The role of nuclear imaging in evaluating cholestatis — an update. Semin Ultrasound 1:134, 1980

28. Zanzi I, Perpignano MC, Margouleff D, et al: Cholescintigraphic abnormality in a case of Kawasaki syndrome. Clin Nucl Med 10:475, 1985

29. Zeman RK, Lee CH, Stahl R, et al: Strategy for the use of biliary scintigraphy in non-iatrogenic biliary trauma. Radiology 151:771, 1984

BILIARY IMAGING

False-Negative Morphine-augmented Studies

COMMON: Dislodgement of a cystic duct stone by increased
intraductal pressure
Gangrenous cholecystitis with relief of cystic duct
obstruction after perforation
Partial cystic duct obstruction
Intermittent dislodgement of obstructing stone
Acute acalculous cholecystitis

REFERENCES

1. Bourekas EC, Tupler RH, Turbiner EH: Morphine-augmented cholescintigraphy with false-negative result and apparent ectopic gallbladder. Clin Nucl Med 17:931, 1992

2. Choy D, Shi E, McLean R, et al: Cholescintigraphy in acute cholecystitis: Use of intravenous morphine. Radiology 151:203, 1984

3. Fig LM, Wahl RL, Stewart RE, et al: Morphine-augmented hepatobiliary scintigraphy in the severely ill: Caution is in order. Radiology 175:467, 1990

4. Fink-Bennett D, Balon H, Robbins T, et al: Morphine-augmented cholescintigraphy: Its efficacy in detecting acute cholecystitis. J Nucl Med 32:1231, 1991

5. Mack JM, Salvin JD, Spencer RP: Two false-negative results using morphine sulfate in hepatobiliary imaging. Clin Nucl Med 14:87, 1989

6. Yeo EE, Low JC, Azizi F: False-negative morphine-augmented cholescintigraphy in patient with gangrenous cholecystitis. Clin Nucl Med 17:929, 1992

BILIARY IMAGING

Decreased Gallbladder Ejection Fraction

COMMON AND
UNCOMMON: Adenomyomatosis
Cholelithiasis
Chronic acalculous cholecystitis
Chronic cholecystitis
Cystic duct syndrome
Gallbladder dyskinesia
Isolated common bile duct obstruction (gallstones,
    stricture, malignancy)
Normal
Sclerosing cholangitis
Sphincter of Oddi dyskinesia

REFERENCES

1. Fink-Bennett D, DeRidder P, Kolozsi WZ, et al: Cholecystokinin chole-scintigraphy: Detection of abnormal gallbladder motor function in patients with chronic acalculous gallbladder disease. J Nucl Med 32:1695, 1991

2. Krishnamurthy GT: Nuclear hepatology: Where is it heading now? J Nucl Med 29:1144, 1988

3. Krishnamurthy S, Krishnamurthy GT: Gallbladder ejection fraction: A decade of progress and future promise. J Nucl Med 32:542, 1992

4. Swayne LC, Heitner D, Rubenstein JB, et al: Differential gallbladder contrac-tility in fundal adenomyomatosis: Demonstration by cholecystokinin cholescintigraphy. J Nucl Med 28:1771, 1987

5. Ziessman HA, Fahey FH, Hixson DJ: Calculation of gallbladder ejection frac-tion: Advantage of continuous sincalide infusion over 3-minute infusion method. J Nucl Med 33:537, 1992

BILIARY IMAGING

Delayed Bowel Activity

COMMON: Choledocholithiasis with incomplete obstruction
Normal
Severe hepatocellular disease

UNCOMMON
AND RARE: Acute cholecystitis
AIDS cholangitis
Ascending cholangitis
Choledochal cyst with incomplete obstruction
Chronic cholecystitis
Intrahepatic cholestasis
Intrahepatic lithiasis
Liver transplant rejection
Narcotics
Neonatal hepatitis
Odditis
Rejection (liver transplant)
Sphincter of Oddi
Stenosis
Tumor involving ampulla of Vater

REFERENCES

1. Freeman LM, Frank MS, Sugarman LA, et al: Evaluation of biliary tract disorders with technetium-99m-HIDA cholescintigraphy. Tex Med 75:39, 1979

2. Freitas JE: Cholescintigraphy in acute and chronic cholecystitis. Semin Nucl Med 12:18, 1982

3. Gelfand MJ, Smith HS, Ryckman FC, et al: Hepatobiliary scintigraphy in pediatric liver transplant recipients. Clin Nucl Med 17:542, 1992

4. Harwood S. Zusmer N, Robbins R, et al: The detection of a choledochal cyst by combined grey-scale ultrasound and ^{131}I-Rose Bengal scintigraphy. Clin Nucl Med 1:113, 1976

5. Itoh H, Murase K, Hamamoto K: Reflux sign in cholescintigraphy after administration of gallbladder contracting agent. J Nucl Med 30:1192, 1989

6. Jacobson AF, Cronin EB, Holman BL: Sequential hepatobiliary scintigraphy demonstrating apparent transient biliary obstruction. J Nucl Med 28:1175, 1987

7. Loken MK, Ascher NL, Boudreau RJ, et al: Scintigraphic evaluation of liver transplant function. J Nucl Med 27:451, 1986

8. Miller JH, Sinatra FR, Thomas DW: Biliary excretion disorders in infants: Evaluation using ^{99m}Tc-PIPIDA. AJR 135:47, 1980

9. Oshiumi Y, Nakayama C, Morita K, et al: Serial scintigraphy of choledochal cysts using ^{131}I-Rose Bengal and ^{131}I-bromsulphalein. AJR 128:769, 1977

10. Patch GG, Morton KA, Arias JM, Datz FL: Naloxone reverses pattern of obstruction of distal common bile duct induced by analgesic narcotics in hepatobiliary imaging. J Nucl Med 32:1270, 1991

11. Pauwels S, Steels M, Piret L, et al: Clinical evaluation of Tc-99m-diethyl-IDA in hepatobiliary disorders. J Nucl Med 19:783, 1978

12. Rosenthall L: Cholescintigraphy in the presence of jaundice using Tc-IDA. Semin Nucl Med 12:53, 1982

13. Rosenthall L, Shaffer EA, Lisbona R, et al: Diagnosis of hepatobiliary disease by ^{99m}Tc-HIDA cholescintigraphy. Radiology 126:467, 1978

14. Shih WJ, DeLand FH, Domstad PA: Demonstrating alcoholic cirrhosis of the liver by Tc-99m BIDA scintigram. Clin Nucl Med 9:444, 1984

15. Weissman HS, Badia J, Sugarman LA, et al: Spectrum of 99m-Tc-IDA cholescintigraphic patterns in acute cholecystitis. Radiology 138:167, 1981

16. Weissman HS, Frank MS, Bernstein LH, et al: Rapid and accurate diagnosis of acute cholecystitis with ^{99m}Tc-HIDA cholescintigraphy. AJR 132:523, 1979

17. Weissman HS, Gliedman ML, Wilk PJ, et al: Evaluation of the postoperative patient with ^{99m}Tc-IDA cholescintigraphy. Semin Nucl Med 12:27, 1982

18. Weissman HS, Rosenblatt R, Sugarman LA, et al: The role of nuclear imaging in evaluating cholestasis — an update. Semin Ultrasound 1:134, 1980

19. Weidman MA, Tan A, Martinez CJ: Fetal sonography and neonatal scintigraphy of a choledochal cyst. J Nucl Med 26:893, 1985

BILIARY IMAGING

Nonvisualization of the Bowel

COMMON: Choledocholithiasis

UNCOMMON: Biliary atresia
Drug-induced cholestasis
Pancreatic carcinoma
Severe hepatocellular disease
Spasm of sphincter of Oddi secondary to morphine

RARE: Bile duct carcinoma
Choledochal cyst with complete obstruction
Dubin-Johnson syndrome
Hematobilia
Inspissated bile syndrome
Ligation of main biliary duct at surgery
Massive tumor
Replacement of liver
Pancreatitis
Perforated ulcer
Portal vein thrombosis
Sepsis

REFERENCES

1. Freeman LM, Frank MS, Sugarman LA, et al: Evaluation of biliary tract disorders with technetium-99m-HIDA cholescintigraphy. Tex Med 75:39, 1979
2. Freitas JE: Cholescintigraphy in acute and chronic cholecystitis. Semin Nucl Med 12:18, 1982
3. Gerhold JP, Klingensmith WC III, Kuni CC, et al: Diagnosis of biliary atresia with radionuclide hepatobiliary imaging. Radiology 146:499, 1983
4. Hughes KS, Marrangoni AG, Thompson DR, et al: Endotoxic shock and its effects on hepatobiliary scanning in dogs. Radiology 148:823, 1983
5. Hughes KS, Marrangoni AG, Turbiner E: Etiology of the obstructive pattern in hepatobiliary imaging. Clin Nucl Med 9:222, 1984
6. Lee RGL, Gregg JA, Koroshetz AM, et al: Sphincter of Oddi stenosis: Diagnosis using hepatobiliary scintigraphy and endoscopic manometry. Radiology 156:793, 1985
7. Miller JH, Sinatra FR, Thomas DW: Biliary excretion disorders in infants: Evaluation using ^{99m}Tc-PIPIDA. AJR 135:47, 1980

8. Noel AW, Velchik MG, Alavi A: The "liver scan" appearance in cholescintigraphy: A sign of complete common bile duct obstruction. Clin Nucl Med 10:264, 1985

9. Oshiumi Y, Nakayama C, Morita K, et al: Serial scintigraphy of choledochal cysts using ^{131}I-Rose Bengal and ^{131}I-bromsulphalein. AJR 128:769, 1977

10. Pauwels S, Steels M, Piret L, et al: Clinical evaluation of Tc-99m-diethyl-IDA in hepatobiliary disorders. J Nucl Med 19:783, 1978

11. Rosenthall L: Cholescintigraphy in the presence of jaundice using Tc-IDA. Semin Nucl Med 12:53, 1982

12. Rosenthall L, Shaffer EA, Lisbona R, et al: Diagnosis of hepatobiliary disease by ^{99m}Tc-HIDA cholescintigraphy. Radiology 126:467, 1978

13. Shanley DJ, Buckner AB, Alexander HG: Scintigraphic duodenal cut off sign in acute pancreatitis. Clin Nucl Med 16:223, 1991

14. Sty JR, Wells RG, Schroeder BA: Comparative imaging — bile-plug syndrome. Clin Nucl Med 12:489, 1987

15. Weissman HS, Frank MS, Bernstein LH, et al: Rapid and accurate diagnosis of acute cholecystitis with ^{99m}Tc-HIDA cholescintigraphy. AJR 132:523, 1979

16. Weissman HS, Gliedman ML, Wilk PJ, et al: Evaluation of the postoperative patient with ^{99m}Tc-IDA cholescintigraphy. Semin Nucl Med 12:27, 1982

17. Weissman HS, Rosenblatt R, Sugarman LA, et al: The role of nuclear imaging in evaluating cholestasis — an update. Semin Ultrasound 1:134, 1980

18. Williamson MR, Rosenberg RD, Davis M, Williamson SL: Hematobilia causing complete biliary obstruction on ^{99m}Tc DISIDA scan. Clin Nucl Med 15:583, 1990

19. Wynchank S, Gulliet J, Leccia F, et al: Biliary atresia and neonatal hepatobiliary scintigraphy. Clin Nucl Med 9:121, 1984

BILIARY IMAGING

Enterogastric Reflux

COMMON: Normal
Acute cholecystitis
Chronic cholecystitis
Postccholecystectomy
Morphine-augmented study
Duodenal ulcer

UNCOMMON
AND RARE: Chronic gastritis
Duodenal hematoma
Pancreatitis
Hepatic abscess
Duodenitis
Scleroderma

REFERENCES

1. Colletti PM, Barakos JA, Siegel ME, et al: Enterogastric reflux in suspected acute cholecystitis. Clin Nucl Med 12:533, 1987

2. Drane WE, Hanner JS: Complete duodenogastric reflux: Scintigraphic sign of significant duodenal pathology. J Nucl Med 30:1568, 1989

3. Mintz A, Rosenson A, Saltiel AA, et al: Duodenal hematoma — a mechanical cause for enterogastric reflux in cholescintigraphy. Clin Nucl Med 16:491, 1991

4. Oates E, Achong DM: Incidence and significance of enterogastric reflux during morphine-augmented cholescintigraphy. Clin Nucl Med 17:926, 1992

5. Sawaf NW, Orzel JA, Weiland FL: Gastroesophageal reflux demonstrated by hepatobiliary imaging in scleroderma. J Nucl Med 28:387, 1987

6. Shih WJ, Coupal JJ, Domstad PA, et al: Disorders of gallbladder function related to duodenogastric reflux in ^{99m}Tc DISIDA hepatobiliary scintigraphy. Clin Nucl Med 12:857, 1987

7. Wang GX, Shih WJ, Tang PL, et al: Duodenogastric reflux demonstrated by cholescintigraphy in peptic ulcer disease and chronic gastritis. Clin Nucl Med 19:100, 1994

BILIARY IMAGING

Rim Sign

COMMON: Acute cholecystitis
Emphysema of the gallbladder
Gallbladder perforation
Gangrenous cholecystitis

UNCOMMON
AND RARE: Adjacent hepatic inflammatory process
Chronic cholecystitis
Hepatic amebic abscess
Prominent porta hepatis

REFERENCES

1. Brachman MB, Tanasescu DE, Ramanna L: Acute gangrenous cholecystitis: Radionuclide diagnosis. Radiology 151:209, 1984

2. Bushnell DL, Perlman SB, Wilson MA, et al: J Nucl Med 27:353, 1986

3. Cawthon MA, Brown DM, Hartshorne MF, et al: Biliary scintigraphy: The "hot rim" sign. Clin Nucl Med 9:619, 1984

4. Meekin CK, Ziessman HA: The prognostic value of increased hepatic activity adjacent to the gallbladder fossa during cholescintigraphy for acute cholecystitis (abstract). J Nucl Med 27:938, 1986

5. Remedios PA, Colletti PM, Ralls, PW: Hepatic amebic abscess: Cholescintigraphic rim enhancement. Radiology 160:395, 1986

6. Shih WJ, Mills BJ, Pulmano C: Prominent porta hepatitis resulting in rim sign appearance on cholescintigraphy. Clin Nucl Med 15:400, 1990

7. Smith R, Rosen JM, Gallo LN, et al: Pericholecystic hepatic activity in cholescintigraphy. Radiology 156:797, 1985

8. Smith R, Rosen JM, Alderson PO: Gallbladder perforation: Diagnostic utility of cholescintigraphy in suggested subacute or chronic cases. Radiology 158:63, 1986

BILIARY IMAGING

Liver Scan Appearance (No Splenic Activity)

COMMON: Choledocholithiasis
Tumor-obstructing duct
    Pancreatic carcinoma
    Cholangiocarcinoma
    Ampullary carcinoma
    Metastatic tumor
Pancreatitis

UNCOMMON
AND RARE: Sepsis
Peritonitis
Hepatocellular disease (hepatitis, cholangitis)
Partial vein thrombosis
Biliary atresia
Dubin-Johnson syndrome
Drug-induced cholestasis

REFERENCES

1. Bar-Meir S, Baron J, Seligson U, et al: ^{99m}Tc HIDA cholescintigraphy in Dubin-Johnson and Rotor syndromes. Radiology 142:743, 1982

2. Egbert RN, Braunstein P, Lyon KP, Miller DR: Total bile duct obstruction — prompt diagnosis by hepatobiliary imaging. Arch Surg 118:709, 1983

3. Ford KB, Porter BA, Stadalnik RC, Brown DW: Functional causes of ductal obstructive pattern on hepatobiliary scans. Clin Nucl Med 12:713, 1987

4. Hughes KS, Marrangoni AG, Turbiner E: Etiology of obstructive pattern in hepatobiliary imaging. Clin Nucl Med 9:222, 1984

5. Klingensmith WC, Ashdown BC: Cholescintigraphy in diagnosis of intrahepatic cholestatis — how specific is it? Clin Nucl Med 16:621, 1991

6. Klingensmith WC, Kuni CC, Fritzberg AR: Cholescintigraphy in extra-hepatic biliary obstruction. Am J Radiol 139:65, 1982

7. Silfen D: Role of hepatobiliary imaging in evaluation and management of patients with common bile duct gallstones. J Nucl Med 32:1261, 1991

BILIARY IMAGING

Splenic Visualization

COMMON AND
UNCOMMON: Accidental mixing of IDA and sulfur colloid in
syringe
Radiopharmaceutical preparation error — reduced
hydrolyzed technetium colloid
Anatomic liver variant creating pseudo-spleen
Hepatocellular dysfunction

REFERENCES

1. Balseiro J, Fratkin MJ, Hirsch JI, Haden HT: Persistent splenic visualization on ^{99m}Tc DISIDA hepatobiliary studies. Clin Nucl Med 15:237, 1990

2. Lecklitner ML, Benedetto AR, Straw JD: Failure of quality control to detect errors in preparation of ^{99m}Tc disofenin (DISIDA). Clin Nucl Med 10:468, 1985

3. Shih WJ, DeLand FH, Domstad PA: Demonstrating alcoholic cirrhosis of liver by ^{99m}Tc BIDA scintigram. Clin Nucl Med 9:444, 1984

4. Vasquez R, Oates E, Helsa R: Pseudosplenic uptake in a DISIDA scan can be a normal liver variant. Clin Nucl Med 12:763, 1987

BILIARY IMAGING

Peripheral Liver Retention with Central Clearing (bull's eye)

COMMON AND
UNCOMMON: Alagille syndrome
Central tumor

REFERENCES

1. Aburano T, Yokoyama K, Takayama T, et al: Distinct hepatic retention of ^{99m}Tc IDA in arteriohepatic dysplasia (Alagille syndrome). Clin Nucl Med 14:874, 1989

2. Ducret RP, Cefalu JB, Alford BA, et al: Hepatocarcinoma in association with Alagille syndrome. Clin Nucl Med 13:920, 1988

BILIARY IMAGING

Intrahepatic Hot Spots

COMMON AND
UNCOMMON: Bile duct cysts secondary to infarcts of polyarteritis
Biloma (trauma)
Caroli's disease
Hepatoma
Hydatid cyst communicating with the biliary system
Intrahepatic calculi
Metastases
Multiple liver abscesses
Postsurgical
Sclerosing cholangitis
Sclerosing form of cholangiocarcinoma

REFERENCES

1. Ament AE, Bick RJ, Miraldi FD, et al: Sclerosing cholangitis: Cholescintigraphy with Tc-99m-labeled DISIDA. Radiology 151:197, 1984

2. Amir A, Jacobs PH, Piepsz A: Unusual cholescintigraphic findings in polyarteritis nodosa. Clin Nucl Med 9:585, 1984

3. Cabrera J, Quintero E, Bruguera M, et al: Diagnosis of Caroli's disease by technetium-99m DISIDA cholescintigraphy: Report of three cases. Clin Nucl Med 10:478, 1985

4. Jackson DE, Floyd JL: Hemobilia: An unusual cause of segmental bile duct obstruction. Clin Nucl Med 11:77, 1986

5. Lee VW, O'Brien MJ, Devereux DF: Hepatocellular carcinoma: Uptake of ^{99m}Tc-IDA in primary tumor and metastasis. AJR 143:57, 1984

6. Padhy AK, Gopinath PG, Basu AK, et al: Hepatobiliary scintigraphy in congenital cystic dilation of biliary tract. Clin Nucl Med 10:703, 1985

7. Padhy AK, Gopinath PG, Basu AK, et al: Scintigraphic findings in a case of hydatid cyst of the liver communicating with the biliary system. Clin Nucl Med 11:281, 1986

8. Weissman HS, Byun KJC, Freeman LM: Role of Tc-99m IDA scintigraphy in the evaluation of hepatobiliary trauma. Semin Nucl Med 13:199, 1983

BILIARY IMAGING

Collection of Bile along Course of Biliary Tree

COMMON AND
   UNCOMMON: Intrahepatic gallbladder
                      Choledochal cyst
                      Bilobed or duplicated gallbladder
                      Uni- or multicystic liver disease with ruptured
                          septum

REFERENCE

1. Gad MA, Krishnamurty GT, Glowniak JV: Identification and differentiation of congenital gallbladder abnormality by quantitative ^{99m}Tc IDA cholescintigraphy. J Nucl Med 33:431, 1992

BILIARY IMAGING

Abnormal Collection of Bile Outside Liver

COMMON: Bile leak

UNCOMMON
AND RARE: Duodenal obstruction
Retroanastomatic herniation
Bowel malrotation
Metastatic hepatoma

REFERENCES

1. Archibeque F, Williamson MR, Rosenberg R, et al: Hepatoma: [99m]Tc DISIDA uptake in primary and metastatic lesions. Clin Nucl Med 14:707, 1989
2. Coupland D, Lentle B, Scudamore C: Malrotation simulating gallbladder perforation on ^{99m}Tc IDA scintigraphy — pitfall to avoid. Clin Nucl Med 16:904, 1991
3. Fortenbery EJ, Blue PW: Pseudobiliary leak. Clin Nucl Med 17:414, 1992
4. Kuy RS, Yen TC, Kuo SJ, Yeh SH: Retroanastomotic herniation mimicking biliary leakage in cholescintigraphic pattern. Clin Nucl Med 12:673, 1987

HEPATIC SCINTIANGIOGRAPHY

Early or Increased Flow to the Liver

COMMON: Chronic liver disease
           Hepatoma
           Lymphoma
           Metastatic disease

UNCOMMON: Abscess
           Adenoma
           Focal nodular hyperplasia
           Following radiation therapy
           Hemangioma and hemangioendothelioma

RARE: Dilated portal vein
           Massive breast shielding

REFERENCES

1. DeNardo GL, Stadalnik RC, DeNardo SJ, et al: Hepatic scintiangiographic patterns. Radiology 111:135, 1974

2. Echevarria RA, Bonanno C: Value of routine abdominal nuclide angiography as part of liver scan. Clin Nucl Med 4:66, 1979

3. Hollerman JJ, Bernstein MA, Froelich JW, et al: Detection of hemangiomas using whole-body imaging with technetium-99m labeled RBCs. Clin Nucl Med 11:716, 1986

4. McLoughlin MJ, Colapinto RF, Gilday DL, et al: Focal nodular hyperplasia of the liver: Angiography and radioisotope scanning. Radiology 107:257, 1973

5. Moinuddin M, Allison JR, Montgomery JH, et al: Scintigraphic diagnosis of hepatic hemangioma: Its role in the management of hepatic mass lesions. AJR 145:223, 1985

6. Noel AW, Heyman S: Scintigraphic findings in infantile hemangioendothelioma. Clin Nucl Med 11:413, 1986

7. Ramanathan P, Ganatra RD, Blau M: Dynamic blood flow studies of space occupying lesions in the liver. J Nucl Med 15:1021, 1974

8. Stadalnik RC, DeNardo SJ, DeNardo GL, et al: Critical evaluation of hepatic scintiangiography for neoplastic tumors of the liver. J Nucl Med 16:595, 1975

9. Stanley P, Gates GF, Eto RT, et al: Hepatic cavernous hemangiomas and hemangioendotheliomas in infancy. AJR 129:317, 1977

10. Waxman AD, Apau R, Siemsen JK: Rapid sequential liver imaging. J Nucl Med 13:522, 1972

11. Witek JT, Spencer RP: Clinical correlation of hepatic flow studies. J Nucl Med 16:71, 1975

HEPATIC SCINTIANGIOGRAPHY

Focally Decreased Flow (Solitary or Multiple)

COMMON: Abscess (amebic or pyogenic)
Cyst (Any etiology)
Extrinsic mass
Hemangioma
Hematoma
Hepatoma
Some metastases

UNCOMMON
AND RARE: Fatty infiltration
Lymphoma
Regenerating nodule

REFERENCES

1. DeNardo GL, Stadalnik RC, DeNardo SJ, et al: Hepatic scintiangiographic patterns. Radiology 111:135, 1974

2. Echevarria RA, Bonanno C: Value of routine abdominal nuclide angiography as part of liver scan. Clin Nucl Med 4:66, 1979

3. Hollerman JJ, Bernstein MA, Froelich JW, et al: Detection of hemangiomas using whole-body imaging with technetium-99m labeled RBCs. Clin Nucl Med 11:716, 1986

4. Moinuddin M, Allison JR, Montgomery JH, et al: Scintigraphic diagnosis of hepatic hemangioma: Its role in the management of hepatic mass lesions. AJR 145:223, 1985

5. Ramanathan P, Ganatra RD, Blau M: Dynamic blood flow studies of space occupying lesions in the liver. J Nucl Med 15:1021, 1974

6. Reeder MM, Felson B: Gamuts in Radiology. Cincinnati, Audiovisual Radiology of Cincinnati, 1975

7. Waxman AD, Apau R, Siemsen JK: Rapid sequential liver imaging. J Nucl Med 13:522, 1972

8. Yeh SH, Shih WJ, Liang JC: Intravenous radionuclide hepatography in the differential diagnosis of intrahepatic mass lesions. J Nucl Med 14:565, 1973

LIVER-SPLEEN SCAN

Hepatomegaly

COMMON: Abscess
Cirrhosis
Cyst (e.g., congenital, traumatic, hydatid)
Fatty infiltration
Hepatitis
Hepatoma
Metastasis
Other primary neoplasm — benign or malignant
Riedel's lobe

UNCOMMON
AND RARE: Acromegaly
Actinomycosis
AIDS
Amyloidosis
Budd-Chiari syndrome
Chronic hemolytic anemia
Collagen vascular diseases
Following chemotherapy
Following splenectomy
Gaucher's disease
Hematoma
Hemochromatosis
Histiocytosis X
Homocystinuria
Kala-azar
Lymphoma
Miliary histoplasmosis
Miliary tuberculosis
Mucopolysaccharidosis (e.g., Hurler's, Hunter's)
Polycystic liver disease
Sarcoidosis
Schistosomiasis
Wolman's disease

REFERENCES

1. Bingham JB, Maisey MN: Unusual scintigraphic appearances of a mobile accessory lobe of the liver. J Nucl Med 19:1235, 1978

2. Cohen GA, Smoak WM, Goldberg LD: Acromegalic cholecystomegaly. J Nucl Med 15:720, 1974

3. Gottschalk A, Potchen EJ (eds): Diagnostic Nuclear Medicine. Baltimore, Williams and Wilkins, 1976

4. Kaplan WD, Drum DE, Lokich JJ: The effect of cancer chemotherapeutic agents on the liver-spleen scan. J Nucl Med 21:84, 1980

5. Meindok H, Langer B: Liver scan in Budd-Chiari syndrome. J Nucl Med 17:365, 1976

6. Reeder MM, Felson B: Gamuts in Radiology. Cincinnati, Audiovisual Radiology of Cincinnati, Inc., 1975

7. Salzman SH, Burke G: The differential diagnosis of giant liver — a review of the clinical significance of massive hepatomegaly. Am J Gastroenterol 47:221, 1967

8. Sham R, Sain A, Silver L: Hypertrophic Riedel's lobe of the liver. Clin Nucl Med 3:79, 1978

9. Smith R: Liver-spleen scintigraphy in patients with acquired immunodeficiency syndrome. AJR 145:1201, 1985

10. Sty JR, Starshak RJ: Scintigraphy in Wolman's disease. Clin Nucl Med 3:397, 1978

11. Waxman AD: Scintigraphic evaluation of diffuse hepatic disease. Semin Nucl Med 12:75, 1982

LIVER-SPLEEN SCAN

Massive Hepatomegaly

COMMON AND
UNCOMMON: Abscess
             Amyloidosis
             Biliary cirrhosis
             Congestive heart failure
             Fatty infiltration
             Hemochromatosis
             Leukemia
             Lymphoma
             Metastatic disease
             Polycystic liver disease

REFERENCES

1. Gottschalk A, Potchen EJ (eds): Diagnostic Nuclear Medicine. Baltimore, Williams and Wilkins, 1976

2. Salzman SH, Burke G: The differential diagnosis of giant liver — a review of the clinical significance of massive hepatomegaly. Am J Gastroenterol 47:221, 1967

LIVER-SPLEEN SCAN

Solitary Defect in the Liver

COMMON: Abscess
Any of false-positive causes
Cyst
Hemangioma
Hepatoma
Metastases

UNCOMMON: Hematoma
Hepatic adenoma
Postsurgical
Pseudotumor in cirrhosis

RARE: Arteriovenous malformation
Fatty infiltration
Focal nodular hyperplasia
Glycogen storage disease
Granuloma
Hydatid cyst
Infarct
Intrahepatic aneurysm
Intrahepatic gallbladder
Localized bile duct obstruction
Lymphoma
Pseudotumor in hepatitis
Radiation
Scleroderma
Thoratrast

REFERENCES

1. Antar MA, Kassamali H, Spencer RP: Sequential loss of splenic and the hepatic function in patient with thorotrast loading. Clin Nucl Med 14:634, 1989

2. Barnett CA, Olson R, Stadalnik RC: Chronic passive congestion of the liver appearing as focal defects on liver imaging. Clin Nucl Med 2:52, 1977

3. Beal W, Soin JS, Burdine JA: Hepatic cavernous hemangioma presenting as an "avascular mass" in a newborn. J Nucl Med 15:902, 1974

4. Beauchamp JM, Gelanger MA, Heitzschman HR: Intrahepatic focal lesion in acute viral hepatitis. J Nucl Med 15:356, 1974

5. Burke TS, Tatum JL: Hepatic infarction detected on ^{99m}Tc sulfur colloid imaging. Clin Nucl Med 15:673, 1990

6. Chandra S, Laor YG: Liver scan in a case of hepatic infarct. J Nucl Med 14:858, 1973

7. Conte PJ: Aortic aneurysm causing multiple liver scan defects. AJR 128:516, 1977

8. Custer JR, Shafer RB: Changes in liver scan following splenectomy. J Nucl Med 16:194, 1975

9. DaCosta H, Gandhi R, Deshmukh S, et al: Hepatosplenic scintigraphy in children with obstructive jaundice. Clin Nucl Med 2:381, 1977

10. Drum DE: Current status of radiocolloid hepatic scintiphotography for space-occupying disease. Semin Nucl Med 12:64, 1982

11. Drum DE: Optimizing the clinical value of hepatic scintiphotography. Semin Nucl Med 8:346, 1978

12. Drum DE, Beard JO: Liver scintigraphic features associated with alcoholism. J Nucl Med 19:154, 1978

13. Drum DE, Beard JO: Scintigraphic criteria for hepatic metastases from cancer of the colon and breast. J Nucl Med 17:577, 1976

14. Groshar D, Jerusalmi J, Gips S, et al: Focal liver defect caused by hydatid cyst in the lung. Clin Nucl Med 10:602, 1985

15. Herbst KD, Corder MP: Radiotheraphy-induced liver scan defects. J Nucl Med 17:425, 1976

16. Herbst KD, Corder MP, Morita ET: Hepatic scan defects following radiotherapy for lymphoma. Clin Nucl Med 3:331, 1978

17. Israel O, Jerushalmi J, Front D: Scintigraphic findings in Gaucher's disease. J Nucl Med 27:1557, 1986

18. Kim E, Mattar AG: Scan findings in a case of splenic infarction due to amyloidosis: Case report. J Nucl Med 17:902, 1976

19. Koenigsberg M, Freeman LM: Intrahepatic focal lesion in acute viral hepatitis. J Nucl Med 14:612, 1973

20. Lee HK, Jones L: Subphrenic abscess mimicking intrahepatic defect in a combined lung-liver scan. Clin Nucl Med 2:207, 1977

21. Lunia S, Barthasarathy KL, Bakshi S, et al: An evaluation of ^{99m}Tc sulphur colloid liver scintiscans and their usefulness in metastatic work-up: A review of 1424 studies. J Nucl Med 16:62, 1975

22. Lutzker LG: Radionuclide imaging of the injured spleen and liver. Semin Nucl Med 13:184, 1983

23. Miller JH, Gates GF, Landing BA, et al: Scintigraphic abnormalities in glycogen storage disease. J Nucl Med 18:596, 1977

24. Myerson P, Prokop E, Sziklas JJ, et al: Scan findings in hepatic adenoma (focal nodular hyperplasia). Clin Nucl Med 1:108, 1976

25. Poshyachinda M, Maturosakul B, Manothaya C: Scintigraphy in a case of pseudocyst of liver: Case report. J Nucl Med 16:825, 1975

26. Salvo AF, Schiller A, Athanasoulis C, et al: Hepatoadenoma and focal nodular hyperplasia: Pitfalls in radiocolloid imaging. Radiology 125:451, 1977

27. Suzuki K, Okuda K, Yoshida T, et al: False-positive liver scan in a patient with hepatic amyloidosis: Case report. J Nucl Med 17:31, 1976

28. Taylor RD, Anderson PM, Winston MA, et al: Diagnosis of hepatic hemangioma using multiple radionuclide and ultrasound techniques. J Nucl Med 17:362, 1976

29. Trackler RT: Liver imaging in hemochromatosis secondary to multiple blood transfusions. Clin Nucl Med 2:128, 1977

30. Velchik MG, Noel AW: False-positive liver scan due to intrahepatic gallbladder detected by cholescintigraphy. Clin Nucl Med 12:50, 1987

31. Weissmann HS, Chun KJ, Frank J: Demonstration of traumatic bile leakage with cholescintigraphy and ultrasonography. AJR 133:843, 1979

32. Winston MA, Shapiro M: Pseudotumors in acute hepatitis. J Nucl Med 15:1039, 1974

LIVER-SPLEEN SCAN

Prominent Porta Hepatis

COMMON: Cirrhosis
Dilated bile ducts
Fibrosis
Metastasis
Normal variant

UNCOMMON
AND RARE: Abscess
Bifurcation of portal vein
Choledochal cyst
Colonic interposition
Cyst of the falciform ligament
Dilated splenic vein
Extrinsic pressure (e.g., pancreatic carcinoma)
Hepatic laceration
Hepatoma
Impression by normal kidney
Infarction
Pancreatic pseudocyst
Ruptured gallbladder
Viral hepatitis

REFERENCES

1. McClelland RR: Focal porta hepatitis scintiscan defects: What is their significance? J Nucl Med 16:1007, 1976
2. Sample FW, Gray RK, Poe ND, et al: Nuclear imaging, tomographic nuclear imaging and gray scale ultrasound in the evaluation of the porta hepatis. Radiology 122:773, 1977
3. Shih W-J, Reba RC, DeLand FH: Causes of focal hepatic portal defect on ^{99m}Tc-sulfur colloid scintigraphy. Semin Nucl Med 13:171, 1983
4. Siegel BA, Alazraki NP, Alderson PO, et al (eds): Nuclear Radiology Syllabus, Second Series. Chicago, Waverly Press, 1978

LIVER-SPLEEN SCAN

Widened Renal Fossa

COMMON: Hepatic abscess
Hepatic tumor (primary or secondary)
Hydronephrosis
Hypernephroma
Polycystic renal disease
Perinephric abscess
Retroperitoneal hematoma

UNCOMMON
AND RARE: Glycogen storage disease
Other tumors (Wilm's, neuroblastoma)
Pancreatitis
Psoas abscess
Pyelonephritis
Retroperitoneal adenopathy and tumor
Subhepatic abscess

REFERENCES

1. Heyman S: Liver-spleen scintigraphy in glycogen storage disease (glycogenosis). Clin Nucl Med 10:839, 1985
2. Lecklitner ML: Liver imaging — the "widened renal fossa" sign in posterior liver scintigraphy. Semin Nucl Med 13:298, 1983

LIVER-SPLEEN SCAN

Multiple Cold Defects

COMMON: Abscess
Any of false-positive causes
Biliary obstruction
Metastases
Polycystic disease
Pseudotumor in cirrhosis

UNCOMMON
AND RARE: Any of causes of solitary defect
Chronic passive congestion
Congenital cystic dilation of the intrahepatic ducts
Intrahepatic lithiasis
Leukemia
Sickle cell anemia

REFERENCES

1. Barnett CA, Olson R, Stadalnik RC: Chronic passive congestion of the liver appearing as focal defects on liver imaging. Clin Nucl Med 2:52, 1977

2. Conte PJ: Aortic aneurysm causing multiple liver scan defects. AJR 128:516, 1977

3. Drum DE: Current status of radiocolloid hepatic scintiphotography for space-occupying disease. Semin Nucl Med 12:64, 1982

4. Drum DE: Optimizing the clinical value of hepatic scintiphotography. Semin Nucl Med 8:346, 1978

5. Drum DE, Beard JO: Liver scintigraphic features associated with alcoholism. J Nucl Med 19:154, 1978

6. Gottschalk A, Potchen EJ (eds): Diagnostic Nuclear Medicine. Baltimore, Williams and Wilkins, 1976

7. Herbst KD, Corder MP: Radiotherapy-induced liver scan defects. J Nucl Med 17:424, 1976

8. Kirchner PT (ed): Nuclear Medicine Review Syllabus. New York, Society of Nuclear Medicine, 1980

9. Leekam RN, Shankar L, Bayley TA: Demonstration of segmental bile duct dilatation on technetium-99m sulfur colloid imaging. Clin Nucl Med 11:735, 1986

10. Lunia S, Parthasarathy KL, Bakshi S, et al: An evaluation of ^{99m}Tc-sulfur colloid liver scintiscans and their usefulness in metastatic workup: A review of 1424 studies. J Nucl Med 16:62, 1975

11. Masuda Y, Sawa H, Kim OH, et al: A case of congenital hepatic fibrosis: Usefulness of hepatobiliary scintigraphy. Clin Nucl Med 5:359, 1980

12. Miller JH, Gates GF, Landing BA, et al: Scintigraphic abnormalities in glycogen storage disease. J Nucl Med 18:596, 1977

13. Samuel AM, Ganatra RD, Ramanathan P: Liver-spleen scan in sickle cell anemia. J Nucl Med 17:851, 1976

14. Smith R: Hepatic scintigraphy of nodular regenerative hyperplasia of the liver (letter to the editor). J Nucl Med 27:563, 1986

15. Sty JR, Sullivan P, Wagner R, et al: Hepatic scintigraphy in Caroli's disease. Radiology 127:732, 1978

16. Suzuki K, Okuda K, Yoshida T, et al: False-positive liver scan in a patient with hepatic amyloidosis: Case report. J Nucl Med 17:31, 1976

17. Winston MA, Shapiro M: Pseudotumors in acute hepatitis. J Nucl Med 15:1039, 1974

18. Yeh SH, Liu OK, Huang MJ: Sequential scintigraphy with technetium-99m pyridoxylideneglutemate in the detection of intrahepatic lithiasis: Concise communication. J Nucl Med 21:17, 1980

LIVER-SPLEEN SCAN

Cold Defect in a Pediatric Patient

COMMON AND
UNCOMMON: Abscess (e.g., chronic granulomatous disease,
neutropenia)
Benign tumor (e.g., hemangioma,
hemangioendothelioma)
Caroli's disease
Choledochal cyst
Cirrhosis (e.g., cystic fibrosis)
Cyst (e.g., polycystic disease)
Hepatoma
Metastasis (e.g., neuroblastoma, Wilms', lymphoma)
Posttraumatic (e.g., hematoma, following surgery or
radiation)
Pseudodefect
Sclerosing cholangitis

REFERENCE

1. Sty JR, Babbitt P: Perforated appendicitis presenting as a focal hepatic defect.
Clin Nucl Med 4:209, 1979

LIVER-SPLEEN SCAN

False-Positive Defect in the Liver

COMMON: Anatomic variations of liver size, shape, and
position
Breast shadow
Gallbladder fossa
Porta hepatis
Rib impression
Riedel's lobe
Thin left lobe

UNCOMMON: Barium in colon
Cirrhosis (pseudotumor)
Congestive heart failure
Dilated biliary radicals
Fossa of the inferior vena cava
Object overlying liver (e.g., breast prosthesis)
Porta hepatis defect (See Gamut)
Right kidney or psoas muscle impression
Scoliosis
Vertebral pressure defect

RARE: Agenesis of the right lobe
Aorta aneurysm
Ascites-caput medusa
Chilaiditi's syndrome
Dextrocardia
Dilated portal vein
Emphysema
Free pertechnetate
Gaseous bowel distension
Hydronephrosis
Hypernephroma
Intrahepatic gallbladder
Lung tumor, pneumonia, or abscess
Pancreatic cancer of pseudocyst
Perinephric abscess
Phototube defect
Pleural fluid
Radiation
Radiographic contrast in the gallbladder

Retroperitoneal lymph nodes
Right-sided adrenal tumor
Splenomegaly
Subdiaphragmatic fluid

REFERENCES

1. Atkins HL, Oster ZH: Visualization of caput medusa in a patient with hepatoma. Clin Nucl Med 11:591, 1986

2. Carollo BR, Leonard JC: False-positive liver scintigraphy secondary to posterior sulcus pulmonary neoplasm. Clin Nucl Med 10:385, 1985

3. Chaudhuri TK: False-positive liver scan caused by dextrogastria. J Nucl Med 17:1109, 1976

4. Covington EE: Pitfalls in liver photoscans. AJR 109:745, 1970

5. Duong RB, Nishiyama H, Volarich DT, et al: Hydronephrosis mimicking metastatic disease on a Tc-99m sulfur colloid liver-spleen scan. Clin Nucl Med 8:225, 1983

6. Eybalin MC, LeBlond R, Chartrand R, et al: Cystic hypernephroma mimicking an hepatic mass. Clin Nucl Med 9:648, 1984

7. Genant HK, Hoffer PB: False-positive liver scan due to lung abscess. J Nucl Med 13:945, 1972

8. Gupta SM, Herrera NE: Retroperitoneal lymphoma appearing as a hepatic mass. Clin Nucl Med 4:343, 1979

9. Izhar M: Pectus excavatum causing a false-positive defect in the liver. Clin Nucl Med 2:392, 1977

10. Joo KG, Carter JE: Extrinsic lesions simulating hepatic masses. Clin Nucl Med 4:128, 1979

11. Kochar AS: Pseudocysts of the pancreas mimicking space-occupying lesions on liver scan. Clin Nucl Med 8:177, 1983

12. Kuhn MJ, Goldfarb CR, Ongseng F: Free technetium simulating a solitary hepatic defect on technetium-99m liver scans. Clin Nucl Med 10:736, 1985

13. McCauley D, Braunstein P: Unusual artifact in lateral liver scans. J Nucl Med 15:1201, 1974

14. Milder MS, Larson SM, Swann SJ, et al: False-positive liver scan due to breast prosthesis. J Nucl Med 14:189, 1973

15. Ozturk E, Narin Y, Pabuccu Y, et al: False-positive space-occupying lesion — apperance in colloid liver scintigraphy due to Chilaiditi's syndrome. Clin Nucl Med 18:159, 1993

16. Perlman SB, Bushnell DL, Polcyn RE: Apparent filling defects of the liver. Clin Nucl Med 9:723, 1984

17. Radin DR, Colletti PM, Ralls PW, et al: Agenesis of right lobe of liver. Radiology 164:639, 1987

18. Ramanna L, Brachman MB, Tanasescu DE, et al: Osteoblastic metastasis or rib cage causing attenuation on liver scan. Clin Nucl Med 10:665, 1985

19. Ramsby GR, Henken EM, Spencer RP: Enlarged portal vein causing abnormality on hepatic dynamic and static images. Clin Nucl Med 3:301, 1978

20. Rossleigh MA, Uren RF, Bernstein L: Focal defects on liver scintigraphy due to right ventricular failure. Clin Nucl Med 9:196, 1984

21. Ryo UY, Pinsky SM: "Artifactitious lesion" on a liver scan caused by an infiltrate in the right lung base. Clin Nucl Med 8:378, 1983

22. Ryo UY, Siddiqui A, Yum HY, et al: Focal defect due to renal impression in anterior liver imaging. Clin Nucl Med 1:64, 1976

23. Shih W-J, Daniel T, DeLand F, et al: False-positive radiocolloid liver image due to a subphrenic abscess. Clin Nucl Med 11:400, 1986

24. Shih W-J, Mandelstam P, Domstad PA, et al: Prominent gaseous distension of bowel causing false-positive technetium-99m sulfur colloid liver scintigram. Clin Nucl Med 10:284, 1985

25. Shih W-J, Nolan NG: False-positive liver scan due to spine deformity. J Nucl Med 21:808, 1980

26. Ueno K, Kabuto H, Rikimaru S: Pulmonary nodules causing false-positive liver scans: Preoperative and postoperative scintigraphic findings in three cases. Clin Nucl Med 9:199, 1984

27. Weinraub JM: False-positive liver scan caused by dilated splenic vein. J Nucl Med 15:142, 1974

28. Williams AG, Christie JH, Mettler FA, et al: Ascites causing a false-positive radionuclide liver image. Clin Nucl Med 8:76, 1983

29. Zwas ST, Braunstein P: Splenic focal defect produced by barium in the colon. Clin Nucl Med 3:202, 1978

LIVER-SPLEEN SCAN

Focal Increased Liver Activity (Hot Spot)

COMMON: Budd-Chiari syndrome
Cirrhosis (regenerating nodules)
Focal nodular hyperplasia
Superior and inferior vena cava obstruction

UNCOMMON
AND RARE: Abscess
Acute cholecystitis
Amyloidosis
Anatomic varient
Constructive pericarditis
Hamartoma
Hemangioma
Hepatoma
Hepatoblastoma
Idiopathic
Injection of colloid in the hepatic vein (through a
central venous catheter)
Irregular fatty infiltration
Pseudo-Budd-Chiari syndrome
Pseudopod of liver extending into a ventral hernia
Tricuspid insufficiency

REFERENCES

1. Benedict KT, Chen PS, Janower ML, et al: Contraceptive-associated hepatic tumor. AJR 132:452, 1979

2. Chayes Z, Koenigsberg M, Freeman LM: The "hot" hepatic abscess. J Nucl Med 15:305, 1974

3. Chhabria PB, Chandnani PC: "Hot spot" on radiocolloid scan of the liver. Clin Nucl Med 1:258, 1976

4. Dhawan VM, Sziklas JJ, Spencer RP: Pseudo-Budd-Chiari syndrome. Clin Nucl Med 3:30, 1978

5. Gooneratne NS, Buse MG, Quinn JL, et al: "Hot spot" on hepatic scintigraphy and radionculide venacavography. AJR 129:447, 1977

6. Greditzer GH, Ho JE, Wolverson M, et al: A benign cause of increased radiocolloid accumulation on a liver scan. AJR 132:289, 1979

7. Hattner RS, Shames DM: Nonspecificity of the radiocolloid hepatic "hot spot" for superior vena caval obstruction. J Nucl Med 15:1041, 1974

8. Helbig HD: Focal iatrogenic increased radiocolloid uptake on liver scan. J Nucl Med 14:354, 1973

9. Henke CE, Wolff JM, Shafer RB: Vascular dynamics in liver scan "hot spot." Clin Nucl Med 3:267, 1978

10. Holmquest DL, Burdine JA: Caval-portal shunting as a cause of a focal increase in radiocolloid uptake in normal livers. J Nucl Med 14:348, 1973

11. Hopkins GB: Superior vena caval obstruction and increased radiocolloid activity on liver scintiphotos. J Nucl Med 14:883, 1973

12. Hughes FA III: The value of hepatic scintiangiography and static liver scans in superior vena caval obstruction: Case report. J Nucl Med 16:626, 1975

13. Imaeda T, Inoue A, Doi H, Ozawa N: Increased focal uptake of ^{99m}Tc stannous phytate in irregular fatty liver demonstrated by SPECT imaging. Clin Nucl Med 15:504, 1990

14. Jackson DE, Floyd JL: An unusual cause of a hot spot on sulfur colloid liver imaging. Clin Nucl Med 11:549, 1986

15. Lee HK: Preferential visualization of the inferior vena cava in the dynamic hepatic flow study of the superior vena cava syndrome. Clin Nucl Med 2:296, 1977

16. Lee KR, Preston DF, Martin NL, et al: Angiographic documentation of systemic portal venous shunting as a cause of a liver scan "hot spot" in superior vena caval obstruction. AJR 127:637, 1976

17. McMullen CT, Montgomery JL: Arteriographic findings of focal nodular hyperplasia of the liver and review of the literature. AJR 117:380, 1973

18. Meindok H, Langer B: Liver scan in Budd-Chiari syndrome. J Nucl Med 17:365, 1976

19. Mikolajkow A, Jasinski WK: Increased focal uptake of radiocolloid by the liver. J Nucl Med 14:175, 1973

20. Miller JH, Greenspan BS: Integrated imaging of hepatic tumors in childhood. Part I. Malignant lesions (primary and metastatic). Radiology 154:83, 1985

21. Morita ET, McCormack KR, Weisberg RL: Further information on a "hot spot" in the liver. J Nucl Med 14:606, 1973

22. Parker LA, Banning B: Focal nodular hyperplasia of the liver: Scintigraphic demonstration with technetium-99m sulfur colloid emission computed tomography. Clin Nucl Med 10:601, 1983

23. Pasquier J, Dorta T: Focal hyperfixation of radiocolloid by the liver. J Nucl Med 15:725, 1974

24. Rogers JV, Mack LA, Freeny PC, et al: Hepatic focal nodular hyperplasia: Angiography, CT, sonography, and scintigraphy. AJR 137:983, 1981

25. Sandler MS, Park CH, Lin D, et al: "Hot spot" on liver scan due to tricuspid atresia. Clin Nucl Med 5:494, 1980

26. Slavin JD, Yoosufani Z, Spencer RP: Hepatic hot spot on both radiocolloid and hepatobiliary imaging in acute cholecystitis. Clin Nucl Med 12:536, 1987

27. Stadalnik RC: "Hot spots" — liver imaging. Semin Nucl Med 9:220, 1979

28. Sty JR, Starshak RJ, Casper JT: Image correlation: Budd-Chiari syndrome. Clin Nucl Med 8:369, 1983

29. Tetalman MR, Kusumi R, Gaughran G, et al: Radionuclide liver spots: Indicator of liver disease or a blood flow phenomenon. AJR 130:291, 1978

30. Thijs LG, Heidendal AK, Huijgens PC, et al: The use of nuclear medicine procedures in the diagnosis of Budd-Chiari syndrome. Clin Nucl Med 3:389, 1978

31. Valdez VA, Herrera NE: Demonstration of superior vena caval obstruction and "hot spot" on liver scan in a case of non-Hodgkin's lymphoma. Clin Nucl Med 3:139, 1978

32. Vincent LM, McCartney WH, Flynn TC: Unusual hepatic uptake pattern of technetium-99m sulfur colloid and technetium-99m HDP in amyloidosis. Clin Nucl Med 11:436, 1986

33. Yeh SDJ, Garcia A, Benua RS: Abnormal radiocolloid and MAA uptake by the liver in superior vena caval obstruction. Clin Nucl Med 2:184, 1977

LIVER-SPLEEN SCAN

Inhomogenous Uptake

COMMON AND
UNCOMMON: Circulatory
      Congestive heart failure (acute myocardial
        infarction, cardiomyopathy, valvular disease)
      Constructive pericarditis
      Extrinsic compression
      Hepatic artery obstruction
      High output states (e.g., thyrotoxicosis, Paget's
        disease, beriberi)
      Hypovolemia
      Increased red cell destruction (e.g., spherocytosis,
        thalessemia major)
      Inferior vena cava and hepatic vein obstruction
      Portal or splenic vein obstruction (e.g., cirrhosis,
        SS disease, etc.)
      Pulmonary embolism
      Pulmonary hypertension
    Infiltrative
      Actinomycosis
      Alcoholic hepatitis
      Alpha-1-antitrypsin deficiency
      Amyloidosis
      Brucellosis
      Celiac disease
      Chronic active hepatitis
      Chronic vitamin A intoxication
      Drugs (e.g., phenothiazines, INH, adriamycin,
        phenobarbital, testosterone, estrogens, oxacillin,
        tetracycline, warfarin)
      Dubin-Johnson syndrome
      Extramedullary hematopoiesis (e.g., myelofibrosis
        with myeloid metaplasia)
      Fatty infiltration (e.g., diabetes, malabsorption
        syndromes, hyperalimentation)
      Gaucher's disease
      Hemochromatosis
      Histoplasmosis
      Hypereosinophilic syndromes
      Hypergammaglobulinemia

Infiltrative (cont'd)
Idiopathic cirrhosis
Infectious mononucleosis
Lead poisining
Leschmaniasis
Leukemia (e.g., chronic myelocytic
lymphocytic, hairy cell)
Liver transplant
Lymphoma, lymphosarcoma, Hodgkin's disease
Malaria
Metastasis
Niemann-Pick disease
Polyarteritis nodosa
Polycystic liver disease
Polycythemia vera
Primary biliary cirrhosis
Sarcoidosis
Schistosomiasis
Syphilis
Thrombocythemia
Ulcerative colitis
Viral hepatitis
Waldenström's macroglobulinemia
Wilson's disease

REFERENCES

1. Gottschalk A, Potchen EJ (eds): Diagnostic Nuclear Medicine. Baltimore, Williams and Wilkins, 1976

2. Harbert JC, Richa AF: Textbook of Nuclear Medicine: Clinical Applications. Philadelphia, Lea and Febiger, 1984

3. Rothfield B (ed): Nuclear Medicine: Hepatolienal. Philadelphia, J.B. Lippincot, 1980

LIVER-SPLEEN SCAN

Lack of Liver Uptake of Sulfur Colloid

COMMON AND
UNCOMMON: Advanced cirrhosis
Familial erythrophagocytic lymphohistiocytosis
Intestinal bypass
Irradiation (usually not complete)
Schistosoma mansoni infestation
Severe hepatitis
Tuberculosis

REFERENCES

1. Antar MA, Sziklas JJ, Spencer RP: Liver imaging during reticuloendothelial failure. Clin Nucl Med 2:293, 1977

2. DeLand FH, Tonkin A: Serial liver scanning as an index of hepatic function following jejunoileal bypass surgery. J Nucl Med 14:390, 1973

3. Hinckle GH, Leonard JC, Krous HF, et al: Absence of hepatic uptake of Tc-99m sulfur colloid in an infant with Coxsackie B$_2$ viral infection. Clin Nucl Med 8:246, 1983

4. O'Brien RP, Schwartz AD, Pearson AD, et al: Reticuloendothelial failure in familial erythrophagocytic lymphohistiocytosis. Pediatrics 81:543, 1972

5. Spencer RP, Knowlton AH: Redistribution of radiocolloid uptake after focal hepatic irradiation. Oncology 32:266, 1975

6. Suresh K, Turner JW, Spencer RP, et al: Hepatic reticuloendothelial "failure" in *Schistosoma mansoni* infestation. Clin Nucl Med 2:163, 1977

LIVER-SPLEEN SCAN

Sulfur Colloid Uptake in the Kidneys

COMMON: Congestive heart failure
Renal transplant — rejection

UNCOMMON: Radiopharmaceutical preparation
Renal transplant — acute tubular necrosis
Sepsis

RARE: Accessory spleen in kidney
Coxsackie viral infection
Disseminated intravascular coagulation
Liver transplant
Sickle cell anemia

REFERENCES

1. Binnur K, Firat G, Sukran T, Metin E: [99m]Tc HMDP uptake by the kidney in sickle cell disease. Clin Nucl Med 17:236, 1992

2. Coleman RE: Renal colloid localization. J Nucl Med 15:367, 1974

3. Dey HM, Spencer RP, Rosenberg RJ, Baldwin RD: Renal uptake of ^{99m}Tc sulfur colloid in disseminated intravascular coagulation. Clin Nucl Med 15:742, 1990

4. Frick MP, Loken MK, Goldberg ME, et al: Use of ^{99m}Tc-sulfur colloid in evaluation of renal transplant complications. J Nucl Med 17:181, 1976

5. Higgins CB, Taketa RM, Taylor A, et al: Renal uptake of ^{99m}Tc-sulfur colloid. J Nucl Med 15:564, 1974

6. Hiltz A, Iles S: Renal accumulation of ^{99m}Tc sulfur colloid. Clin Nucl Med 14:118, 1989

7. Jackson GL: Renal accumulation of ^{99m}Tc-SC. Clin Nucl Med 2:176, 1977

8. Klingensmith WC III, Ryerson TW, Corman JL: Lung uptake of ^{99m}Tc-sulfur colloid in organ transplantation. J Nucl Med 14:757, 1973

9. Kuni CC, Klingensmith WC III: Renal uptake of ^{99m}Tc-sulfur colloid in liver transplant patients. Clin Nucl Med 4:335, 1979

10. Mikhael MA, Evens RG: Phagocytic capability of the kidney: A possible mechanism for renal uptake of colloid in liver-spleen scanning. J Nucl Med 16:709, 1975

11. Shook DR, Shafer RB: Renal uptake of ^{99m}Tc-sulfur colloid. Clin Nucl Med 1:224, 1976

12. Tiu S, Klein B, Kramer EL, Sanger JJ: Renal uptake in liver scan. Semin Nucl Med 16:80, 1986

LIVER-SPLEEN SCAN

Sulfur Colloid Uptake by the Lungs

COMMON: Childhood (faint uptake is normal)
Cirrhosis
Hypercoagulable state
Malignancy (e.g., metastases, malignant lymphoma)
Radiopharmaceutical preparation

UNCOMMON: Bacterial infection without abscess (e.g.,
tuberculosis)
Collagen vascular disease
Histiocytosis X
Intraabdominal abscess
Mucopolysaccharidosis type II (Hunter's)

RARE: Amyloidosis
Anemia
Breast carcinoma uptake simulating lung uptake
Budd-Chiari syndrome
Chronic passive congestion of the liver
Elevated aluminum levels
Estrogen administration
Fatty liver disease of pregnancy
Heat stroke
Hepatic infarction
Malaria
Myelofibrosis
Pseudo-Budd-Chiari syndrome
Transplants (e.g., liver, spleen, bone marrow)
Viral infection (infectious mononucleosis, Lassa
fever, toxoplasmosis)

REFERENCES

1. Blend MJ, Dondalski M: Diffuse lung uptake of ^{99m}Tc sulphur colloid associated with fatty liver disease of pregnancy. Clin Nucl Med 12:287, 1987

2. Bobinet DD, Sevrin R, Zurbriggen MT, et al: Lung uptake of ^{99m}Tc-sulfur colloid in patient exhibiting presence of AL3+ in plasma. J Nucl Med 15:1220, 1974

3. Bowen BM, Coates G, Garnett ES: Technetium-99m-sulfur colloid lung scan in patients with histiocytosis X. J Nucl Med 16:332, 1975

4. Calandra JD, Ryerson TW, Cahill E: Uptake of ^{99m}Tc sulfur colloid by a breast carcinoma. Clin Nucl Med 14:432, 1989

5. Garty I, Tal I, Kaynan A: Tc-99m colloid lung uptake in a rare case of toxoplasmosis with liver involvement. Clin Nucl Med 9:310, 1984

6. Gillespie PJ, Alexander JL, Edelstyn GA: High concentration of ^{99m}Tc-sulfur colloid found during routine liver scan in lungs of patient with advanced breast cancer. J Nucl Med 14:711, 1973

7. Hammes CS, Landry AJ, Bunker SR, et al: Diffuse lung uptake of Tc-99m sulfur colloid in infectious mononucleosis (letter to the editor). J Nucl Med 24:1083, 1983

8. Imarisio JJ: Liver scan showing intense lung uptake in neoplasia and infection. J Nucl Med 16:188, 1975

9. Jacobson AF, Marks MA, Kaplan WD: Increased lung uptake on ^{99m}Tc sulfur colloid liver-spleen scans in patients with hepatic venoocclusive disease following bone marrow transplantation. J Nucl Med 31:372, 1990

10. Keyes JW, Wilson GS, Wuinonest JD: An evaluation of lung uptake of colloid during liver imaging. J Nucl Med 14:687, 1973

11. Klingensmith WC III, Lovett VJ: Lung uptake of ^{99m}Tc-sulfur colloid secondary to intraperitoneal endotoxin. J Nucl Med 15:1028, 1974

12. Klingensmith WC III, Ryerson TW: Lung uptake of ^{99m}Tc-sulfur colloid. J Nucl Med 14:201, 1973

13. Klingensmith WC III, Tsan MF, Wagner HN: Factors affecting the uptake of ^{99m}Tc-sulfur colloid by the lung and kidney. J Nucl Med 17:681, 1976

14. Klingensmith WC III, Yang SL, Wagner HN: Lung uptake of Tc-99m-sulfur colloid in liver and spleen imaging. J Nucl Med 19:31, 1978

15. Marigold JH, Clarke SEM, Gaunt JI, et al: Lung uptake of Tc-99m-tin colloid in a patient with Lassa fever (letter to the editor). J Nucl Med 24:750, 1983

16. Mikhael MA, Evens RG: Migration and embolization of macrophages to the lung — a possible mechanism for colloid uptake in the lung during liver scanning. J Nucl Med 16:22, 1975

17. Polga JP, Holstein G, Spencer RP: Radiocolloid redistribution and multiple splenic infarcts in myelofibrosis. Clin Nucl Med 8:335, 1983

18. Stadalnik RC: Diffuse lung uptake of Tc-99m-sulfur colloid. Semin Nucl Med 10:106, 1980

19. Stewart CA, Hung GL, Siegel ME, McHutchison JG: Unusual pattern of lung uptake of ^{99m}Tc sulfur colloid seen on liver scan of patient with pulmonary tuberculosis. Clin Nucl Med 14:271, 1989

20. Tonami N, Taki J, Hisada K, et al: Diffuse lung uptake of technetium-99m tin colloid in heat stroke: Case report. Clin Nucl Med 10:769, 1985

21. Turner JW, Syed IB, Hanc RP: Lung uptake of ^{99m}Tc-sulfur colloid during liver scanning. J Nucl Med 15:460, 1974

22. Turner JW, Syed IB, Hanc RP: Retention of ^{99m}Tc-sulfur colloid in the lungs. J Nucl Med 16:249, 1975

23. Wilf LH, Ziessman HA, Marion LI, et al: ^{99m}Tc sulfur colloid diffuse lung uptake and its resolution in acute fatty liver of pregnancy. Clin Nucl Med 12:951, 1987

24. Ziessman HA: Lung uptake of ^{99m}Tc-sulfur colloid in falciparum malaria: Case report. J Nucl Med 17:794, 1976

LIVER-LUNG SCAN

Separation Between Liver and Lung Activity

COMMON: Right lower lobe pneumonia, atelectasis, or pleural
effusion
Subphrenic abscess

UNCOMMON
AND RARE: Ascites
Bile
Cardiomegaly (left side)
Colonic interposition
Ectopic kidney
Emphysema
Fibrous adhesions
Hematoma
Hepatic cirrhosis
Hepatic polycystic disease
Intraperitoneal free air
Pulmonary cyst
Pulmonary embolism
Right diaphragm paralysis
Tumor (mets, hepatoma)

REFERENCES

1. Alter AJ, Farrer PA: The perihepatic halo in liver scintiangiographic perfusion studies: A sign of ascites. J Nucl Med 15:396, 1974

2. Berg GR: False positive liver-lung scan caused by intraperitoneal free air. Clin Nucl Med 6:386, 1981

3. Gottschalk A, Potchen EJ (eds): Diagnostic Nuclear Medicine. Baltimore,- Williams and Wilkins, 1976

4. Lecklitner ML: Liver-lung imaging — discontinuity of activity in liver-lung scintigraphy. Semin Nucl Med 13:391, 1983

5. Rocha AF, Harbert JC: Textbook of Nuclear Medicine: Clinical Applications. Philadelphia, Lea and Febiger, 1979

6. Salamanca JE, Stadalnik RC, DeNardo GL: Clinical assessment of combined organ imaging in the diagnosis of subphrenic abscess. Clin Nucl Med 3:113, 1978

7. Strakosch CR, Cooper RA, Wiseman JC, et al: High ectopic kidney presenting as an abnormal liver-lung scan: Case report. J Nucl Med 18:274, 1977

8. Yeh EL, Ruetz PP, Meade RC: Separation of lung-liver scintiphotos due to ascites — a false-positive test for subdiaphragmatic abscess. J Nucl Med 13:249, 1972

LIVER-SPLEEN SCAN

Splenomegaly

COMMON: Amyloidosis
Anemia (e.g., sickle cell, thalassemia, hemolytic)
Cirrhosis
Congestive heart failure
Extramedullary hematopoiesis
Hematoma
Leukemia
Lymphoma
Myelofibrosis

UNCOMMON
AND RARE: AIDS
Bacterial infection (e.g., subacute bacterial
endocarditis, military tuberculosis, brucellosis,
etc.)
Benign tumor (e.g., hamartoma, fibroma)
Cystic lymphangioma
Dermoid and epidermoid cyst
Dysgammaglobulinemia
Felty's syndrome
Fungal infection (e.g., histoplasmosis)
Gaucher's disease
Hemangioma
Hemochromatosis
Hemorrhagic pseudocyst
Histiocytosis X
Infarct
Juvenile rheumatoid arthritis
Lupus erythematosis
Metastatic disease (e.g., breast, lung, melanoma,
islet cell tumor)
Multiple myeloma
Narcotic addiction
Niemann-Pick disease
Osteopetrosis
Pancreatic pseudocyst involving the spleen
Parasites (e.g., malaria, schistosomiasis, hydatid cyst,
kala-azar)
Polyarteritis nodosa
Polycythemia vera

Psoriasis
Sarcoidosis
Sarcoma (e.g., angiosarcoma)
Serum sickness
Splenic vein obstruction (e.g., thrombosis,
    pancreatic tumor)
Viral infection (e.g., infectious mononucleosis,
    cytomegalic inclusion disease)
Wolman's disease

REFERENCES

1. Drum DE, Beard JO: Liver scintigraphic features associated with alcoholism. J Nucl Med 19:154, 1978

2. Gottschalk A, Potchen EJ (eds): Diagnostic Nuclear Medicine. Baltimore, Williams and Wilkins, 1976

3. Groshar D, Israel O, Front D: Spleen imaging — enlargement of the spleen. Semin Nucl Med 13:295, 1983

4. Hanelin J, Carlson DH: A case of pancreatic pseudocyst extending into the spleen with associated subcapsular hemorrhage. Clin Nucl Med 3:232, 1978

5. Larson SM, Tuell SH, Moores KD, et al: Dimensions of the normal adult spleen and prediction of spleen weight. J Nucl Med 12:123, 1971

6. Moniot AL: Liver-spleen scintiscan in kala-azar: Case report. J Nucl Med 16:1128, 1975

7. Reeder MM, Felson B: Gamuts in Radiology. Cincinnati, Audiovisual Radiology of Cincinnati, Inc., 1975

8. Spencer RP: The spleen in psoriasis. Clin Nucl Med 2:119, 1977

LIVER-SPLEEN SCAN

Mild Splenomegaly

COMMON AND
UNCOMMON: Acute infection
Congestive heart failure
Lupus erythematosus
Metastatic disease
Other causes of splenomegaly
Polyarteritis nodosa
Rheumatoid arthritis
Subacute bacterial endocarditis
Thrombocytopenia purpura

REFERENCE

1. Gottschalk A, Potchen EJ (eds): Diagnostic Nuclear Medicine. Baltimore, Williams and Wilkins, 1976

LIVER-SPLEEN SCAN

Moderate Splenomegaly

COMMON AND
UNCOMMON: Cirrhosis
Hemolytic anemias
Hepatitis — acute and chronic
Hodgkin's disease
Infectious mononucleosis
Other causes of splenomegaly
Other lymphomas
Polycythemia vera
Sickle cell anemia (early)

REFERENCE

1. Gottschalk A, Potchen EJ (eds): Diagnostic Nuclear Medicine. Baltimore, Williams and Wilkins, 1976

LIVER-SPLEEN SCAN

Massive Splenomegaly

COMMON: Chronic myeloid leukemia
Myeloid metaplasia

UNCOMMON
AND RARE: Amyloidosis
Banti's disease
Cirrhosis
Gaucher's disease
Kala-azar
Lymphoma
Multiple cysts of the liver
Niemann-Pick disease
Schistosomiasis
Thalassemia major

REFERENCES

1. Gottschalk A, Potchen EJ (eds): Diagnostic Nuclear Medicine. Baltimore, Williams and Wilkins, 1976
2. Larson SM, Tuell SH, Moores KD, et al: Dimensions of the normal adult spleen and prediction of spleen weight. J Nucl Med 12:123, 1971
3. Moniot AL: Liver-spleen scintiscan in kala-azar: Case report. J Nucl Med 16:1128, 1975

LIVER-SPLEEN SCAN

Decreased Spleen Size

COMMON AND
    UNCOMMON: Celiac disease
                 Dermatitis herpatiformis
                 Fanconi's anemia
                 Sickle cell disease
                 Thyrotoxicosis
                 Ulcerative colitis

REFERENCE

1. Sty JR, Conway JJ: The spleen: Development and functional evaluation. Semin Nucl Med 15:276, 1985

LIVER-SPLEEN SCAN

Cold Defect in the Spleen

COMMON: Hematoma
Hepatic walk (left lobe of liver creating
  pseudodefect)
Infarct
Lymphoma
Prominent hilum

UNCOMMON: Artifacts (e.g., metallic object, barium in colon,
  breast, left arm)
Metastasis (e.g., melanoma, islet cell, lung, breast)
Other extrinsic masses (e.g., sarcoma)
Pancreatic pseudocyst
Splenic artery aneurysm

RARE: Abscess
Accessory spleen
Amyloidosis
Arteriovenous malformation
Benign tumors (e.g., hemangioma, fibroma,
  hamartoma)
Congenital fissure
Congenital thinning
Cyst
Hepatic walk
Idiopathic
Sarcoidosis
Upside down spleen

REFRENCES

1. Brown JJ, Sumner TE, Crowe JE: Preoperative diagnosis of splenic abscess by ultrasonography and radionuclide scanning. J Nucl Med 20:1221, 1979

2. Chaudhuri TK: Identical splenic imaging in three different entities: An approach to differential diagnosis. Clin Nucl Med 2:441, 1977

3. Chaudhuri TK, Bobbitt JV: Marked enlargement of the left lobe of the liver causing a false-positive spleen image. Radiology 119:169, 1976

4. Dickerman JD, Clements JP: Abnormal spleen scan following MOPP therapy in a patient with Hodgkin's disease: Case report. J Nucl Med 16:457, 1975

5. Evans GW, Kieran JH: Radionuclide imaging in the diagnosis of splenic trauma. Clin Nucl Med 2:32, 1977

6. Garfunkel F: Epidermoid cyst of the spleen: Case report. J Nucl Med 17:196, 1976

7. Hinton AA, Sandler MP, Shaff MI: Pseudo defect of spleen in adolescent with fever of unknown origin. Clin Nucl Med 12:471, 1987

8. Kim EE: Focal splenic defect. Semin Nucl Med 9:320, 1979

9. Levison ED, Dhawan V, Spencer RP: "Hollow spleen" in histiocytic lymphoma. J Nucl Med 18:1144, 1977

10. Lindfors KK, Meyer JE, Palmer EL III, et al: Scintigraphic findings in large-cell lymphoma of the spleen: Concise communication. J Nucl Med 25:969, 1984

11. Mall JC, Kaiser JA: CT diagnosis of splenic laceration. AJR 134:265, 1980

12. McCullough RW, Moonan D, Schatz S, et al: Congenital spleen thinning mimicking space-occupying lesions. Clin Nucl Med 11:262, 1986

13. Moinuddin M, Rockett JF: Splenic cysts demonstrated on radionuclide angiogram. Clin Nucl Med 3:449, 1978

14. Parker JA, Popky GL, Younis MT: Use of the spleen scan in evaluation of pancreatic pseudocyst. Clin Nucl Med 1:137, 1976

15. Russell CD, Jones AE, Johnston GS, et al: Arteriographically confirmed focal defect in colloid spleen scan with no gross pathologic lesion: Case report. J Nucl Med 17:376, 1976

16. Ryo UV: An artifact that simulates an infarction on a posterior view spleen scan. J Nucl Med 16:99, 1975

17. Shapiro H, Roswig DM, Spencer RP: Splenic rotation to the "upside down" configuration. Clin Nucl Med 9:361, 1984

18. Simpson AJ, Salzman AJ, Astin JK: Inversion of the spleen — scintigraphic features. J Nucl Med 18:1145, 1977

19. Slavin JD, Vento JA, Spencer RP: False-positive spleen imaging: Splenic cleft and accessory spleen. Clin Nucl Med 11:509, 1986

20. Spencer RP, Gupta SM: Radionuclide studies of the spleen in trauma and iatrogenic disorders. Semin Nucl Med 15:305, 1985

21. Spencer RP, Karimeddini MK: "Swiss cheese" spleen. Clin Nucl Med 5:323, 1980

22. Thijs LG, Van Heukelem HA, Hoitsma HF, et al: Detection of epidermoid cysts of the spleen using a combined isotopic and ultrasonic investigation. Clin Nucl Med 2:443, 1977

23. Wilson DG, Lieberman LM: Unusual splenic band: Appearance on liver-spleen scan. Clin Nucl Med 8:270, 1983

LIVER-SPLEEN SCAN

Absence of Splenic Visualization

COMMON: Following splenectomy

UNCOMMON
AND RARE: All causes of functional asplenia
Asplenia syndrome
Isolated asplenia

REFERENCE

1. Graves DS, Stadalnik RC: Anatomic and functional asplenia — absence of the splenic image during ^{99m}Tc-sulfur colloid scintigraphy. Semin Nucl Med 12:95, 1982

LIVER-SPLEEN SCAN

Functional Asplenia

COMMON: Sickle cell anemia

UNCOMMON
AND RARE: AIDS-related complex
Amyloidosis
Celiac artery thrombosis
Celiac sprue
Chronic aggressive hepatitis
Congenital heart disease
Following thoratrast
Graft-versus-host disease
Hemoglobin SC disease
Lymphocytic lymphoma
Malignant mastocytosis
Metastases
Multiple myeloma
Nephrotic syndrome
Pancreatic pseudocyst (splenic vein occlusion?)
Polycythemia vera
Rheumatoid arthritis
Sarcoidosis
Sarcoma
Splenic artery, vein, or both being occluded
Subdiaphragmatic splenic transposition
Systemic lupus erythematosus
Thalassemia
Torsion of wandering spleen

REFERENCES

1. Al-Eid MA, Tutschka PJ, Wagner HN Jr, et al: Functional asplenia in patients with chronic graft-versus-host disease: Concise communication. J Nucl Med 24:1123, 1983

2. Armas RR: Clinical studies with spleen-specific radiolabeled agents. Semin Nucl Med 15:260, 1985

3. Dhawan V, Antar MA, Spencer RP: Functional asplenia with few Howell-Jolly bodies. Clin Nucl Med 2:106, 1977

4. Dhawan V, Spencer RP, Pearson HA, et al: Functional asplenia in the absence of circulating Howell-Jolly bodies. Clin Nucl Med 2:395, 1977

5. Goergen TG, Taylor A, Alazraki N: Lack of gallium uptake in primary hepatic amyloidosis. AJR 126:1246, 1976

6. Groshar D, Israel O, Barzilai A, et al: The value of scintigraphy in the evaluation of a wandering spleen. Clin Nucl Med 11:42, 1986

7. Kamdar N, Zanzi I, Kroop S, et al: Reversible functional asplenia in systemic lupus erythematosus. Clin Nucl Med 16:760, 1991

8. Lernau OZ, Baron J, Nissan S: Torsion of the spleen with incomplete infarction: Case report. J Nucl Med 18:1208, 1977

9. Mathews J, Sziklas JJ, Spencer RP: Functional asplenia and uptake of bone imaging agent in angiosarcoma of spleen. Clin Nucl Med 10:527, 1985

10. Park CH, Wecsler PI, Lin D, et al: Splenic scan findings in sickle cell hemoglobin C disease. J Nucl Med 21:43, 1980

11. Rao BR, Winebright JW, Dresser TP: Functional asplenia after thoratrast adminstration. Clin Nucl Med 4:437, 1979

12. Roth J, Brudler O, Hanze E: Functional asplenia in malignant mastocytosis. J Nucl Med 26:1149, 1985

13. Siddiqui AR: Functional hyposplenia in child with AIDS-related complex. Clin Nucl Med 14:840, 1989

14. Silberstein EB, DeLong S, Cline J: Tc-99m diphosphonate and sulfur colloid uptake by the spleen in sickle disease: Interrelationship and clinical correlates: Concise communication. J Nucl Med 25:1300, 1984

15. Spencer RP, Dhawan V, Suresh K, et al: Causes and temporal sequence of onset of functional asplenia in adults. Clin Nucl Med 3:17, 1978

16. Spencer RP, Pearson HA: Splenic radiocolloid uptake in the presence of circulating Howell-Jolly bodies. J Nucl Med 15:294, 1974

17. Yucel AE, Durak H, Bernay I, et al: Functional asplenia and portal hypertension in patient with primary splenic hemangiosarcoma. Clin Nucl Med 15:324, 1990

LIVER-SPLEEN SCAN

Increased Splenic Uptake (Shunting)

COMMON AND
UNCOMMON: Diffuse hepatic involvement
             Cirrhosis
             Fatty infiltration
             Hepatitis
             Widespread hepatic metastases
             Systemic tumor
             Carcinoma without hepatic involvement
             Recurrent melanoma
             Reticuloendothelial system overstimulation
             Chronic granulomatous diseases
             Septicemia
             Circulatory
             Congestive heart failure
             Hematopoietic
             Anemia — especially iron deficiency
             Felty's syndrome
             Myeloproliferative disorders
             Endocrine
             Diabetes
             Technical
             Patient position

REFERENCES

1. Bases RE, Krakoff IH: Enhanced reticuloendothelial phagocytic activity in myeloproliferative diseases. J Reticuloendothel Soc 2:1, 1965

2. Bekerman C, Gottschalk A: Diagnostic significance of the relative uptake of liver compared with spleen in ^{99m}Tc-sulfur colloid scintiphotography. J Nucl Med 12:237, 1971

3. Eddleston AL, Blendis LM, Osborn SB, et al: Significance of increased splenic uptake on liver scintiscanning. Gut 10:711, 1969

4. Gould L, Collica C, Comprecht RF, et al: Scintiphotography in congestive heart failure. JAMA 219:1734, 1972

5. Harvey WC, Kopp DT, Podoloff DA, et al: Reversed liver-spleen ratio and the normal liver-spleen scintigram. J Reticuloendothel Soc 19:19, 1976

6. Kaplan WD, Drum DE, Lokich JJ: The effect of cancer chemotherapeutic agents on the liver-spleen scan. J Nucl Med 21:84, 1980

7. Koh HK, Sober AJ, Kopf A, et al: Prognosis in stage 1 malignant melanoma: Seven-year follow-up study of splenic radiocolloid uptake as predictor of death. J Nucl Med 25:1183, 1984

8. Lin DS: "Hot" spleen on Tc-99m sulfur colloid images. Clin Nucl Med 8:237, 1983

9. Makler PT, Goldstein HA, Velchik MG, et al: Variation of the spleen-liver activity ratio due to a change in position. Clin Nucl Med 9:85, 1984

10. Nathanson L, Kahn P: Splenic uptake of Tc-99m-sulfur colloid in malignant melanoma. J Nucl Med 18:1040, 1977

11. Shih W-J, Domstatd PA, Li CY, et al: Radiocolloid scintigraphy in Felty's syndrome. AJR 146:181, 1986

12. Sober AJ, Mintzis MM, Lew RA, et al: The significance of augmented radiocolloid uptake by the spleen in patients with malignant melanoma. J Nucl Med 20:1232, 1979

13. Wilson GA, Keyes JW Jr: The significance of the liver-spleen uptake ratio in liver scanning. J Nucl Med 15:593, 1974

LIVER-SPLEEN SCAN

Decreased Splenic Uptake

COMMON: Hodgkin's disease
           Other lymphomas

UNCOMMON: Amyloidosis
           Leukemia (e.g., chronic lymphocytic, chronic
             granulocytic)
           Multiple myeloma
           Mycosis fungoides
           Pancreatic carcinoma

RARE: Sickle cell anemia in crisis
           Subacute bacterial endocarditis

REFERENCES

1. Bekerman C, Gottschalk A: Diagnostic significance of the relative uptake of liver compared with spleen in ^{99m}Tc-sulfur colloid scintiphotography. J Nucl Med 12:237, 1971

2. Tantum JL, Burke TS, Frathin MF, et al: Relative decreased splenic uptake of Tc-99m-sulfur colloid in patients with pancreatic carcinoma. Clin Nucl Med 7:1, 1982

3. Wilson GA, Keyes JW: The significance of the liver-spleen uptake ratio in liver scanning. J Nucl Med 15:593, 1974

LIVER-SPLEEN SCAN

Splenic Hot Spot

COMMON AND
UNCOMMON: Hamartoma
Hemangioma
Redundant tissue

REFERENCES

1. Gulenchyn KY, Dover MR, Kelly S: Splenic hemangioma presenting as a "hot spot" on radiocolloid scintigraphy. J Nucl Med 27:804, 1986
2. Okada J, Yoshikawa K, Uno K, et al: Increased activity on radiocolloid scintigraphy in splenic hamartoma. Clin Nucl Med 15:112, 1990
3. Spencer RP: Splenic "hot spot" due to redundant tissue. Clin Nucl Med 8:239, 1983

LIVER-SPLEEN SCAN

Displaced Spleen

COMMON: Dilatation of stomach or colon
Positional changes
Wandering spleen

UNCOMMON
AND RARE: Diaphragm paralysis
Extrinsic mass
Abscess
Aneurysm
Cyst
Pancreatic pseudocyst
Tumor (gastric, intestinal, pancreatic,
retroperitoneal sarcoma)
Hyperinflated left lung
Idiopathic

REFERENCE

1. Moreno AJ, Spicer MJ, Farnum GD, et al: The displaced spleen. Semin Nucl
Med 16:216, 1986

LIVER-SPLEEN SCAN

Uptake in Abdomen Outside Liver, Spleen

COMMON: Accessory spleen

UNCOMMON
AND RARE: Kidney (See Gamut)
Extramedullary hematopoiesis
Tumor (malignant fibrous histiocytoma,
hemangiopericytoma, leiomyosarcoma)

REFERENCES

1. Lundy MM, Blue PW, Crawford GJ, Parker SH: Abdominal hemangiopericytoma scintigraphically simulating accessory spleen. Clin Nucl Med 13:812, 1988

2. Palestro CJ, Klein M, Kim CK, et al: ^{111}In-labeled leukocyte and ^{99m}Tc sulfur colloid uptake by malignant fibrous histiocytoma: Phagocytosis by tumor cells? J Nucl Med 31:1548, 1990

3. Yang SO, Lee MC, Koh CS, et al: Jejunal leiomyosarcoma detected by ^{99m}Tc sulfur colloid gastrointestinal bleeding scan. Clin Nucl Med 15:327, 1990

LIVER-SPLEEN SCAN

Disparate Imaging with Sulfur Colloid and IDA:
Decreased Activity with S.C. and Normal or
Increased Activity in Iminodiacetic Acid (IDA) Image

COMMON: Cirrhosis
Dilated gallbladder
Dilated hepatic duct
Focal nodular hyperplasia
Hepatic adenoma
Hepatoma
Intrahepatic gallbladder

UNCOMMON: Bile leak
Following radiation
Hepatitis
Hypervitaminosis A

RARE: Caroli's disease
Choledochal cyst
Cystadenoma
Familial erythrophagocytic lymphohistiocytosis
Hemochromatosis
Hepatic duct diverticulum
Intestinal bypass
Wilson's disease

REFERENCES

1. Antar MA, Sziklas JJ, Spencer RP: Liver imaging during reticuloendothelial failure. Clin Nucl Med 2:293, 1977

2. Bierssck HJ, Thelen M, Torres JF, et al: Focal nodular hyperplasia of the liver as established by 99m-Tc-sulfur colloid and HIDA scintigraphy. Radiology 137:187, 1980

3. DeNardo SJ, Bell GB, DeNardo GL, et al: Diagnosis of cirrhosis and hepatitis by quantitative hepatic and other reticuloendothelial clearance rates. J Nucl Med 17:449, 1976

4. Gainey MA, Faerber EN: Disparate hepatic imaging with technetium-99m sulfur colloid and disofenin in Wilson's disease. J Nucl Med 26:368, 1985

5. Herbst KD, Corder MP, Morita ET: Hepatic scan defects following radiotherapy for lymphoma. Clin Nucl Med 3:331, 1978

6. Horisawa M, Goldstein G, Waxman A, et al: The abnormal hepatic scan of chronic liver disease: Its relationship to hepatic hemodynamics and colloid extraction. Gastroenterology 71:210, 1976

7. Kipper MS, Reed KR, Contardo M: Visualization of hepatic adenoma with Tc-99m di-isopropyl IDA. J Nucl Med 25:986, 1984

8. Klingensmith WC III, Koep LJ, Fritzberg AR: Bile leak into a hepatic abscess in a liver transplant: Demonstration with ^{99m}Tc-diethyl iminodiacetic acid. AJR 131:889, 1978

9. Knopf DR, McClees EC, Fajman WA, et al: Discordant hepatic uptake of ^{99m}Tc sulfur colloid and ^{99m}Tc-DISIDA in hemochromatosis. AJR 141:563, 1983

10. Lamki L: A dichotomy in hepatic uptake of ^{99m}Tc-IDA and ^{99m}Tc-colloid. Semin Nucl Med 12:92, 1982

11. Park H-M, Ransburg R, Roth C, et al: Scintigraphic dissociation of reticulo-endothelial and hepatocyte function in chronic vitamin A hepatoxicity. Clin Nucl Med 10:364, 1985

12. Rao BK, Pastakia B, Lieberman LM: Evaluation of focal defects of ^{99m}Tc sulfur colloid scans with new hepatobiliary agents. Radiology 136:497, 1980

13. Salvo AF, Schiller A, Athanasoulis C, et al: Hepatoadenoma and focal nodular hyperplasia: Pitfalls in radiocolloid imaging. Radiology 125:451, 1977

14. Schey WL, Pinsky SM, Lipshutz HS, et al: Hepatic duct diverticulum simulating a choledochal cyst. AJR 128:318, 1977

15. Sty JR, Sullivan P, Wagner R, et al: Hepatic scintigraphy in Caroli's disease. Radiology 127:732, 1978

16. Ueno K, Haseda Y: Concentration and clearance of ^{99m}Tc-pyridoxyline isoleucine by a hepatoma. Clin Nucl Med 5:196, 1980

17. Vincent LM, McCartney WH, Mauro MA, et al: Discordant hepatic uptake between Tc-99m sulfur colloid and Tc-99m DISIDA in hypervitaminosis A. J Nucl Med 24:207, 1984

18. Wardle N, Andersen A, James O: Kupffer cell phagocytosis in relation to BSP clearance in liver and inflammatory bowel diseases. Dig Dis Sci 25:414, 1980

LIVER-SPLEEN SCAN

Disparate Imaging with Sulfur Colloid and IDA: Normal Activity with S.C. and Decreased Activity in IDA Image

COMMON: Hepatitis

UNCOMMON
AND RARE: Cholangioma causing segmental biliary obstruction
Following irradiation (early)
Stauffer's syndrome

REFERENCES

1. Aburano T, Taniguchi M, Hisada K, et al: Discordant hepatic uptake of ^{99m}Tc HIDA and ^{99m}Tc colloid in a patient with segmental biliary obstruction. Clin Nucl Med 13:599, 1988
2. Lamki L: A dichotomy in hepatic uptake of ^{99m}Tc-IDA and ^{99m}Tc-colloid. Semin Nucl Med 12:92, 1982

ESOPHAGEAL TRANSIT

Delayed

COMMON AND
UNCOMMON: Achalasia
Barrett's esophagus
Chagas' disease
Chronic idiopathic intestinal pseudo-obstruction
Diabetes mellitus
Diffuse esophageal spasm
Hypertensive lower esophageal sphincter
Hypothyroidism
Nonspecific esophageal motor disorders
Nutcracker esophagus
Obstruction
Reflux esophagitis
Scleroderma

REFERENCES

1. Benjamin SB, O'Donnell JK, Hancock J, et al: Prolonged radionuclide transit in "nutcracker esophagus": Dig Dis Sci 28:775, 1983

2. Blackwell JN, Hannan WJ, Adam RD, et al: Radionuclide transit studies in the detection of oesophageal dysmotility. Gut 24:421, 1983

3. Blue PW: Scintigraphic evaluation of dysphagia. Clin Nucl Med 7:489, 1981

4. Datz FL: The role of radionuclide studies in esophageal disease. J Nucl Med 25:1040, 1984

5. Drane WE, Johnson DA, Hagan DP, Cattau EL: Nutcracker esophagus: Diagnosis with radionuclide esophageal scintigraphy vs manometry. Radiology 163:244, 1987

6. Dubois A, Castel DO (eds): Esophageal and Gastric Emptying. Boca Raton, CRC Press, 1984

7. Guillet J, Wynchank S, Basse-Cathalinat B, et al: Pediatric esophageal scintigraphy: Results of 200 studies. Clin Nucl Med 9:427, 1983

8. Holloway RH, Drosin G, Lange RC, et al: Radionuclide esophageal emptying of a solid meal to quantitate results of therapy in achalasia. Gastroenterology 84:771, 1983

9. Karvelis KC, Drane WE, Johnson DA, Silverman ED: Barrett esophagus: Decreased esophageal clearance shown by radionuclide esophageal scintigraphy. Radiology 162:97, 1987

10. McCallum RW: Radionuclide scanning in esophageal disease. J Clin Gastroenterol 4:67, 1982

11. McKinney MK, Brady CE III, Weiland FL: Radionuclide esophageal transit: An evaluation of therapy in achalasia. South Med J 76:1136, 1983

12. Malmud LS, Fisher RS: Radionuclide studies of esophageal transit and gastro-esophageal reflux. Semin Nucl Med 12:104, 1982

13. Malmud LS, Fisher RS: Scintigraphic evaluation of disorders of the esophagus, stomach and duodenum. Med Clin NA 65:1291, 1981

14. Russell COH, Hill LD, Holmes ER III, et al: Radionuclide transit: A sensitive screening test for esophageal dysfunction. Gastroenterology 80:887, 1981

15. Tolin RD, Malmud LS, Reilley J, et al: Esophageal scintigraphy to quantitate esophageal transit (quantitation of esophageal transit). Gastroenterology 76:1402, 1979

GASTRIC EMPTYING

Rapid

COMMON AND
UNCOMMON: Drugs
Dumping syndrome
Duodenal ulcers without outlet obstruction
Enterogastric reflux gastritis
Hyperthyroidism
Zollinger-Ellison syndrome

REFERENCES

1. Bateman DN, Kahn C, Davies DS: Concentration effect studies with oral metoclopramide. Br J Clin Pharmacol 8:179, 1979

2. Donovan IA, Gunn IF, Brown A, et al: A comparison of gastric emptying before and after vagotomy with antrectomy and vagotomy with pyloroplasty. Surgery 76:729, 1974

3. McLoughlin JC, Green WER, Buchanan KD: Gastric emptying of ingested acid and its effect on plasma gastrin and secretin in duodenal ulcer subjects. Gastroenterology 13:313, 1978

4. Mayer EA, Thomson JB, Jehn D, et al: Gastric emptying and sieving of solid food and pancreatic and biliary secretion after solid meals in patients with truncal vagotomy and antrectomy. Gastroenterology 83:184, 1982

5. Metgzer WH, Cano R, Sturdevant AL: Effect of metoclopramide in chronic gastric retention after gastric surgery. Gastroenterology 71:30, 1976

6. Urbain JLC, Vantrappen G, Janssens J, et al: Intravenous erythromycin dramatically accelerates gastric emptying in gastroparesis diabeticorum and normals and abolishes emptying discrimination between solids and liquids. J Nucl Med 31:1490, 1990

GASTRIC EMPTYING

Delayed

COMMON: Diabetes mellitus
           Postsurgical
           Females
           Drugs

UNCOMMON
AND RARE: Acute gastroenteritis
             Age
             Amyloidosis
             Anorexia nervosa
             Brain tumor
             Chronic idiopathic intestinal pseudoobstruction
             Gastric outlet obstruction (ulcer, tumor, etc.)
             Gastritis
             Gastroesophageal reflux
             Hypothyroidism
             Idiopathic gastroparesis
             Muscular dystrophy
             Obesity
             Pernicious anemia
             Poliomyelitis
             Pyloric stenosis
             Pylorospasm
             Scleroderma
             Technical
             Uremia

REFERENCES

1. Carrio I, Notivol R, Estorch M, et al: Gender-related differences in gastric emptying. J Nucl Med 29:573, 1988

2. Chaudhuri TK, Chaudhuri TK: Gastric emptying: A physiological and pharmacological test. In RP Spenser (ed.): Interventional Nuclear Medicine. Orlando, Fla., Grune and Stratton, 1984, p 287

3. Christian PE, Datz FL, Moore JG: Gastric emptying studies in morbidly obese before and after gastroplasty. J Nucl Med 27:1686, 1986

4. Christian PC, Datz FL, Sorenson JA, et al: Technical factors in gastric emptying studies. J Nucl Med 24:264, 1983

5. Datz FL, Christian PE, Moore JA: Sex-related differences in gastric emptying. J Nucl Med 27:904, 1986

6. Domstad PA, Shih WJ, Humphries L, et al: Radionuclide gastric emptying studies in patients with anorexia nervosa. J Nucl Med 28:816, 1987

7. Dubois A, Castell DO (eds): Esophageal and Gastric Emptying. Boca Raton, CRC Press, 1984

8. Feldman M, Smith HJ, Simon TR: Gastric emptying of solid radiopaque markers: Studies in health subjects and diabetic patients. Gastroenterology 87:895, 1984

9. Fox S, Behar J: Pathogenesis of diabetic gastroparesis: A pharmacologic study. Gastroenterology 78:757, 1980

10. Glowniak JV, Wahl RL: Patient motion artifacts on scintigraphic gastric emptying studies. Radiology 154:537, 1985

11. Maddern GJ, Horowitz M, Jamieson GG, et al: Abnormalities of esophageal and gastric emptying in progressive systemic sclerosis. Gastroenterology 87:922, 1984

12. Moore JG, Christian PE, Taylor AT, et al: Gastric emptying measurements: Delayed and complex emptying patterns without appropriate correction. J Nucl Med 26:1206, 1985

13. Rees WDE, Miller LJ, Malagelada J-R: Dyspepsia, antral motor dysfunction and gastric stasis of solids. Gastroenterology 78:360, 1980

14. Rhodes JB, Robinson RG, McBride N: Sudden onset of slow gastric emptying of food. Gastroenterology 77:569, 1979

15. Rosen PR, Treves S: The relationship of gastroesophageal reflux and gastric emptying in infants and children: Concise communication. J Nucl Med 25:571, 1984

16. Schulze-Delrieu K: The study of gastric stasis: Static no longer (editorial). Gastroenterology 78:867, 1980

17. Seibert JJ, Byrne WJ, Euler AR: Gastric emptying in children: Unusual patterns detected by scintigraphy. AJR 141:49, 1983

18. Shih W-J, DeLand FH, Domstad A, et al: Scintigraphic findings in primary amyloidosis of the heart and stomach. Clin Nucl Med 10:466, 1985

19. Szilagyi A, Stern J, Armanious S, Brem S: Gastroparesis secondary to medulloblastoma of posterior fossa. Clin Nucl Med 12:864, 1987

20. Urbain JL, Penninckx F, Siegel JA, et al: Effect of proximal vagotomy and roux-en-Y diversion on gastric emptying kinetics in asymptomatic patients. Clin Nucl Med 15:688, 1990

21. Singh A, Barthel J: Delayed gastric emptying associated with gastric bezoar. Semin Nucl Med XVIII:173, 1988

GALLIUM IMAGING

Focal Uptake

COMMON: Abscess
Arthritis
Bronchogenic carcinoma
Cellulitis
Intestinal activity — normal
Lymphoma — Hodgkin's and non-Hodgkin's
Osteomyelitis
Other malignant tumors
Physiologic breast activity
Pneumonia
Pyelonephritis
Sarcoidosis
Surgical wound or scar
Thymus in children
Tuberculosis

UNCOMMON: Acute cholecystitis
Chronic cholecystitis
Crohn's disease
Dermatomyositis
Diverticulitis
Fracture
Gallbladder empyema
Hematoma
Infected pancreatic pseudocyst
Injection sites
Pancreatitis
Peritonitis
Postoperative synthetic graft infection
Pseudomembranous colitis
Stomach
Ulcerative colitis

RARE: Acne vulgaris
Actinomycosis
Acute panniculitis
Aggressive fibromatosis
Bite
Breast augmentation

Castleman's disease
Cerebritis
Congenital adrenal hyperplasia
Corynebacterium parvum immunotherapy
Cryptococcus
Dissecting aortic aneurysm
Epididymo-orchitis
Gastritis
Hashimoto's thyroiditis
Hepatoblastoma
Heterotopic bone
Hypopharynx — secondary to tear production
Incarcerated hernia
Inflammatory pseudotumor
Leiomyoma
Leukemia
Mesenteric adenitis
Multiple myeloma
Muscular dystrophy
Mycotic aneurysm
Myositis ossificans
Neurogenic arthropathy
Paget's disease
Periarteritis nodosa
Polyostatic fibrous dysplasia
Pulmonary embolism
Retroperitoneal fibrosis
Rhabdomyolysis
Rheumatoid pachymeningitis
Sporotrichosis
Starch peritonitis
Subacute bacterial endocarditis
Subacute thyroiditis
Syphilis
Thrombophlebitis
Tuberous sclerosis
Venous occlusion (spleen)

REFERENCES

1. Ackerman L, Reyes CV, Freeman ML, et al: Gallium-67 uptake in hepatic angiosarcoma. J Nucl Med 25:677, 1984

2. Adler S, Parthasarathy KL, Bakshi SP, et al: Gallium-67-citrate scanning for the localization and staging of lymphomas. J Nucl Med 16:255, 1975

3. Auringer ST, Scott MD, Sumner TE: Inflammatory pseudotumor: A gallium-avid mobile mesenteric mass. J Nucl Med 32:1614, 1991

4. Bekerman C, Schulak JA, Kaplan EL, et al: Parathyroid adenoma imaged by Ga-67-citrate scintigraphy: Case report. J Nucl Med 18:1096, 1977

5. Bekerman C, Vyas MI: Renal localization of ^{67}Ga-citrate in renal amyloidosis: Case reports. J Nucl Med 17:899, 1976

6. Campeau RJ, LaCorte WS: Abnormal splenic uptake of gallium-67 citrate in a case of infectious mononucleosis. Clin Nucl Med 10:355, 1985

7. Cancroft ET, Montorfano D, Goldfarb R: Metastases to bone from malignant thymoma detected by technetium-phosphate and gallium-67 scintigraphy. Clin Nucl Med 3:312, 1978

8. Carter JE, Joo KG: Gallium accumulation in intramuscular injection sites. Clin Nucl Med 4:304, 1979

9. Causey DA, Fajman WA, Perdue GD, et al: [67]Ga scintigraphy in postoperative synthetic graft infections. AJR 134:1041, 1980

10. Choy D, Murray IP, Ford JC: Gallium scintigraphy in acute panniculitis. J Nucl Med 22:973, 1981

11. Creagh MF, Nunan TO: Positive ^{67}Ga citrate uptake in patient with polyostotic fibrous dysplasia. Clin Nucl Med 13:241, 1988

12. Dey HM, Karimeddini MK, Ciesielski TE, et al: Radiogallium hot spleen in Trousseau's syndrome with splenic vein occlusion. Clin Nucl Med 11:640, 1986

13. Eikman EA, Tenorio LE, Frank BA, et al: Gallium-67 accumulation in the stomach in patients with postoperative gastritis. J Nucl Med 21:706, 1980

14. Farrer PA: Gallium-67 imaging in acute epididymoorchitis. Clin Nucl Med 5:417, 1980

15. Freeman LM (ed): Nuclear Medicine Annual 1980. New York, Raven Press, 1980

16. Garcia OM, Sarma D: Gallium scanning in a patient with sarcoidosis. Clin Nucl Med 8:557, 1983

17. Gates GF: The gallium "bone scan" in acute leukemia. J Nucl Med 20:854, 1979

18. Geslien GE, Thrall JH, Johnson MC: Gallium scanning in acute amebic abscess. J Nucl Med 15:561, 1974

19. Glynn TP: Marked gallium accumulation in neurogenic arthropathy. J Nucl Med 22:1016, 1982

20. Gram ED, Almaria HE, Brownstein S: ^{67}Ga-citrate accumulation in breasts of a postabortion patient. Clin Nucl Med 2:406, 1977

21. Grassi CJ, Lee RGL, Pezzuit RT, et al: Accumulation of Ga-67 citrate in an inguinal hernia simulating scrotal pathology. Clin Nucl Med 9:111, 1984

22. Haden HT, Lippman HR: Gallium localization in dissecting aortic aneurysm. Clin Nucl Med 13:569, 1988

23. Halpern S, Hagan P: Gallium-67-citrate imaging in neoplastic and inflammatory disease. In Freeman LM, Weissmann HS (eds): Nuclear Medicine Annual 1980. New York, Raven Press, 1980

24. Heidendal GA, Roos P, Thijs LG, et al: Evaluation of cold areas on the thyroid scan with ^{67}Ga-citrate. J Nucl Med 16:793, 1975

25. Higgins WL, Marano GD: Gallium imaging of rheumatoid pachymeningitis. Clin Nucl Med 11:350, 1986

26. Hoffer P: Status of Gallium-67 in tumor detection. J Nucl Med 21:394, 1980

27. Hoffer P, Beckerman C, Henkin RE: Gallium-67 Imaging. New York, John Wiley and Sons, Inc., 1978

28. Hopkins GB, Kan M, Schwartz LJ: Myocardial involvement in secondary syphilis detected by ^{67}Ga scintigraphy. Clin Nucl Med 2:208, 1977

29. Ishimura J, Fukuchi M: Marked uptake of ^{67}Ga citrate in giant leiomyoma uteri. Clin Nucl Med 16:129, 1991

30. Iwase M, Shimizu Y, Kitahara H, et al: Parathyroid carcinoma visualized by gallium-67 citrate scintigraphy. J Nucl Med 27:63, 1986

31. Jones B, Abbruzzese AA, Hill TC, et al: Gallium-67-citrate scintigraphy in ulcerative colitis. Gastrointest Radiol 5:267, 1980

32. Joo KG, Landsberg R, Parthasarthy KL, et al: Abnormal gallium scan in regional enteritis. Clin Nucl Med 3:134, 1978

33. Joseph U, Jhingran SG, Johnson PC: Gallium-67 imaging and Crohn's disease. J Nucl Med 20:903, 1979

34. Kennedy TD, Martin NL, Robinson RG: Identification of an infected pseudocyst of the pancreas with ^{67}Ga-citrate: Case report. J Nucl Med 16:1132, 1975

35. Kipper MS, Taylor A, Ashburn WL: Gallium-67-citrate uptake in a case of acne vulgaris. Clin Nucl Med 6:409, 1981

36. Klaas KK, Gregg DC, Sty JR: ^{67}Ga imaging of cervical collar sign in periarteritis nodosa. Clin Nucl Med 19:155, 1994

37. Leonard JC, Humphrey GB, Vanhoutte JJ: Positive ^{67}Ga-citrate scans in patients receiving Corynebacterium parvum. Clin Nucl Med 3:370, 1978

38. Leibowich S, Tumeh SS: ^{67}Ga imaging and computed tomography in early retroperitoneal fibrosis. Clin Nucl Med 13:829, 1988

39. Lepanto PB, Rosenstock J, Littman P, et al: Gallium-67 scans in children with solid tumors. AJR 126:179, 1976

40. Lorberbym M, Sarkar SD, Speiser P, et al: Bilateral adrenal uptake of ^{67}Ga citrate in patient with congenital adrenal hyperplasia. Clin Nucl Med 15:849, 1990

41. MacMahon H, Vyborny C, Sephardari S, et al: Gallium accumulation in the stomach: A frequent incidental finding. Clin Nucl Med 10:719, 1985

42. McNeill JA, Llaurado JG: Innocent intramural gastric uptake of gallium-67 in a case of AIDS. Clin Nucl Med 11:123, 1986

43. Mackey JK, Alexieva-Jackson B, Fetters DV, et al: Bone and gallium scan findings in malignant fibrous histiocytoma. Clin Nucl Med 12:17, 1987

44. Michal JA, Coleman E: Localization of ^{67}Ga-citrate in a mycotic aneurysm. AJR 129:1111, 1977

45. Miller JH: Accumulation of Gallium-67 in costochondritis. Clin Nucl Med 5:362, 1980

46. Moinuddin M, Rockett JF: Gallium imaging in inflammatory diseases. Clin Nucl Med 1:271, 1976

47. Moreno AJ, Brazier JM, Baker FJ, et al: Gallium-67 citrate localization in disseminated sporotrichosis. Clin Nucl Med 10:424, 1985

48. Moreno AJ, Weisman IM, Yedinak MA, et al: Gallium-67 citrate scintigraphy in pulmonary embolism. Clin Nucl Med 10:626, 1985

49. Moreno AJ, Yedinak MA, Spicer MJ, et al: Myositis ossificans with Ga-67 citrate positivity. Clin Nucl Med 10:40, 1985

50. Myerson PJ, Berg GR, Spencer RP, et al: Gallium-67 spread to the anterior pararenal space in pancreatitis: Case report. J Nucl Med 18:893, 1977

51. Myerson PJ, Myerson D, Spencer RP: Anatomic patterns of Ga-67 distribution in localized and diffuse peritoneal inflammation. Case report. J Nucl Med 18:977, 1977

52. Newcomer AD, Wahner HW: Gallium scan: Clue to diagnosis of starch peritonitis. Clin Nucl Med 4:465, 1979

53. Nishiyama H, Morand TM, Siewert VJ: Extensive skeletal involvement detected by ^{67}Ga citrate in patient with multiple myeloma. Clin Nucl Med 13:179, 1988

54. Norris S, Erlich MG, Keim DE, et al: Early diagnosis of disc space infection using Gallium-67. J Nucl Med 19:384, 1978

55. Ohta H, Endo K, Konishi J, et al: Scintigraphic evaluation of aggressive fibromatosis. J Nucl Med 31:1632, 1990

56. Park CH, Miller FJ, Lipton A, et al: Incidentally detected thrombosed vein during ^{67}Ga-citrate scanning. AJR 126:1249, 1976

57. Parthasarathy KL, Bakshi SP, Parikh S: Localization of metastatic adrenal carcinoma utilizing ^{67}Ga-citrate. Clin Nucl Med 3:24, 1978

59. Rashad FA, Miraldi FD, Bellon EM: Gallium-67 uptake in tuberous sclerosis. Clin Nucl Med 4:242, 1979

60. Rheingold OJ, Tedesco FJ, Block FE, et al: ^{67}Ga-citrate scintiscanning in active inflammatory bowel disease. Dig Dis Sci 24:363, 1979

61. Schleissner LA, Mishkin FS: Gallium imaging in sarcoid dactylitis. Clin Nucl Med 10:106, 1986

62. Seder J, Hattner RS: Incidental localization of ^{67}Ga-citrate in an incarcerated inguinal hernia. Clin Nucl Med 3:411, 1978

63. Seder J, Shimshak R, Williams R: Reversible ^{67}Ga-citrate uptake in the thyroid with subacute thyroiditis. Clin Nucl Med 4:158, 1979

64. Smith WP, Robinson RG, Gobuty AH: Positive whole body ^{67}Ga scintigraphy in dermatomyositis. AJR 133:126, 1979

65. Stansby G, Hilson A, Hamilton G: Gallium scintigraphy in diagnosis and management of multifocal Castleman's disease. Br J Radiol 64:165, 1991

66. Steinbach JJ: Abnormal ^{67}Ga-citrate scan of the abdomen in tuberculous peritonitis: Case report. J Nucl Med 17:272, 1976

67. Sziklas JJ, Vento JA, Spencer RP, et al: Radiogallium accumulation in heterotopic bone. Clin Nucl Med 10:376, 1985

68. Teates CD, Preston DF, Boyd CM: Gallium-67-citrate imaging in head and neck tumors: Report of a cooperative group. J Nucl Med 21:622, 1980

69. Tenenzapf MJ, Thanawala S, Dunn EK: Gallium scanning in rhabdomyolysis. Clin Nucl Med 6:425, 1981

70. Wahner HW, Goellner JR, Hoagland HC: Giant lymph node hyperplasia resembling abdominal abscess on gallium scan. Clin Nucl Med 3:19, 1978

71. Waxman AD, Siemsen JK: Gallium gallbladder scanning in cholecystitis. J Nucl Med 16:148, 1975

72. Waxman AD, Siemsen JK, Singer F: Gallium scanning in Paget's disease of bone: A superior parameter in following the response to calcitonin therapy. J Nucl Med 18:621, 1977

73. Winchell HS: Gallium-67 scanning of tuberous peritonitis. J Nucl Med 17:1020, 1976

74. Winston MA, Retzky M: ^{67}Ga concentration in mesenteric adenitis. Clin Nucl Med 2:427, 1977

75. Yeh EL, Tisdale PL, Zielonka JS: Gastric gallium-67 uptake in gastritis. Clin Nucl Med 8:605, 1983

GALLIUM IMAGING

Skin Uptake

COMMON: Infection
Surgical scar or wound

UNCOMMON: Acne vulgaris
Cutaneous sarcoidosis
Exfoliative erythroderma

RARE: Leprosy
Lymphocytic lymphoma
Mycobacterium avium-intracellulare septicemia
Mycosis fungoides
Polyarteritis nodosa

REFERENCES

1. Acio ER, Balasubramanian N, Vieras F, Smith JJ: [67]Ga localization in herpetic skin lesion. Clin Nucl Med 13:667, 1988

2. Alexander JE, Siebert JJ, Lowe BA: Cutaneous uptake of ^{67}Ga in polyarteritis nodosa. Clin Nucl Med 12:883, 1987

3. Allwright SJ, Chapman PR, Antico VF, Gruenewald SM: Cutaneous gallium uptake in patients with AIDS with *Mycobacterium avium-intracellulare* septicemia. Clin Nucl Med 13:506, 1988

4. Beck RN, Blumhardt R, Bennett W, et al: Gallium-67 scintigraphy in well-differentiated lymphocytic lymphoma of the skin. Clin Nucl Med 10:589, 1985

5. Drane WE, Karvelis K, Buck JL, et al: The "3-D effect" of diffuse skin involvement by mycosis fungoides on gallium imaging. Clin Nucl Med 11:264, 1986

6. Glickstein MF, Velchik MG: Gallium uptake in cutaneous sarcoidosis. Clin Nucl Med 11:119, 1986

7. Klaas KK, Gregg DC, Sty JR: [67]Ga imaging of cervical collar sign in periarteritis nodosa. Clin Nucl Med 19:155, 1994

8. Primeau M, Carrier L, Verrault JM, et al: [67]Ga uptake in cutaneous lepromatous lesions. Clin Nucl Med 13:924, 1988

9. Taillefer R, Danais S, Dumont M: Gallium-67 scintigraphy: The beard sign. Clin Nucl Med 8:271, 1983

10. Wheeland RG, Leonard JC, Ellis DL: Gallium scintigraphy in exfoliative erythroderma. Clin Nucl Med 10:887, 1985

GALLIUM IMAGING

Salivary Gland Uptake

COMMON: Nodal uptake in Hodgkin's simulating parotid
uptake
Previous head and neck irradiation
Sarcoidosis
Sjögren's syndrome

UNCOMMON: Idiopathic (has been seen in patients with
carcinomas such as lung, pancreas, esophagus,
abdominal abscess, etc.)
Sialadenitis
Uremia

RARE: Alcoholism
Chronic graft-versus-host disease
Collagen vascular disease
Mumps parotitis
Neoplasia
Sialography

REFERENCES

1. Bekerman C, Hoffer PB: Salivary gland uptake of ^{67}Ga-citrate following radiation therapy. J Nucl Med 17:685, 1976

2. Hardoff R, Nachtigal D: Unilateral ^{67}Ga uptake in submandibular salivary gland following sialography. Clin Nucl Med 14:65, 1989

3. Heyman S: The uptake of Gallium-67-citrate by the parotid glands in a uremic patient. Clin Nucl Med 5:404, 1980

4. Higashi T, Shindo J, Everhart R, et al: [99m]Tc pertechnetate and ^{67}Ga imaging in salivary gland disease. Clin Nucl Med 14:504, 1989

5. Hoffer PB, Beckerman C, Henkin RE: Gallium-67 Imaging. New York, John Wiley and Sons, 1978

6. Logic JR, Ball GV, Tauxe WN: Uptake of 67-gallium in parotid glands of patients with Sjögren's syndrome. J Nucl Med 17:530, 1976

7. Lubat E, Kramer EL: Gallium-67 citrate accumulation in parotid and submandibular glands in sarcoidosis. Clin Nucl Med 10:593, 1985

8. Mishkin FS, Maynard WP: Lacrimal gland accumulation of [67]Ga. J Nucl Med 15:630, 1974

9. Oren VO, Uszler JM, White J: Diagnosis of uveoparotid fever by ⁶⁷Ga-citrate imaging. Clin Nucl Med 3:127, 1978

10. Rose J: Increased salivary gland uptake of ⁶⁷Ga-citrate 36 months after radiation therapy. J Nucl Med 18:495, 1977

11. Wiener SN, Patel BP: ⁶⁷Ga-citrate uptake by the parotid glands in sarcoidosis. Radiology 130:753, 1979

12. Yamauchi K, Noguchi K, Suzuki Y, Nagao T: ⁶⁷Ga uptake in salivary glands in chronic graft-vs-host disease after bone marrow transplant. Clin Nucl Med 14:330, 1989

GALLIUM IMAGING

Diffuse Thyroid Uptake

COMMON AND
UNCOMMON: Amiodarone-induced hyperthyroidism
Sarcoidosis
Thyroiditis — subacute and chronic

REFERENCES

1. Moreno AJ, Brown JM, Spicer MJ, et al: Thyroid localization of Ga-67 citrate. Semin Nucl Med 15:224, 1985
2. White WB, Spencer RP, Sziklas JJ, et al: Incidental finding of intense thyroid radiogallium activity during febrile illness. Clin Nucl Med 10:71, 1985

GALLIUM IMAGING

Focal Thyroid Uptake

COMMON AND
UNCOMMON: Leiomyosarcoma
Lymphoma
Metastases
Parathyroid adenoma
Thyroid carcinoma
Thyroiditis

REFERENCES

1. Moreno AJ, Brown JM, Spicer MJ, et al: Thyroid localization of Ga-67 citrate. Semin Nucl Med 15:224, 1985
2. White WB, Spencer RP, Sziklas JJ, et al: Incidental finding of intense thyroid radiogallium activity during febrile illness. Clin Nucl Med 10:71, 1985

GALLIUM IMAGING

Myocardial Uptake

COMMON AND
UNCOMMON: Abscess
Amyloidosis
Bacterial endocarditis
Hypersensitivity angiitis
Idiopathic congestive cardiomyopathy
Kawasaki's disease
Metastases (e.g., angiosarcoma, lung lymphoma,
melanoma)
Myocardial infarction
Myocarditis
Pericarditis (e.g., mixed bacterial, histoplasmosis,
rheumatoid arthritis, tuberculosis)
Postpericardiotomy syndrome
Sarcoidosis
Severe heart failure
Syphilis
Transplant rejection

REFERENCES

1. Alpert LI, Welch P, Fisher N: Gallium-positive Lyme disease myocarditis. Clin Nucl Med 10:617, 1985

2. Braun SD, Lisbona R, Novales-Diaz JA, et al: Myocardial uptake of ^{99m}Tc-phosphate tracer in amyloidosis. Clin Nucl Med 4:244, 1979

3. Hopkins GB, Kan M, Schwartz LJ: Myocardial involvement in secondary syphilis detected by ^{67}Ga scintigraphy. Clin Nucl Med 2:208, 1977

4. Huang T-Y: Gallium-67 imaging in dilated cardiomyopathy secondary to viral infection. Clin Nucl Med 10:432, 1985

5. Moinuddin M, Rockett JF: Gallium imaging in inflammatory diseases. Clin Nucl Med 1:271, 1976

6. Moreno AJ, Brown JM, Spicer MJ, et al: Gallium-67 citrate localization in the heart secondary to constrictive pericarditis with myocardial fibrosis. J Nucl Med 25:66, 1984

7. O'Brien K, Barnes D, Martin RH, Rae JR: Gallium-SPECT in detection of prosthetic valve endocarditis and aortic ring abscess. J Nucl Med 32:1791, 1991

8. O'Connel JB, Robinson JA, Henkin RE, et al: Immunosuppressive therapy in patients with congestive cardiomyopathy and myocardial uptake of Gallium-67. Circulation 64:780, 1981

9. O'Connell JB, Henkin RE, Robinson JA, et al: Gallium-67 imaging in patients with dilated cardiomypathy and biopsy-proven myocarditis. Circulation 70:58, 1984

10. Paspa P, Movahed A: Cardiac blood pool visualization by ^{67}Ga scintigraphy at 48 hours in patient with severe heart failure. Clin Nucl Med 18:80, 1993

11. Reeves WC, Jackson GL, Flickinger FW, et al: Radionuclide imaging of experimental myocarditis. Circulation 63:640, 1981

12. Robinson JA, O'Connell J, Henkin RE, et al: Gallium-67 imaging in cardiomyopathy. Ann Intern Med 90:198, 1979

13. Shah PJ, Shreeve WW: Uptake of Ga-67 in the cardiac region in hypersensitivity angiitis. Clin Nucl Med 6:547, 1981

14. Shreiner DP, Krishnaswami V, Murphy JH: Unsuspected purulent pericarditis detected by gallium-67 scanning: A case report. Clin Nucl Med 6:411, 1981

15. Spies SM, Meyers SN, Barresi V, et al: A case of myocardial abscess evaluated by radionuclide techniques: Case report. J Nucl Med 18:1089, 1977

16. Sty JR, Chused MJ, Dorrington A, et al: Ga-67 imaging: Kawasaki disease. Clin Nucl Med 6:112, 1981

17. Taillefer R, Lemieux RJ, Picard D, et al: Gallium-67 imaging in pericarditis secondary to tuberculosis and histoplasmosis. Clin Nucl Med 6:413, 1981

18. Tajima T, Naito T, Dohi Y, et al: Ga-67 and Tl-201 imaging in sarcoidosis involving the myocardium. Clin Nucl Med 6:120, 1981

19. Yamamoto S, Bergsland J, Michalek SM, et al: Uptake of myocardial imaging agents by rejecting and nonrejecting cardiac transplants. A comparative clinical study of ^{201}Tl, ^{99m}Tc, and ^{67}Ga. J Nucl Med 30:1464, 1989

GALLIUM IMAGING

Symmetrical Breast Uptake

COMMON: Drugs (including oral contraceptives)
Hormone therapy
Menarche
Postabortion
Postpartum
Pregnancy

UNCOMMON: Gynecomastia
Obesity
Renal failure

RARE: Breast augmentation
Choriocarcinoma
Idiopathic galactorrhea
Neonate
Non-African Burkitt's lymphoma

REFERENCES

1. Boxen I: Intense bilateral breast uptake of ^{67}Ga. J Nucl Med 29:1606, 1988
2. Chandramouly BS, Tiu S, Castronuovo JJ: Uptake of gallium in the breasts. Semin Nucl Med 14:50, 1984
3. Desai AG, Intenzo C, Park C, Green P: Drug-induced gallium uptake in breasts. Clin Nucl Med 12:703, 1987
4. Firman K, Howman-Giles R: Breast uptake of ^{67}Ga in a neonate. Clin Nucl Med 17:213, 1992
5. Fram ED, Almaria HH Jr, Brownstein S: ^{67}Ga citrate accumulation in breasts of a postabortion patient. Clin Nucl Med 2:406, 1977
6. Freeman LM (ed): Nuclear Medicine Annual 1980. New York, Raven Press, 1980
7. Hoffer PB, Beckerman CS, Henkin RE: Gallium-67 Imaging. New York, John Wiley and Sons, 1978
8. Joffer P: Status of Gallium-67 tumor detection. J Nucl Med 21:394, 1980
9. Kosuda S, Kawahara S, Tamura K, et al: ^{67}Ga uptake in diethylstilbestrol-induced gynecomastia — experience with six patients. Clin Nucl Med 15:879, 1990
10. Lopez OL, Rodriguez Maisano E: Ga-67 uptake postcesarean section. Clin Nucl Med 9:103, 1984

11. Palestro CJ, Chau P, Goldsmith SJ: [67]Ga uptake after breast and hip augmentation with silicone. Clin Nucl Med 17:897, 1992

12. Teates CD, Bray ST, Williamson BRJ: Tumor detection with ^{67}Ga citrate: A literature survey (1970–1978). Clin Nucl Med 3:456, 1978

---

*Note all these are symmetrical and bilateral.

GALLIUM IMAGING

Asymmetrical Breast Uptake

COMMON: Abscess
Breastfeeding
Carcinoma
Cystosarcoma phylloides
Fibroadenoma
Granuloma
Hematoma

UNCOMMON
AND RARE: Drug abuse-injection sites
Lymphoma
Malignant cystic mesodermal tumor
Metastases to breast
Postmastectomy (contralateral breast)

REFERENCES

1. Chandramouly BS, Tiu S, Castronuovo JJ: Uptake of gallium in the breasts. Semin Nucl Med 14:50, 1984

2. Fram ED, Almaria HH Jr, Brownstein S: ^{67}Ga citrate accumulation in breasts of a postabortion patient. Clin Nucl Med 2:406, 1977

3. Freeman LM (ed): Nuclear Medicine Annual 1980. New York, Raven Press, 1980

4. Hoffer PB, Bekerman CS, Henkin RE: Gallium-67 Imaging. New York, John Wiley and Sons, 1978

5. Joffer P: Status of gallium-67 tumor detection. J Nucl Med 21:394, 1980

6. Swayne LC: ^{67}Ga detection of intramammary injection sites secondary to intravenous drug abuse. Clin Nucl Med 14:693, 1989

GALLIUM IMAGING

Diffuse Renal Uptake (Unilateral or Bilateral)

COMMON: Abscess (esp. perinephric)
Normal
Pyelonephritis
Recent transplant

UNCOMMON
AND RARE: Acute renal failure
Acute tubular necrosis
Amyloidosis
Chemotherapy
Congestive heart failure
Interstitial nephritis
Leukemia
Lymphoma
Metastasis (e.g., melanoma, leukemia, lymphoma)
Nephrotic syndrome
Obstruction
Rejection
Saturated iron binding sites (hemochromatosis,
multiple blood transfusions)
Severe hepatocellular disease
Tuberculosis
Ureterosigmoidostomy
Vasculitis
Wegner's granulomatosis

REFERENCES

1. Alazraki N, Sterkel B, Taylor A Jr: Renal gallium accumulation in the absence of renal pathology in patients with severe hepatocellular disease. Clin Nucl Med 8:200, 1983

2. Garcia JE, Van Nostrand D, Howard WH III, et al: The spectrum of gallium-67 renal activity in patients with no evidence of renal disease. J Nucl Med 25:575, 1984

3. Johnson PM, Fawwaz RA, Hardy MA, et al: Sequential Ga-67 imaging in diagnosis of renal allograft rejection. J Nucl Med 20:630, 1979

4. Kawamura J, Itoh H, Yoshida O, et al: "Hot spot" on Ga-67-citrate scan in a case of renal cell carcinoma. Clin Nucl Med 5:471, 1980

5. Long SE, Sonnemaker RE, Burdine JA: Renal accumulation of ^{67}Ga-citrate. Semin Nucl Med 14:52, 1984

6. Mendez G, Morillo G, Alonso M, et al: Gallium-67 radionuclide imaging in acute pyelonephritis. AJR 134:17, 1980

7. Sauerbrunn BJ, Andrews GA, Hubner KF: Ga-67-citrate imaging in tumors of the genitourinary tract: Report of a cooperative study. J Nucl Med 19:470, 1978

8. Sterkel BB, Alazraki NA, Taylor A: Persistent renal uptake of gallium in the absense of renal pathology in patients with severe hepatocellular disease. J Nucl Med 21:67, 1980

GALLIUM IMAGING

Bilateral Diffuse Renal Uptake

COMMON AND
UNCOMMON: Acute renal failuire
Acute tubular necrosis
Amyloidosis
Any cause of vasculitis
Bilateral carcinoma (primary or metastatic)
Bilateral obstruction
Chemotherapy
Interstitial nephritis
Leukemia
Lymphoma
Metastasis
Multiple transfusions
Nephrotic syndrome
Normal
Pyelonephritis
Saturated iron binding
Severe hepatocellular disease
Tuberculosis
Ureterosigmoidostomy
Wegener's granulomatosis

REFERENCES

1. Bekerman C, Vyas MI: Renal localization of ^{67}Ga-citrate in renal amyloidosis: Case reports. J Nucl Med 17:899, 1976

2. Edeburn GF, Treves ST: Gallium scan findings following multiple blood transfusions in an infant with erythroblastosis fetalis. Clin Nucl Med 12:70, 1987

3. Fawwaz RA, Johnson PM: Renal localization of radiogallium — a retrospective study. J Nucl Med 18:595, 1977

4. Freeman LM (ed): Nuclear Medicine Annual 1980. New York, Raven Press, 1980

5. Hauser MF, Alderson PO: Gallium-67 imaging in abdominal disease. Semin Nucl Med 8:251, 1978

6. Kumar B, Coleman RE: Significance of delayed ^{67}Ga localization in the kidneys. J Nucl Med 17:872, 1976

7. Long SE, Sonnemaker RE, Burdine JA: Renal accumulation of ^{67}Ga-citrate. Semin Nucl Med 14:52, 1984

8. Sterkel BB, Alazraki NP, Taylor A: Persistent renal uptake of gallium in the absence of renal pathology in patients with severe hepatocellular disease. J. Nucl Med 21:67, 1980

9. Taylor A, Nelson H, Vasquez M, et al: Renal gallium accumulation in rats with antibiotic-induced nephritis: Clinical implications. Concise communication. J Nucl Med 21:646, 1980

10. Wood B, Sharma J, Germann D, et al: Gallium citrate Ga-67 imaging in non-infectious interstitial nephritis. Arch Intern Med 138:1665, 1978

GALLIUM IMAGING

Focal Unilateral Renal Uptake

COMMON: Abscess (renal or perinephric)

UNCOMMON: Acute focal bacterial nephritis (acute lobar
            nephronia)
            Acute pyelonephritis
            Renal cell carcinoma

RARE: Actinomycosis
        Nephrolithiasis
        Sarcoidosis
        Wilms' tumor

REFERENCE

1. Long SE, Sonnemaker RE, Burdine JA: Renal accumulation of ^{67}Ga-citrate. Semin Nucl Med 14:52, 1984

GALLIUM IMAGING

Focal Bilateral Renal Uptake

COMMON AND
UNCOMMON: Leukemia
Lymphoma
Metastases (melanoma)
Nephrolithiasis
Tuberculosis

REFERENCE

1. Long SE, Sonnemaker RE, Burdine JA: Renal accumulation of ^{67}Ga-citrate. Semin Nucl Med 14:52, 1984

GALLIUM IMAGING

Focal Liver Uptake

COMMON: Abscess (pyogenic or amebic)
Hepatoma
Metastases

UNCOMMON
AND RARE: Acute cholecystitis
Budd-Chiari syndrome
Cholangiocarcinoma
Cirrhosis (pseudotumor)
Hepatoblastoma
Sarcoidosis

REFERENCE

1. Garty I, Horovitz I, Keynan A: The use of gallium-67 liver imaging for the early diagnosis of Budd-Chiari syndrome. J Nucl Med 25:320, 1984
2. Tanasescu DE, Waxman AD, Hurvitz C: Scintigraphic findings mimicking focal nodular hyperplasia in case of hepatoblastoma. Clin Nucl Med 16:236, 1991

GALLIUM IMAGING

Decreased Hepatic Uptake

COMMON: Chemotherapy
Blood transfusions (iron overload)

UNCOMMON
AND RARE: Bile peritonitis
Liver failure
Liver replacement by non-Ga-67-avid lesions

REFERENCES

1. Bekerman C, Pavel DG, Bitran J, et al: The effects of inadvertent administration of antineoplastic agents prior to Ga-67 injection: Concise communication. J Nucl Med 25:430, 1984

2. Ensslen RD, Jackson FI, Reid AM: Bone and gallium scans in mastocytosis: Correlation with count rates, radiography, and microscopy. J Nucl Med 24:586, 1983

3. Lentle BC, Penney H, Ensslen RD: A generalized increase in uptake of gallium-67 in bone. Semin Nucl Med 14:143, 1984

4. Moreno AJ, Swaney JJ, Spicer MJ, et al: The gallium-67 citrate bone scan. Clin Nucl Med 10:594, 1985

5. Roswig DM, Spencer RP: Decreased hepatic concentration of radiogallium — ^{67}Ga. Semin Nucl Med 14:57, 1984

GALLIUM IMAGING

Liver Rim Sign

COMMON AND
UNCOMMON: Acute cholecystitis
Amebic abscess
Necrotic liver metastasis
Primary liver cell carcinoma
Pyogenic abscess

REFERENCES

1. Deroo MJK: Scintigraphic appearance of necrotic liver metastasis identical with that of amebic abscesses. J Nucl Med 16:250, 1975

2. Geslien GE, Thrall JH, Johnson MC: Gallium scanning in acute hepatic amebic abscess. J Nucl Med 15:561, 1974

3. Hauser MF, Alderson PO: Gallium-67 imaging in abdominal disease. Semin Nucl Med 8:251, 1978

4. Hoffer PB, Bekerman C, Henkin RE (eds): Gallium-67 Imaging. New York, John Wiley and Sons, 1978

5. James O, Wood EJ, Sherlock S: ⁶⁷Gallium scanning in the diagnosis of liver disease. Gut 15:404, 1974

6. Maze M, Wood J: Uptake of ⁶⁷Ga in space-occupying lesions in the liver. J Nucl Med 16:443, 1975

7. Staab EV, McCartney WH: Role of Gallium-67 in inflammatory disease. Semin Nucl Med 8:219, 1978

GALLIUM IMAGING

Ring Sign Outside of Liver

COMMON AND
UNCOMMON: Abscess
Infected pancreatitic pseudocyst
Inflammatory bowel disease
Periephric abscess
Radiation enteritis
Splenic and perisplenic abscess

REFERENCES

1. Lin DS: "Ring" sign in gallium-67 abdominal imaging. Semin Nucl Med 13:181, 1983
2. Smith SM, Park CH: The perisplenic halo of Ga-67 citrate: A sign of perisplenic abscess. Clin Nucl Med 10:93, 1985

GALLIUM IMAGING

Diffuse Abdominal Uptake

COMMON: Inflammatory bowel disease
Normal bowel uptake
Peritonitis (bacterial, starch)

UNCOMMON
AND RARE: Diffuse lymphoma
Generalized bowel or peritoneal activity
Hypoproteinemia
Mesenteric adenitis
Metastases
Pancreatitis
Peritoneal mesothelioma
Vasculitis

REFERENCES

1. Ammann W, Kassen BO: Diffuse abdominal gallium uptake. Semin Nucl Med 16:214, 1986

2. Armas RR, Goldsmith SJ: Gallium scanning in peritoneal mesothelioma. AJR 144:563, 1985

3. Kim EE, Gobuty A, Gutierrez C: Diffuse abdominal uptake of Ga-67 citrate in a patient with hypoproteinemia. J Nucl Med 24:508, 1983

4. LaManna MM, Saluk PH, Zekavat PP, et al: Gallium localization in peritonitis: Two case reports. Clin Nucl Med 9:25, 1984

5. Winzelberg GG: Focal gallium uptake in the liver. Semin Nucl Med 14:55, 1984

GALLIUM IMAGING

Stomach Uptake

COMMON AND
UNCOMMON: Gastritis
Gastric carcinoma
Lymphoma
Coarse gastric mucosa

REFERENCES

1. Eikman EA, Tenorio LE, Frank BA, et al: [67]Ga accumulation in stomach in patients with postoperative gastritis. J Nucl Med 211:706, 1980

2. Hardoff R, Quitt M, Agahai E: Gastric visualization by ^{67}Ga scintigraphy and coarse gastric mucosa in patient with Hodgkin's disease in remission. Clin Nucl Med 16:124, 1991

3. Que L, McCartney W, Haukins A, et al: Lymphomatous involvement of stomach, demonstrated by ^{67}Ga citrate. Dig Dis Sci 19:271, 1974

4. Teates CD, Bray ST, Williamson BRJ: Tumor detection with ^{67}Ga citrate. Clin Nucl Med 3:456, 1978

5. Wahner HW, Brown ML, Dickson ER: Gallium accumulation in stomach: A false-positive scan suggesting abscess. J Nucl Med 20:577, 1979

GALLIUM IMAGING

Diffuse Increased Osseous Uptake

COMMON AND
UNCOMMON: Blood transfusion (iron overload)
Chemotherapy
Chronic anemia — any cause
Hyperparathyroidism
Leukemia
Mastocytosis
Pediatric patient
Radiopharmaceutical
Tumor (prostate, breast)

REFERENCES

1. Bekerman C, Pavel DG, Bitran J, et al: The effects of inadvertent administration of antineoplastic agents prior to Ga-67 injection: Concise communication. J Nucl Med 25:430, 1984

2. Ensslen RD, Jackson FI, Reid AM: Bone and gallium scans in mastocytosis: Correlation with count rates, radiography, and microscopy. J Nucl Med 24:586, 1983

3. Lentle BC, Penney H, Ensslen RD: A generalized increase in uptake of gallium-67 in bone. Semin Nucl Med 14:143, 1984

4. Moreno AJ, Swaney JJ, Spicer MJ, et al: The gallium-67 citrate bone scan. Clin Nucl Med 10:594, 1985

GALLIUM IMAGING

Altered Biodistribution

COMMON AND
UNCOMMON: Drugs (scandium, desferoxamine, gadolinium, iron
dextran)
Mutliple transfusions
Elevated serum aluminum levels

REFERENCES

1. Brown SJ, Slizofski WJ, Dadparvar S: Altered biodistribution of ^{67}Ga in patient with aluminum toxicity treated with desferoxamine. J Nucl Med 31:115, 1990

2. Engelstad B, Luk SS, Hattner RS: Altered ^{67}Ga citrate distribution in patients with multiple red blood cell transfusions. Am J Roentgenol 139:755, 1982

3. Hattner RS, White DL: [67]Ga/stable gadolinium antagonism: MRI contrast agent markedly alters normal biodistribution of [67]Ga. J Nucl Med 31:1844, 1990

4. Oster ZH, Larson SM, Wagner HN: Possible enhancement of ^{67}Ga citrate imaging by iron dextran. J Nucl Med 17:356, 1976

5. Sephton R, Martin JJ: Modification of distribution of ^{67}Ga in man by administration of iron. Br J Radiol 53:572, 1980

GALLIUM AND SULFUR COLLOID LIVER IMAGING

Disparate Results

COMMON AND
UNCOMMON: Abscess — amebic
Abscess — pyogenic
Hepatoma
Some metastases (e.g., Hodgkin's, melanoma)

RARE: Actinomycosis
Hepatic adenoma

REFERENCES

1. Belanger MA, Beauchamp JM, Heitzschman HR: Gallium uptake in benign tumor of liver: Case report. J Nucl Med 16:470, 1975
2. Lunia S, Chodos RB, Sundaresh R: Actinomycosis of the liver and Ga-67-citrate scintigraphy. Clin Nucl Med 1:263, 1976

GALLIUM AND SULFUR COLLOID LIVER IMAGING

Matched Results

COMMON AND
UNCOMMON: Cysts
Fibrosis
Most benign tumors
Occasional metastases

REFERENCES

1. Gottschalk A, Potchen EJ: Diagnostic Nuclear Medicine. Baltimore, William and Wilkins, 1976

2. Waxman AD, Richmond R, Juttner H, et al: Correlation of contrast angiography and histologic pattern with gallium uptake in primary liver cell carcinoma: Non-correlation with alpha-feto protein: Concise communication. J Nucl Med 21:324, 1980

3. Yeh SDJ, Leeper RD, Benua RS: Multi-radionuclide studies of filling defects in liver and spleen of patients with cancer. J Nucl Med 16:583, 1975

SALIVARY GLAND IMAGING

Cold Defect

COMMON: Carcinoma
Pleomorphic adenoma (mixed cell tumor)

UNCOMMON: Abscess
Other adenomas

RARE: Cyst
Lymphoma
Metastatic disease
Sarcoidosis

REFERENCES

1. Chaudhuri TK, Stadalnik RC: Salivary gland imaging. Semin Nucl Med 10:400, 1980

2. Mishkin FS: Radionuclide salivary gland imaging. Semin Nucl Med 11:258, 1981

3. Parret J, Peyrin JO: Radioisotopic investigations in salivary pathology. Clin Nucl Med 4:250, 1979

4. Zwas ST, Rubenstein I: The value of dual radionuclide studies in solitary parotid gland sarcoidosis. Clin Nucl Med 9:359, 1984

SALIVARY GLAND IMAGING

Hot Nodules

COMMON: Warthin's tumor (papillary cystadenoma lymphomatosum)

UNCOMMON
AND RARE: Oxyphilic adenoma
Pleomorphic adenoma (mixed cell tumor)

REFERENCES

1. Chaudhuri TK, Stadalnik RC: Salivary gland imaging. Semin Nucl Med 10:400, 1980

2. Hannum JS, Harrill JA, Maynard CD: ^{99m}Tc-sodium pertechnetate scanning of a cystadenoma of the larynx: A case report. Clin Nucl Med 1:230, 1976

3. Mishkin FS: Radionuclide salivary gland imaging. Semin Nucl Med 11:258, 1981

SALIVARY GLAND IMAGING

Diffuse Increased Uptake

COMMON: Acute parotitis (mumps, bacterial, alcoholic, etc.)
Chronic recurrent parotitis

UNCOMMON
AND RARE: Large Warthin's tumor
Partial obstruction of a major duct

REFERENCES

1. Chaudhuri TK, Stadalnik RC: Salivary gland imaging. Semin Nucl Med 10:400, 1980
2. Mishkin FS: Radionuclide salivary gland imaging. Semin Nucl Med 11:258, 1981

SALIVARY GLAND IMAGING

Unilateral Decreased Uptake

COMMON: Chronic recurrent sialoadenitis
Following radiation therapy
Idiopathic
Mumps parotitis
Obstructive sialolithiasis
Other infections (mycobacterial, catscratch fever,
    Cytomegalovirus, etc.)
Postsurgical
Posttraumatic

UNCOMMON
AND RARE: Congenital agenesis

REFERENCES

1. Abdel-Dayem HM: Congenital absence of submaxillary gland detected on ^{99m}Tc-pertechnetate thyroid imaging. Clin Nucl Med 3:442, 1978

2. Boedecker RA, Sty JR, Thompson N: Salivary gland scintigraphy in atypical mycobacterium infection. Clin Nucl Med 4:202, 1979

3. Chaudhuri TK, Stadalnik RC: Salivary gland imaging. Semin Nucl Med 10:400, 1980

4. Mishkin FS: Radionuclide salivary gland imaging. Semin Nucl Med 11:258, 1981

5. Parret J, Peyrin JO: Radioisotopic investigations in salivary pathology. Clin Nucl Med 4:250, 1979

SALIVARY GLAND IMAGING

Bilateral Decreased Uptake

COMMON: Acute suppurative parotitis
Aging
Other collagen
Sjögren's syndrome
Vascular diseases

UNCOMMON
AND RARE: Multicentric sialoangiectasis
Neonatal hypothyroidism

REFERENCES

1. Chaudhuri TK, Stadalnik RC: Salivary gland imaging. Semin Nucl Med 10:400, 1980

2. Mishkin FS: Radionculide salivary gland imaging. Semin Nucl Med 11:258, 1981

3. Parret J, Peyrin JO: Radioisotopic investigations in salivary pathology. Clin Nucl Med 4:250, 1979

4. Spencer RP, Karimenddini KK: Decreased salivary gland accumulation of pertechnetate in neonatal hypothyroidism. J Nucl Med 22:96, 1981

SALIVARY GLAND IMAGING

Salivary Gland Enlargement

COMMON: Mumps parotitis
Obstructive sialolithiasis
Suppurative sialitis
Tumor

UNCOMMON
AND RARE: Alcoholism
Cirrhosis
Diabetes mellitus
Ductal stricture
Hyperlipoproteinemia
Hypothyroidism
Lactation
Malnutrition
Mikulicz's disease
Pregnancy
Sarcoidosis
Sjögren's syndrome

REFERENCES

1. Mishkin FS: Radionuclide salivary gland imaging. Semin Nucl Med 11:258, 1981
2. Reeder MM, Felson B: Gamuts in Radiology. Cincinnati, Audiovisual Radiology of Cincinnati, Inc., 1975

SALIVARY GLAND IMAGING

Displacement of Gland

COMMON: Adjacent soft tissue tumors
Lymph node enlargement
Tumor of mandible

UNCOMMON
AND RARE: Carotid body tumor

REFERENCES

1. Chaudhuri TK, Stadalnik RC: Salivary gland imaging. Semin Nucl Med 10:400, 1980
2. Mishkin FS: Radionuclide salivary gland imaging. Semin Nucl Med 11:258, 1981

6

Genitourinary

RENAL SCINTIANGIOGRAPHY

Focally Increased Flow

COMMON AND
UNCOMMON: Abscess
Arteriovenous malformation
Bleeding
Extrarenal tumor (renal cell carcinoma metastases,
    etc.)
Focal pyelonephritis
Gastric activity simulating a mass
Hamartoma
Malignant renal tumor, primary or metastatic
    (e.g., hypernephroma)
Pheochromocytoma simulating renal mass
Prominent spleen in normal patient
Renal artery pseudoaneurysm
Tuberous sclerosis
Unilateral agenesis with spleen simulating mass
Uterus/menstruation in transplant patient

REFERENCES

1. Aburano T, Taniguchi M, Hisada K, et al: Renal artery pseudoaneurysm
   demonstrated on radionuclide scintiscan. Clin Nucl Med 19:25, 1994

2. Ball JD, Cowan RJ, Maynard CD: Splenic simulation of a renal mass (letter to the editor). J Nucl Med 17:1104, 1976

3. Bekier A, Bandhauer K: An artifact in dynamic imaging of the kidneys with ^{131}I-o-iodohippurate. J Nucl Med 15:135, 1974

4. Bihl H, Sautter-Bihl ML, Riedasch G: Extrarenal abnormalities in ^{99m}Tc DTPA renal perfusion studies due to hypervascularized tumors. Clin Nucl Med 13:590, 1988

5. Bloss RS, McConnell RW, McConnell BG, et al: Demonstration by radionuclide imaging of possible vascular steal from a renal transplant. J Nucl Med 20:1053, 1979

6. Feldman N, Makler PT, Velchik MG: Visualization of the uterus on evaluation of transplanted kidneys. Clin Nucl Med 11:62, 1986

7. Freeman LM, Meng CH, Bernstein RG, et al: Rapid sequential renal blood flow scintiphotography. Radiology 92:918, 1969

8. Orzel JA, Jaffers GJ: Menstruation: A hazard in radionuclide renal transplant evaluation. Clin Nucl Med 11:409, 1986

9. Rosenthall L: Radionuclide diagnosis of malignant tumors of the kidney. AJR 101:662, 1967

10. Rosenthall L, Reid EC: Radionuclide distinction of vascular and nonvascular lesions of the kidney. Can Med Assoc J 98:1165, 1968

11. Simon H: Metastatic and recurrent hypernephroma demonstrated by isotope angiography. Clin Nucl Med 2:214, 1977

RENAL SCINTIANGIOGRAPHY

Focally Decreased Flow

COMMON: Abscess
Cyst (simple, hydatid, multilocular, polycystic disease)
Hematoma
Infarct
Necrotic neoplasm (e.g., hypernephroma, Wilms')

UNCOMMON
AND RARE: Benign tumor (e.g., adenoma, fibroma, lipoma)
Metastasis (including lymphoma)
Xanthogranulomatous pyelonephritis

REFERENCES

1. Ash JM, Gilday DL: Renal nuclear imaging and analysis in pediatric patients. Urol Clin North Am 7:201, 1980

2. Ball JD, Cowan RJ, Maynard CD: Splenic simulation of a renal mass. J Nucl Med 17:1104, 1976

3. Bloss RS, McConnell RW, McConnell BG, et al: Demonstration by radionuclide imaging of possible vascular steal from a renal transplant. J Nucl Med 20:1053, 1979

4. Kennedy TD, Robinson RG, Lee KR, et al: Segmental renal infarction in a transplanted kidney: Identification by ^{131}I-hippuran and ^{99m}TcO$_4$ scintigraphy. Clin Nucl Med 1:122, 1976

5. Levinson ED, Baldwin RD, Spencer RP: Renal sinus lipomatosis: a cause of medullary "non-filling." J Nucl Med 20:1105, 1979

6. Merton DF, Vogel JM, Adelman RD, et al: Renovascular hypertension as a complication of umbilical arterial catheterization. Radiology 126:751, 1978

7. Mettler FA, Christie JH: The scintigraphic pattern of acute renal vein thrombosis. Clin Nucl Med 5:468, 1980

8. Petrocelli RD, Wetzel RA: Radionuclide detection of a pheochromocytoma. J Nucl Med 16:234, 1975

9. Reeder MM, Felson B: Gamuts in Radiology. Cincinnati, Audiovisual Radiology of Cincinnati, 1975

10. Shoulin M: Radionuclide screening for renovascular hypertension. J Nucl Med 21:104, 1980

11. Simon H: Metastatic and recurrent hypernephroma demonstrated by isotope angiography. Clin Nucl Med 2:214, 1977

12. Singh A, Cohen WN: Renal allograft rejection: Sonography and scintigraphy. AJR 135:73, 1980

RENAL SCINTIANGIOGRAPHY

Early Appearance of IVC after Arm Injection

COMMON AND
UNCOMMON: Extracardiac shunt
                          Tricuspid insufficiency

REFERENCES

1. Jacobson AF, Whitley MA, Harrison SD, Cerqueira MD: Massive tricuspid regurgitation identified on renal flow scintigraphy. Clin Nucl Med 16:767, 1991

2. Slavin JD, Friedman NC, Spencer RP: Inferior vena cava filling after upper extremity injection in tricuspid insufficiency. Clin Nucl Med 18:363, 1992

RENAL IMAGING

Body-Background Defects in Renal Transplants

COMMON AND
UNCOMMON: Abscess
Bowel, air, fluid, or barium filled
Cortical necrosis
Full urinary bladder (early)
Hematoma
Hydronephrosis
Lymphocele
Mock lesions between major blood vessels and
    vascular structures (early)
Nonperfused kidney (e.g., arterial thrombosis, severe
    rejection)
Urinoma

REFERENCES

1. Becker JA, Kutcher R: Urologic complications of renal transplantation. Semin Roentgenol 13:341, 1978
2. Blumhardt R, Growcock G, Lasher H: Cortical necrosis in a renal transplant. AJR 141:95, 1983
3. Burt RW, Reddy RK: Evaluation of nuclear imaging for detecting posttransplant fluid collection. AJR 133:91, 1979
4. Corcoran RJ, Thrall JH, Kaminski RJ, et al: Body-background defects with ^{99m}Tc-DPTA after renal transplantations: Case reports. J Nucl Med 17:696, 1976

RENAL IMAGING

Unilateral Renal Enlargement

COMMON: Compensatory hypertrophy
Cyst (simple, multicystic, polycystic disease)
Duplicated pelvocalyceal system
Hydronephrosis
Idiopathic
Neoplasm (e.g., hypernephroma, metastasis, angiomyolipoma)
Renal vein thrombosis

UNCOMMON
AND RARE: Abscess
Acute pyelonephritis
Acute transplant rejection
Crossed fused renal ectopy
Hematoma

REFERENCES

1. Davidson AJ: Radiologic Diagnosis of Renal Parenchymal Disease. Philadelphia, W.B. Saunders, 1977
2. Mettler FA, Christie JH: The scintigraphic pattern of acute renal vein thrombosis. Clin Nucl Med 5:468, 1980
3. Reeder MM, Felson B: Gamuts in Radiology. Cincinnati, Audiovisual Radiology of Cincinnati, 1975

RENAL IMAGING

Bilateral Renal Enlargement

COMMON: Bilateral duplication of the pelvocalyceal system
Bilateral hydronephrosis
Proliferative/necrotizing/inflammatory disorders
  Acute glomerulonephritides
  Acute interstitial nephritis
  Allergic angiitis
  Diabetic glomerulosclerosis
  Goodpasture's syndrome
  Polyarteritis nodosa
  Schönlein-Henoch purpura
  Systemic lupus erythematosis
  Thrombotic thrombocytopenic purpura
  Wegener's granulomatosis
Polycystic renal disease

UNCOMMON
AND RARE: Acromegaly
Acute tubular necrosis
Amyloidosis
Bilateral renal vein thrombosis
Bilateral simple cysts
Bilateral tumor (e.g., hypernephromas, metastases, hamartomas)
Cirrhosis
Glycogen storage disease
Hemophilia
Leukemia
Lymphoma
Medullary sponge kidney
Multiple myeloma
Polycystic kidney disease
Renal cortical necrosis
Sarcoidosis
Sickle cell anemia

REFERENCES

1. Ash JM, Gilday DL: Renal nuclear imaging and analysis in pediatric patients. Urol Clin North Am 7:201, 1980

2. Davidson AJ: Radiologic Diagnosis of Renal Parenchymal Disease. Philadelphia, W.B. Saunders, 1977

3. Ekelund L: Radiologic findings in renal amyloidosis. AJR 129:851, 1977

4. Mettler FA, Christie JH: The scintigraphic pattern of acute renal vein thrombosis. Clin Nucl Med 5:468, 1980

5. Reeder MM, Felson B: Gamuts in Radiology. Cincinnati, Audiovisual Radiology of Cincinnati, 1975

6. Segal MC, Lecky JW, Slasky BS: Diabetes millitus: The predominant cause of bilateral renal enlargement. Radiology 153:341, 1984

7. Sty JR, Babbit DP, Sheth KJ: Scintigraphy in pediatric urinary tract lymphoma. Clin Nucl Med 3:422, 1978

8. Tracey KP, Metcalf JB, McEwan AJB: Autosomal recessive (infantile) polycystic kidney disease demonstrated by [99mTc] DMSA renal imaging. Clin Nucl Med 17:833, 1992

RENAL IMAGING

Unilateral Decrease in Renal Size

COMMON: Congenital hypoplastic or dysplastic kidney
Postinflammatory atrophy
Postobstructive atrophy
Renal artery stenosis (e.g., arteriosclerosis,
fibromuscular dysplasia, thrombosis)

UNCOMMON
AND RARE: Chronic renal infarction
Radiation nephritis

REFERENCES

1. Davidson AJ: Radiologic Diagnosis of Renal Parenchymal Disease. Philadelphia, W.B. Saunders, 1977
2. Reeder MM, Felson B: Gamuts in Radiology. Cincinnati, Audiovisual Radiology of Cincinnati, 1975

RENAL IMAGING

Bilateral Decrease in Renal Size

COMMON: Arteriolar nephrosclerosis
Bilateral renal artery stenosis (e.g., atherosclerosis, fibromuscular dysplasia)
Chronic glomerulonephritis
Postinflammatory atrophy
Postobstructive atrophy

UNCOMMON
AND RARE: Amyloidosis (late)
Chronic interstitial nephritis
Collagen vascular disease (e.g., systemic lupus erythematosus, polyarteritis nodosa, scleroderma)
Gouty nephritis
Hereditary nephropathies (e.g., Alport's syndrome, medullary cystic disease)
Kimmelsteil-Wilson disease
Renal cortical necrosis (late)
Senile atrophy

REFERENCES

1. Davidson AJ: Radiologic Diagnosis of Renal Parenchymal Disease. Philadelphia, W.B. Saunders, 1977
2. Reeder MM, Felson B: Gamuts in Radiology. Cincinnati, Audiovisual Radiology of Cincinnati, 1975

RENAL IMAGING

Nonvisualization of One Kidney

COMMON: Multicystic kidney
Neoplasm
Obstructive uropathy
Postnephrectomy
Renal artery occlusion (e.g., thrombosis, trauma, stenosis)
Renal vein occlusion (e.g., thrombosis, tumor)

UNCOMMON
AND RARE: Crossed fused ectopia and other congenital anomalies
Fractured kidney
Pyelonephritis
Severe rejection (transplant)
Tumor displacing kidney anteriorly (posterior view)
Unilateral renal agenesis

REFERENCES

1. Davidson AJ: Radiologic Diagnosis of Renal Parenchymal Disease. Philadelphia, W.B. Saunders, 1977

2. Demonico FL, McKusick KA, Cosimi AB, et al: Differentiation between renal allograft rejection and acute tubular necrosis by renal scan. AJR 128:625, 1977

3. Howard WH, Bunker SR, Karl RD, et al: Unilateral renal agenesis and other causes of the solitary photopenic renal fossa. Clin Nucl Med 10:270, 1985

4. Lin DS: "Missing" One Kidney. Semin Nucl Med XXI:167, 1991

5. McDonald P, Tarar R, Gilday D, et al: Some radiologic observations in renal vein thrombosis. AJR 120:268, 1974

6. Reeder MM, Felson B: Gamuts in Radiology. Cincinnati, Audiovisual Radiology of Cincinnati, 1975

7. Shanahan WSM, Slingensmith WC III, Weil R III: Increased perinephric activity in ^{99m}Tc-DTPA studies of renal transplants. Radiology 131:487, 1979

8. Suresh K, Puri S, Spencer RP: "Nonvisualized" kidney during ^{99m}Tc-DTPA study due to anterior displacement by tumor. Clin Nucl Med 2:454, 1977

9. Wulfeck DW, Smith HS, Silberstein EB: Incidental finding of crossed renal ectopia diagnosed on bone scan. Clin Nucl Med 16:441, 1991

10. Yeh EL, Pohlmann G, Meade RC: Spleen simulating vascular renal mass in left renal agenesis. Clin Nucl Med 2:194, 1977

RENAL IMAGING

Bilateral Nonvisualization

COMMON: Acute and chronic renal failure — any etiology
Technical (wrong photopeaks, infiltrated dose, etc.)

UNCOMMON
AND RARE: Acute tubular necrosis
Bilateral complete obstruction
Bilateral renal artery occlusion
Bilateral renal cortical necrosis
Bilateral renal vein occlusion
Glomerulonephritis

REFERENCES

1. Kim CK, Fine EJ, Blaufox MD: Nonvisualization of both kidneys with ^{131}I orthoiodohippurate scintigraphy. Semin Nucl Med XVIII:68, 1988

2. McDonald P, Tarar R, Gilday D, et al: Some radiologic observations in renal vein thrombosis. Am J Roentgenol 120:268, 1974

3. Reeder MM, Felson B: Gamuts in Radiology. Cincinnati, Audiovisual Radiology of Cincinnati, 1975

4. Sherman RA, Blaufox MD: Obstructive uropathy in patients with nonvisualization on renal scan. Nephron 25:82, 1980

5. Staab EV, Hopkins J, Patton DA, et al: Use of radionuclide studies in prediction of function in renal failure. Radiology 106:146, 1973

RENAL IMAGING

Phantom Kidney (Postnephrectomy or Agenesis)

Left
COMMON: Free radiopharmaceutical in stomach
Mesenteric vessels
Spleen

UNCOMMON
AND RARE: Colon

Right
COMMON AND
UNCOMMON: Duodenum
Liver
Malposition of jejunum

REFERENCES

1. Chu DDM, Belzberg AS: Phantom kidney on renal scintigraphy. Clin Nucl Med 16:62, 1991
2. Lin DS: Phantom kidney on perfusion renal imaging. Semin Nucl Med 14:59, 1984
3. Tauxe WN, Dubovsky EV (eds): Nuclear Medicine in Clincal Urology and Nephrology. Norwalk, Connecticut, Appleton-Century-Crofts, 1985

RENAL IMAGING

Space-Occupying Lesions

COMMON AND
UNCOMMON: Abscess
Benign tumor (e.g., hamartoma, adenoma)
Calculus
Cyst (e.g., simple, hydatid, multilocular)
Extrinsic mass (e.g., pheochromocytoma,
gallbladder)
Gallstone (anterior view)
Hematoma
Hydronephrosis
Infarct
Malrotation
Metastases (e.g., lung, lymphoma)
Multicystic disease
Polycystic disease
Position-related false positive
Primary malignant tumor (e.g., hypernephroma,
Wilms')
Pyelonephritis (acute, chronic,
xanthogranulomatous)
Radiation
Renal pseudotumor
Renal sinus lipomatosis
Tuberous sclerosis (angiomyolipomas)

REFERENCES

1. Alexieva-Jackson B, Fetters DV, Cole RL, et al: Gallbladder simulating renal fracture during technetium-99m glucoheptonate evaluation for renal trauma. Clin Nucl Med 11:363, 1985

2. Blatt CJ, Hayt DB, Freeman LM: Radionuclide imaging of the kidney in tuberous sclerosis. J Nucl Med 15:478, 1974

3. Conway JJ: Role of scintigraphy in urinary tract infection. Semin Nucl Med XVIII:308, 1988

4. Davidson AJ: Radiologic Diagnosis of Renal Parenchymal Disease. Philadelphpia, W.B. Saunders, 1977

5. Enlander D, Weber PM, dos Remedios LV: Renal cortical imaging in 35 patients: Superior quality with ^{99m}Tc-DMSA. J Nucl Med 15:743, 1974

6. Gentili AM, Miron SD, Bellon EM: Gallstone simulating renal lesion on skeletal scintigraphy. Clin Nucl Med 18:830, 1992

7. Kennedy TD, Robinson RG, Lee KR, et al: Segmental renal infarction in a transplanted kidney: Identification by ^{131}I-hippuran and ^{99m}TcO$_4$-scintigraphy. Clin Nucl Med 1:122, 1976

8. Lams P, Gerlock AJ, Rusu J: Arteriography: Aid to urography in determining etiology and diagnosis of renal pseudotumors. AJR 133:149, 1979

9. Lang EK, Sullivan J, Frentz G: Renal trauma: Radiological studies. Comparison of urography, computed tomography, angiography and radionuclide studies. Radiology 154:1, 1985

10. Leonard JC, Allen EW, Goin J, et al: Renal cortical imaging and the detection of renal mass lesions. J Nucl Med 20:1018, 1979

11. Levinson ED, Baldwin RD, Spencer RP: Renal sinus lipomatosis: A cause of medullary "non-filling." J Nucl Med 20:1105, 1979

12. Older RA, Konobkin M, Workman J, et al: Accuracy of radionuclide imaging in distinguishing renal masses from normal variants. Radiology 136:443, 1980

13. Rao GM, Nagesh KG, Guruprakash GH: Position-related false-positive renal imaging. Clin Nucl Med 5:318, 1980

14. Reeder MM, Felson BJ: Gamuts in Radiology. Cincinnati, Audiovisual Radiology of Cincinnati, 1975

15. Rosenthall L, Ammann W: Renal trauma. Sem Nucl Med 13:238, 1983

16. Sfakianakis GN, Sfakianaki ED: Nuclear medicine in pediatric urology and nephrology. J Nucl Med 29:1287, 1988

17. Sty JR, Babbit DP, Sheth KJ: Scintigraphy in pediatric urinary tract lymphoma. Clin Nucl Med 3:422, 1978

18. Sty JR, Oechler H: Tc-99m-glucoheptonate renal imaging. Congenital mesoblastic nephroma. J Nucl Med 21:809, 1980

19. Sty JR, Starshak RJ, Sheth KJ: Demonstration of a radionuclide pattern in pheochromocytomas in children. Clin Nucl Med 3:193, 1978

20. Ueno K, Rikimaru S, Miyagi T, et al: False-positive technetium-99m DMSA renal imaging in two cases of malrotated kidney. Clin Nucl Med 10:504, 1985

RENAL IMAGING

Rim Sign (Increased Rim of Activity Surrounding Photopenia)

COMMON AND
 UNCOMMON   Hematoma
            Lymphocele
            Multicystic kidney
            Renal vein thrombosis
            Severe hydronephrosis
            Transplant rejection

REFERENCES

1. Fortenbery EJ, Blue PW, VanNostrand D, Anderson JH: Lymphocele: Spectrum of scintigraphic findings in lymphoceles associated with renal transplant. J Nucl Med 31:1627, 1990

2. Howman-Giles R, Gett M, Roy P: Renal subcapsular rim sign: Radionuclide pattern. Clin Nucl Med 11:285, 1986

3. Rothfeld B, Spees EK, Goldman SM: An unusual combination of findings in renal transplantation. Clin Nucl Med 10:575, 1985

RENAL IMAGING

Photopenic Defect in a Transplanted Kidney

COMMON: Abscess
          Cyst
          Dilated collecting system
          Hematoma
          Infarct
          Pyelonephritis

UNCOMMON
AND RARE: Artifact (coins in pocket, etc.)
            Bowel (air, fluid or barium-filled)
            Tumor
            Urinoma

REFERENCES

1. Sanchez FW, Gordon L, Curry NS: Photopenic defect within transplanted kidney. Semin Nucl Med 14:342, 1984
2. Tauxe WN, Dubovsky EV (eds): Nuclear Medicine in Clinical Urology and Nephrology. Norwalk, Connecticut, Appleton-Century-Crofts, 1985

RENAL IMAGING

Flattened Renogram

COMMON: Chronic renal disease (e.g., glomerulonephritis,
                 diabetic nephropathy)
                 Cyst
                 Dehydration
                 Hypovolemia
                 Obstruction (esp. with parenchymal damage)
                 Pyelonephritis
                 Rejection
                 Renal artery stenosis
                 Tumor

UNCOMMON
AND RARE: Hypoplastic kidney
                 Postextracorporeal shock wave lithotripsy
                 Recent contrast angiogram
                 Severe cyclosporine toxicity

REFERENCES

1. Bomanji J, Boddy SAM, Britton KE, et al: Radionuclide valuation pre- and
    post-extracorporeal shock wave lithotripsy for renal calculi. J Nucl Med 28:1284,
    1987

2. Dubovsky EV, Russell CD: Radionuclide valuation of renal transplants. Semin
    Nucl Med XVIII: 181, 1988

3. Lin DS: "Flattened" pattern in ^{131}I-hippuran renogram. Semin Nucl Med 14:62,
    1984

4. Tauxe WN, Dubovsky EV (eds): Nuclear Medicine in Clinical Urology and
    Nephrology. Norwalk, Connecticut, Appleton-Century-Crofts, 1985

RENAL IMAGING

Continually Rising Renogram

COMMON: Acute tubular necrosis
Congenital dilatation of collecting system
Cortical necrosis
Dehydration
Obstruction
Rejection
Renal artery stenosis

UNCOMMON
AND RARE: Ileal conduit
Neurogenic bladder
Overhydration
Recent intravenous pyelogram or angiogram
Severe cyclosporine toxicity

REFERENCES

1. Lin DS: "Obstructive" pattern in an ^{131}I-hippuran renogram of a transplanted kidney. Semin Nucl Med 14:64, 1984

2. Tauxe WN, Dubovsky EV (eds): Nuclear Medicine in Clinical Urology and Nephrology. Norwalk, Connecticut, Appleton-Century Crofts, 1985

RENAL IMAGING

Flip-Flop Phenomenon with Hippuran

COMMON: Unilateral or asymmetrical obstruction
Unilateral renal artery stenosis

UNCOMMON
AND RARE: Unilateral renal vein thrombosis
Unilateral severe renal disease from any etiology

REFERENCES

1. Fine EJ, Scharf SC, Blaufox MD: Role of nuclear medicine in evaluating hypertensive patient. In: Freeman LM (ed): Nucl Med Ann 1984, New York, Raven Press, 1984, pp 32-58

2. Shih WJ, DeLand FH, Domstad PA: Flip-flop phenomenon in radiohippuran renal imaging: A sign of obstructive uropathy. Clin Nucl Med 11:707, 1986

3. Shih WJ, Loh F, Domstad PA: Flip-flop phenomenon seen in ^{131}I hippuran renal scintigraphy. Semin Nucl Med XVIII 269, 1988

RENAL IMAGING

False-positive Captopril Scan for Renovascular Hypertension

COMMON AND
UNCOMMON: Glomerulonephropathy
Hypotension during study
Volume depletion

REFERENCE

1. Dondi M, Franchi R, Levorato M, et al: Evaluation of hypersensitive patients by means of captopril-enhanced renal scintigraphy with ^{99m}Tc DTPA. J Nucl Med 30:615, 1989

2. Fommii E, Ghione S, Bertelli P, et al: Renal scintigraphy captopril test: Comparison of scintigraphic and angiographic data and preliminary observations in chronic glomerulonephritis. J Nucl Med 29:907, 1988

3. Geyskes GG, Oei HY, Puylaert CBAJ, Mees EJD: Renovascular hypertension identified by captopril-induced changes in renogram. Hypertension 9:451, 1987

4. Pelsang RE, Rezai K: Abnormal captopril renogram in patient without renovascular hypertension. Clin Nucl Med 17:303, 1992

RENAL IMAGING

Persistent Ureteral Activity

COMMON AND
UNCOMMON: Blind-ending ureteral duplication
Localized urinary rupture (e.g., tumor obstruction)
Physiologic
Ureteral diverticulum
Ureteral obstruction
Urinary fistula posttransplant

REFERENCES

1. Dublin AB, Stadalnik RC, DeNardo GL, et al: Scintigraphic imaging of a blind-ending ureteral duplication. J Nucl Med 16:208, 1975

2. Hadin HT, Stacy WK, Wolf JS. et al: Scintiphotography in diagnosis of urinary fistula after renal transplantation. J Nucl Med 16:612, 1975

3. Spigos DG, Tan W, Pavel DG, et al: Diagnosis of urine extravasation after renal transplantation. AJR 129:409, 1977

RENAL IMAGING

False-positive Urinoma Following Transplantation

COMMON: Rejection

UNCOMMON
AND RARE: Vesicoduodenal reflux following combined renal-
pancreatic transplant

REFERENCES

1. Anderson CM, Datz FL, Morton KA, et al: Study of frequency of rejection mimicking urinoma on ^{99m}Tc DTPA imaging of renal transplants. J Nucl Med 34:249, 1993
2. Wilson KM, Gordon L: Potential false-positive urinary leak from vesicoduodenal reflux in combined renal-pancreatic transplant. Clin Nucl Med 17:828, 1992

RENAL IMAGING

Bladder Deformity

COMMON: Enlarged prostate
Foley balloon

UNCOMMON: Bladder wall lesion (abscess, hematoma, tumor)
Enlarged uterus
Impacted fecal material
Intraluminal lesion (calculus, clot)
Lymphocele
Pelvic mass (abscess, hematoma, lymphadenopathy
tumor)
Postoperative deformity
Urinoma

RARE: Colonic distention
Extrauterine pregnancy
Hirschprung's disease
Pelvic lipomatosis
Retroperitoneal lesion (fibrous, tumor)
Ureterocele

REFERENCE

1. Bilchik TR, Spencer RP: Bladder variants noted on bone and renal imaging. Clin Nucl Med 18:60, 1993

2. Gosfield E, Siegel A: Renal scintigraphy in patient with pelvic lipomatosis. Clin Nucl Med 17:630, 1992

3. Lin DS: Urinary tract imaging — urinary bladder deformity. Semin Nucl Med 13:386, 1983

RENAL IMAGING

Sulfur Colloid Uptake in the Kidneys

COMMON: Renal transplant — rejection

UNCOMMON: Congestive heart failure
Hemolytic uremic syndrome
Radiopharmaceutical preparation
Renal transplant — acute tubular necrosis
Sepsis

REFERENCES

1. Granato DB, Salimi Z, George EA, et al: Recurrent hemolytic uremic syndrome in renal transplant recipient. Clin Nucl Med 13:171, 1988

2. Johnson PM, Fawwaz RA, Hardy MA, et al: Sequential Ga-67 imaging in diagnosis of renal allograft rejection. J Nucl Med 20:630, 1979

3. Kawamura J, Itoh H, Yoshida O, et al: "Hot spot" on Ga-67-citrate scan in a case of renal cell carcinoma. Clin Nucl Med 5:471, 1980

4. Mendez G, Morillo G, Alonso M, et al: Gallium-67 radionuclide imaging in acute pyelonephritis. AJR 134:17, 1980

5. Sauerbrunn BJ, Andrews GA, Hubner KF: Ga-67-citrate imaging in tumors of the genitourinary tract: Report of a cooperative study. J Nucl Med 19:470, 1978

RENAL IMAGING

DTPA Uptake Outside the Genitourinary System

COMMON AND
UNCOMMON: Abdominal hemangiomatosis
Breast carcinoma
Chordoma
Desmoid
Extramedullary plasmacytoma of the
retroperitoneum
Goodpasture's syndrome
Gout
Graves' disease (ophthalmopathy and pretibial
edema)
Gravid uterus
Gynecomastia
Hepatic hemangioma
Histiocytoma
Inflammatory bowel disease
Keloid
Leukemia
Myositis ossificans
Neurofibroma
Paget's disease
Retroperitoneal abscess
Soft-tissue sarcoma
Spinal compression fractures
Spinal metastases (renal cell, leukemia, etc.)
Spleen due to contiguous inflammation
Tampon
Thrombosis
Urinoma
Urinothorax
Uterine leiomyoma

REFERENCES

1. Aburano T, Yokoyama K, Michigishi T, et al: ^{99m}Tc DTPA uptake in extramedullary plasmacytoma of retroperitoneum. Clin Nucl Med 13:903, 1988

2. Alevizaki-Harhalaki M, Alevizaki C, Georgiou E, et al: Increased Tc-99m DTPA uptake in active Graves' opthalmopathy and pretibial myxoedema (letter to the editor). J Nucl Med 24:174, 1983

3. DuCret RP, Drake DG, Murray BL, et al: Detection of abdominal hemangiomatosis during ^{99m}Tc DTPA renal imaging. Clin Nucl Med 13:471, 1988

4. Elgazzar AH, Mahmoud AR, Abdel-Dayem HM: ^{99m}Tc DTPA uptake in uterine leiomyoma. Clin Nucl Med 13:29, 1988

5. Goshen E, Meiller I, Lantsberg S, et al: Radionuclide imaging of soft tissue masses with ^{99m}Tc DTPA. Clin Nucl Med 16:636, 1991

6. Goshen E, Meller I, Quastel MR: Localization of ^{99m}Tc DTPA in chordoma. Clin Nucl Med 17:812, 1992

7. Griffith D, Alexander M, Gelman R, Kotlyarov E: Normal uptake in gravid uterus on ^{99m}Tc DTPA imaging. Clin Nucl Med 17:736, 1992

8. Moreno AJ, Rodriguiz AA, Fredericks P, et al: Uptake of ^{99m}Tc DTPA in hepatic hemangioma. Clin Nucl Med 12:408, 1987

9. Oster ZH: Removable hot spot. Clin Nucl Med 13:376, 1988

10. Oster ZH, Atkins HL: Increased pulmonary technetium-99m DTPA accumulation in a patient with Goodpasture's syndrome. Clin Nucl Med 10:724, 1985

11. Pedell L, Fink-Bennett D: Technetium-99m DTPA splenic uptake. J Nucl Med 22:798, 1981

12. Ralston MD, Wilkinson RH: Bilateral urinothorax identified by ^{99m}Tc DTPA renal imaging. J Nucl Med 27:56, 1986

13. Shih WJ, Wierzbinski B, Magoun S, Ryo UY: ^{99m}Tc DTPA localized in gynecomastia secondary to orchiectomy and estrogen therapy in patient with carcinoma of prostate. Clin Nucl Med 13:306, 1988

14. Siddiqui AR: Localization of technetium-99m DTPA in neurofibroma (letter to the editor). J Nucl Med 27:143, 1986

15. Slavin JD, Mack JM, Spencer RP: Delayed accumulation (flip-flop) of ^{99m}Tc DTPA in leiomyosarcoma. Clin Nucl Med 13:654, 1988

16. Sty JR, Wells RG: ^{99m}Tc glucoheptonate imaging — retroperitoneal abscess. Clin Nucl Med 15:270, 1990

RENAL IMAGING

Diffuse Pulmonary DTPA Uptake

COMMON AND
UNCOMMON: Congestive heart failure in renal insufficiency
patient
Coronary artery disease in renal insufficiency patient
Goodpasture's syndrome

REFERENCES

1. Intenzo CM, Park CH, Kim SM: ^{99m}Tc DTPA diffuse pulmonary uptake in patients with coronary artery disease and renal insufficiency. Clin Nucl Med 17:945, 1992

2. Oster ZH, Atkins HL: Increased pulmonary ^{99m}Tc DTPA accumulation in patient with Goodpasture's syndrome. Clin Nucl Med 10:724, 1985

3. Wilson FMA, Smith FW: Unexplained ^{99m}Tc DTPA uptake by lung. Clin Nucl Med 12:487, 1987

RENAL IMAGING

DTPA Uptake in the Spine and Other Osseous Structures

COMMON AND
UNCOMMON: Augmented hematopoiesis
Compression fracture
Leukemia
Myositis ossificans
Paget's disease
Spinal metastases

REFERENCES

1. Kilkenny TE, Strauss EB, Rhodes C: Spinal compression fractures demonstrated on renal scan. Clin Nucl Med 15:205, 1990

2. Rousseau G, Shih WJ: Bone marrow visualization during ^{99m}Tc DTPA renal imaging in septicemia and disseminated intravascular coagulation. Clin Nucl Med 13:958, 1988

3. Zuckier LS, Weissmann HS, Kaplun L, et al: Significance of skeletal uptake detected on radionuclide renal perfusion studies. Clin Nucl Med 12:448, 1987

RENAL IMAGING

DSMA Uptake Outside the Normal Genitourinary System

COMMON AND
  UNCOMMON: Amyloidosis
              Brain tumor
              Breast carcinoma
              Chondrosarcoma
              Ewing's sarcina
              Fracture
              Head and neck squamous cell carcinoma
              Liposarcoma
              Lung carcinoma
              Malignant fibrous histiocytoma
              Maligant melanoma
              Medullary thyroid carcinoma
              Mycosis fungoides
              Myocardial infarction
              Osteogenic sarcoma
              Periodontal disease
              Pheochromocytoma
              Postradiation therapy
              Postsurgical therapy
              Prostate carcinoma
              Renal cell carcinoma
              Spindle cell sarcoma
              Supernumerary kidney

REFERENCES

1. Adams BK, Fataar A, Byrne MJ, et al: Pentavalent ^{99m}Tc (V)-DMSA uptake in pheochromocytoma in patient with Sipple's syndrome. J Nucl Med 31:106, 1990

2. Conrad GR, Loes DJ: Ectopic supernumerary kidney — functional assessment using radionuclide imaging. Clin Nucl Med 12:253, 1987

3. Endo K, Ohta H, Torizuka K, et al: ^{99m}Tc (V)-DMSA in imaging medullary thyroid carcinoma. J Nucl Med 28:252, 1987

4. Halkar RK, Patel MC, Khammash NF: Spindle cell sarcoma showing concentration of ^{99m}Tc sodium pertechnetate and ^{99m}Tc (V) DMSA. Clin Nucl Med 15:126, 1990

5. Hoefnagel CA, Delprat CC, Zanin D, van der Schoot JB: New radionuclide tracers for diagnosis and therapy of medullary thyroid carcinoma. Clin Nucl Med 13:159, 1988

6. Kao CH, Wang SJ, Wey SP, et al: Detection of nasopharynx carcinoma in [99m]Tc (V) dimercaptosuccinic acid SPECT imaging. Clin Nucl Med 18:321, 1993

7. Kashyap R, Babbar A, Sahai I, et al: [99m]Tc (V) DMSA imaging — a new approach to studying mestastases from breast carcinoma. Clin Nucl Med 17:119, 1992

8. Kobayashi H, Sakahara H, Hosono M, et al: Pentavalent ^{99m}Tc dimercaptosuccinic acid SPECT of metastatic renal cell carcinoma in scalp and brain. Clin Nucl Med 19:136, 1994

9. Lette J, Monier D, Ledoux R, Levasseur A: False-positive ^{99m}Tc pentavalent DMSA uptake in imaging medullary carcinoma of the thyroid. Clin Nucl Med 16:136, 1991

10. Lyons KP, Milne N, Karlsberg RP, et al: Myocardial infarct imaging in patients with [99m]Tc 2,3-dimercaptosuccinic acid — superiority of ^{99m}Tc pyrophosphate. Clin Nucl Med 12:514, 1987

11. Mojiminiyi OA, Udelsman R, Soper NDW, et al: Pentavalent ^{99m}Tc DMSA scintigraphy — Prospective evaluation of its role in management of patients with medullary carcinoma of thyroid. Clin Nucl Med 16:259, 1991

12. Ohta H, Endo K, Kanoh T, et al: [99m]Tc(V) DMSA uptake in amyloidosis. J Nucl Med 30:2049, 1989

13. Ohta H, Hatabu H, Endo K, et al: [99m]Tc(V) DMSA accumulation in thyroid amyloidosis. Clin Nucl Med 16:778, 1991

14. Ohta H, Okada T, Furukawa Y, et al: [99m]Tc(V) DMSA uptake in cardiac amyloidosis. Clin Nucl Med 16:673, 1991

15. Watkinson JC, Lazarus CR, Mistry R, Shaheen OH: [99m]Tc(V) dimercaptosuccinic acid uptake in patients with head and neck squamous carcinoma: Experience in imaging. J Nucl Med 30:174, 1989

16. Wulfrank DA, Schelstraeta KH, Small F, Fallais CJ: Analogy between tumor uptake of [99m]Tc(V) dimercaptosuccinic acid (DMSA) and ^{99m}Tc MDP. Clin Nucl Med 14:588, 1989

TESTICULAR IMAGING

Increased Activity Unilaterally — Dynamic and/or Static Images

COMMON: Epididymoorchitis
            Following trauma
            Missed torsion

UNCOMMON: Abscess
            Gumma
            Neoplasm
            Postsurgical
            Spontaneous or manually detorsed testicle
            Testicular neoplasm
            Varicocele

RARE: Acute torsion of testicular appendages
            Anaphylactoid purpura
            Phoechromocytoma

REFERENCES

1. Boedecker RA, Sty JR, Jona JZ: Testicular scanning as a diagnostic aid in evaluating scrotal pain. J Pediatr 94:760, 1979

2. Datta NS, Mishkin FS: Radionuclide imaging in intrascrotal lesions. JAMA 231:1060, 1975

3. Dunn EK, Macchia RJ, Solomen NA: Scintigraphic pattern in missed testicular torsion. Radiology 139:175, 1981

4. Freeman LM(ed): Nuclear Medicine Annual 1981. New York, Raven Press, 1981

5. Holder LE, Matire JR, Holmes ER III, et al: Testicular radionuclide angiography and static imaging: Anatomy, scintigraphic interpretation and clinical idications. Radiology 125:739, 1977

6. Holder LE, Melloul M, Chen D: Current status of radionuclide scrotal imaging. Semin Nucl Med 11:232, 1981

7. Lawrence D, Mishkin F: Radionuclide imaging in epididymoorchitis. J Urol 112:387, 1974

8. Melloul MM, Garty BZ: Radionuclide scrotal imaging in anaphylactoid purpura. Clin Nucl Med 18:298, 1993

9. Mishkin FS: Increased scrotal activity. Semin Nucl Med 11:315, 1981

10. Winston MA, Handler SJ, Pritchard JH: Ultrasonography of the testis — correlation with radiotracer perfusion. J Nucl Med 19:615, 1978

TESTICULAR IMAGING

Decreased Activity Unilaterally — Dynamic and/or Static Images

COMMON: Acute torsion
Hematocele
Hydrocele

UNCOMMON
AND RARE: Epidermoid cyst of testes
Hernia
Spermatocele
Testicular infarction secondary to vascular causes
other than acute torsion
Torsion of appendix testis

REFERENCES

1. Chen DCP, Holder LE, Melloul M: Radionuclide scrotal imaging: Further experiences with 210 patients. Part 1. Anatomy, pathophysiology, and methods. J Nucl Med 24:735, 1983

2. Chen DCP, Holder LE, Melloul M: Radionuclide scrotal imaging: Further experience with 210 patients. Part 2. Results and discussion. J Nucl Med 24:841, 1983

3. Dunn EK, Macchia RJ, Chauhan PS, et al: Scintiscan for acute intrascrotal conditions. Clin Nucl Med 11:381, 1986

4. Freeman LM (ed): Nuclear Medicine Annual 1981. New York, Raven Press, 1981

5. Fischman AJ, Palmer EL, Scott JA: Radionuclide imaging of sequential torsions of appendix testis. J Nucl Med 28:119, 1987

6. Garty I, Chaimovitch G, Wajsman S, et al: The radionuclide scintigraphic appearance in a rare case of epidermoid cyst of the testis. Clin Nucl Med 9:582, 1984

7. Hahn LC, Nadel NS, Gitter MH, et al: Testicular scanning: A new modality for the preoperative diagnosis of testicular torsion. J Urol 113:60, 1975

8. Holder LE, Matire JR, Holmes ER III, et al: Testicular radionuclide angiography and static imaging: Anatomy, scintigraphic interpretation, and clinical indications. Radiology 125:739, 1977

9. Holder LE, Melloul M, Chen D: Current status of radionuclide scrotal imaging. Semin Nucl Med 11:232, 1981

10. Mishkin FS: Lucent scrotal contents. Semin Nucl Med 11:317, 1981

TESTICULAR IMAGING

Bullseye Sign — Dynamic and Static Images

COMMON: Abscess
Hematocele
Hematoma
Missed torsion

UNCOMMON: Hernia
Hydrocele
Spermatocele

RARE: Collagen vascular disease
Epididymal cyst
Epididymoorchitis
Infarcted adrenal rest
Periappendiceal abscess extension via patent process
vaginalis
Postorchiectomy
Scrotal hydrops
Seminoma
Testicular infarction other than torsion (e.g.,
infection, mass impinging on vascular supply,
postoperative)

REFERENCES

1. Barrett FR, Buozas DJ: The lady-bug sign of scrotal hydrops. Clin Nucl Med 1:35, 1976

2. Dunn EK, Macchia RJ, Solomon NA: Scintigraphic pattern in missed testicular torsion. Radiology 139:175, 1981

3. Freeman LM (ed): Nuclear Medicine Annual 1981. New York, Raven Press, 1981

4. Holder LE, Matire JR, Holmes ER, et al: Testicular radionuclide angiography and static imaging: Anatomy, scintigraphic interpretation and clinical indications. Radiology 125:739, 1977

5. Holder LE, Melloul M, Chen D: Current status of radionuclide scrotal imaging. Semin Nucl Med 11:232, 1981

6. Melton JW, Chung CJ, Gordon L: Pseudobullseye sign of testicle — Window to peritoneum. Clin Nucl Med 16:604, 1991

7. Mishkin FS: Bullseye sign in scrotal imaging. Semin Nucl Med 11:316, 1981

8. Mishkin FS: Differential diagnostic features of the radionuclide scrotal image. AJR 128:127, 1977

9. Nagle C, Clark K, Browning D, et al: Testicular ischemia and infarction following herniorrhaphy or varicocelectomy: Evauation by radionuclide imaging. Clin Nucl Med 14:243, 1989

10. Turetsky DB, Wilf LH: Epididymal cyst simulating missed torsion by scrotal scintigraphy. Clin Nucl Med 15:846, 1990

11. Vieras F, Kuhn CR: Nonspecificity of the "rim sign" in the scintigraphic diagnosis of missed testicular torsion. Radiology 146:519, 1983

12. Williamson MR, Archibeque F, Eisenberg B, et al: ^{99m}Tc pyrophosphate localization in chest wall muscles after bench pressing. Clin Nucl Med 14:546, 1989

7

Cardiovascular

PERFUSION IMAGING

Cold Defect at Rest

COMMON: Myocardial infarction, acute or old

UNCOMMON
AND RARE: Anomalous origin of the left coronary artery
Calcified mitral valve annulus
Cardiomyopathies (congestive or restrictive, see
   Gamut)
Cocaine use
Constrictive pericarditis
Coronary artery fistula
Coronary artery spasm
Following bypass surgery
Idiopathic
Left bundle branch block
Leg flexion
Motion artifact
Myocarditis
Normal (e.g., apex)
Orbit-related variation in spatial resolution
Peritoneal fluid
Sarcoidosis
Severe coronary artery disease with normal or only
   mildly abnormal left ventricular wall motion

Soft tissue attenuation
Stable angina
Tumor (e.g., bronchogenic carcinoma, benign
   tumors)
Unstable angina

REFERENCES

1. Bailey IK, Come PC, Kelly DT, et al: Thallium-201 myocardial perfusion imaging in aortic valve stenosis. Am J Cardiol 40:889, 1977

2. Berger BC, Watson DD, Burwell LR, et al: Redistribution of thallium at rest in patients with stable and unstable angina and the effect of coronary artery bypass surgery. Circulation 60:1114, 1979

3. Blumhardt R, Telepak RJ, Hartshorne MF, et al: Thallium imaging of benign cardiac tumor. Clin Nucl Med 8:297, 1983

4. Bodenheimer MM, Banka VS, Helfant RH: Nuclear cardiology. II. The role of myocardial perfusion imaging using thallium-201 in diagnosis of coronary heart disease. Am J Cardiol 45:674, 1980

5. Bulkley BH, Hutchins GM, Bailey I, et al: Thallium-201 imaging and gated cardiac blood pool scans in patients with ischemic and idiopathic congestive cardiomyopathy. A clinical and pathologic study. Circulation 55:753, 1977

6. Bull U, Niendorf HP, Strauer BE, et al: Evaluation of myocardial function with the ^{201}thallium scintimetry in various diseases of the heart. A correlative study based on 100 patients. Eur J Nucl Med 1:125, 1976

7. Daspit SG, Stemple DR, Doherty PW, et al: Unusual findings in ^{201}Tl myocardium scintigraphy: The "hot heart" sign. Clin Nucl Med 2:1, 1977

8. DiCarlo LA, Botvinick EH, Canhasi BS, et al: Value of noninvasive assessment of patients with atypical chest pain and suspected coronary spasm using ergonovine infusion and thallium-201 scintigraphy. Am J Cardiol 54:744, 1984

9. Esquerre JP, Coca FJ, Martinez SJ, Guiraud RF: Prone decubitus: A solution to inferior wall attenuation in ^{201}Tl myocardial tomography. J Nucl Med 30:398, 1989

10. Feiglin D, Huckell V, Staniloff H, et al: Demonstration of segmental thallium perfusion defects in cardiomyopathies having normal coronary arteries. J Nucl Med 19:704, 1978

11. Fernandes J, Rutkowski M, Sanger JJ: Anomalous origin of left coronary artery — use of thallium perfusion scans in evaluating successful revascularization. Clin Nucl Med 17:177, 1992

12. Finley JP, Howman-Giles R, Gilday D, et al: Thallium-201 myocardial imaging in anomalous left coronary artery arising from the pulmonary artery: Applications before and after medical and surgical treatment. Am J Cardiol 42:676, 1978

13. Fischer DR, Beerman LB, Park SC, et al: Diagnosis of intracardiac rhabdomyoma by two-dimensional echocardiography. Am J Cardiol 53:978, 1984

14. Geckle WJ, Frank TL, Links JM, Becker LC: Correction for patient and organ movement in SPECT: Application to exercise ^{201}Tl cardiac imaging. J Nucl Med 29:441, 1988

15. Gerson MC, Noble RJ, Wann LS, et al: Noninvasive documentation of Prinzmetal's angina. Am J Cardiol 43:329, 1979

16. Gewirtz H, Beller GA, Strauss HW, et al: Transient defects of resting thallium scans in patients with coronary artery disease. Circulation 59:707, 1979

17. Goldman MR, Boucher CA: Value of radionuclide imaging techniques in assessing cardiomyopathy. Am J Cardiol 46:1232, 1980

18. Gutgesell HP, Pinsky WW, DePuey EG: Thallium-201 myocardial perfusion imaging in infants and children. Value in distinguishing anomalous left coronary artery from congestive cardiomyopathy. Circulation 61:596, 1980

19. Helmer S, Abghari R, Stone AJ, Lee CC: Detection of benign cardiac fibroma on ^{201}Tl imaging in an adult. Clin Nucl Med 12:365, 1987

20. Keyes JW: SPECT and artifacts — in search of imaginary lesion. J Nucl Med 32:875, 1991

21. Kinney EL, Jackson GL, Reeves WC, et al: The prevalence of sarcoid heart disease detected by thallium scanning. Am J Cardiol 43:436, 1979

22. Lo H-M, Tseng Y-Z, Tseng C-D, et al: Intercardiac goiter: A cause of right ventricular outflow obstruction and successful operative therapy. Am J Cardiol 53:976, 1984

23. Lubell DL, Goldfarb CR: Metastatic cardiac tumor demonstrated by [201]thallium scan. Chest 78:98, 1980

24. McGowan RL, Welch TG, Zaret BL, et al: Noninvasive myocardial imaging with potassium-43 and rubidium-81 in patients with left bundle branch block. Am J Cardiol 38:422, 1976

25. McKillop JH: Thallium-201 scintigraphy (medical progress). West J Med 133:26, 1980

26. McKillop JH, Murray RG, Bessent RG, et al: The significance of the abnormal rest thallium-201 myocardial image in coronary artery disease. Eur J Nucl Med 4:83, 1979

27. McLaughlin PR, Doherty PW, Martin RP, et al: Myocardial imaging in a patient with reproducible variant angina. Am J Cardiol 39:126, 1977

28. Maniawski PJ, Morgan HT, Wackers FJT: Orbit-related variation in spatial resolution as source of artifactual defects in ^{201}Tl SPECT. J Nucl Med 32:871, 1991

29. Maseri A, Parodi O, Severi S, et al: Transient transmural reduction of myocardial blood flow, demonstrated by thallium-201 scintigraphy, as a cause of variant angina. Circulation 54:280, 1976

30. Maseri A, Severi S, de Nes M, et al: "Variant" angina: One aspect of a continuous spectrum of vasospastic myocardial ischemia — pathogenetic mechanisms, estimated incidence and clinical and coronary arteriographic findings in 138 patients. Am J Cardiol 42:1019, 1978

31. Meller J, Goldsmith SJ, Rudin A, et al: Spectrum of exercise thallium-201 myocardial perfusion imaging in patients with chest pain and normal coronary angiograms. Am J Cardiol 43:717, 1979

32. Okada RD, Boucher CA, Strauss, HW, et al: Exercise radionuclide imaging approaches to coronary artery disease. Am J Cardiol 46:1188, 1980

33. Oster ZH, Som P, Wang GJ, Weber DA: Imaging of cocaine-induced global and regional myocardial ischemia. J Nucl Med 32:1569, 1991

34. Petrozzo PJ, Woodard ML, Vitullo DA, et al: Use and diagnostic significance of ^{201}Tl SPECT imaging in case of anomalous left coronary artery. Clin Nucl Med 13:629, 1988

35. Plankey MW, Carlk MW, Strickland MD: [201]TlSPECT artifact associated with leg flexion. J Nucl Med Technol 19:31, 1991

36. Poe ND, Eber LM, Norman AS, et al: Myocardial images in nonacute coronary and noncoronary heart diseases. J Nucl Med 18:18, 1977

37. Rab ST, Alazraki NP, Krawcyznska EG: Peritoneal fluid causing inferior attenuation on SPECT ^{201}Tl myocardial imaging in women. J Nucl Med 29:1860, 1988

38. Silverman KJ, Hutchins GM, Buikley GH: Cardiac sarcoid: A clinicopathologic study of 84 unselected patients with systemic sarcoidosis. Circulation 58:1204, 1978

39. Strich G, Braunstein P, Bridges R, et al: Thallium-201 SPECT imaging of myocardial contusion. J Nucl Med 27:998, 1986

40. Sty JR: Atlas of pediatric nuclear cardiology. Part II. Clin Nucl Med 5:424, 1980

41. Taki J, Nakajima K, Bunko H, et al: Cardiac sarcoidosis demonstrated by ^{201}Tl and ^{67}Ga SPECT imaging. Clin Nucl Med 15:636, 1990

42. Tamaki N, Yonekura Y, Kadota K, et al: Thallium-201 myocardial perfusion imaging in myocarditis. Clin Nucl Med 10:562, 1985

43. Wackers FJ: Thallium-201 myocardial scintigraphy in acute myocardial infarction and ischemia. Semin Nucl Med 10:127, 1980

44. Wackers FJ, Lie KI, Lie KL: Thallium-201 scintigraphy in unstable angina pectoris. Circulation 57:738, 1978

45. Wagoner LE, Movahed A, Reeves WC: Myocardial imaging artifacts caused by mitral valve annulus calcification. Clin Nucl Med 16:94, 1991

46. Yuen Green MS, Yen CK, Lim AD, Lull RJ: [99m]Tc sestamibi myocardial imaging at rest for evaluation of cocaine-induced myocardial ischemia and infarction. Clin Nucl Med 17:923, 1992

PERFUSION IMAGING

Cold Defect with Exercise

COMMON: Coronary artery disease

UNCOMMON
AND RARE: Acute ventricular dilatation
Any cause of a resting defect
Aortic stenosis and aortic insufficiency
Coronary artery spasm
Following bypass surgery
Heart creep with chronic obstructive pulmonary
  disease
Heart creep with exercise
Idiopathic
Idiopathic hypertrophic subaortic stenosis
Left bundle branch block
Malalignment artifact
Mitral valve prolapse
Motion artifact
Myocardial bridges
Physiologic
Sarcoidosis

REFERENCES

1. Ahmad M, Merry SL, Haibach H, et al: Thallium-201 scintigraphic evidence of ischemia in patients with myocardial bridges. Am J Cardiol 45:482, 1980

2. Bailey IK, Come PC, Kelly DT, et al: Thallium-201 myocardial perfusion imaging in aortic valve stenosis. Am J Cardiol 40:889, 1977

3. Berger BC, Abramowitz R, Park CH, et al: Abnormal thallium-201 scans in patients with chest pain and angiographically normal coronary arteries. Am J Cardiol 52:365, 1983

4. Bodenheimer MM, Banka VS, Helfant RH: Nuclear cardiology. II. The role of myocardial perfusion imaging using thallium-201 in diagnosis of coronary heart disease. Am J Cardiol 45:674, 1980

5. Braat SH, Brugada P, Bär FW, et al: Thallium-201 exercise scintigraphy and left bundle branch block. Am J Cardiol 55:224, 1985

6. Cooper R, Puri S, Francis CK, et al: Role of coronary artery disease and collateral circulation in redistribution of thallium-201. Clin Nucl Med 5:292, 1980

7. DePuey EG, Guertler-Krawczynska E, Robbins WL: 201Tl SPECT in coronary artery disease patients with left bundle branch block. J Nucl Med 29:1479, 1988

8. Dunn RF, Wolff L, Wagner S, et al: The inconsistent pattern of thallium defects: A clue to the false-positive perfusion scintigram. Am J Cardiol 48:224, 1981

9. Feiglin D, Huckell V, Staniloff H, et al: Demonstration of segmental thallium perfusion defects in cardiomyopathies having normal coronary arteries. J Nucl Med 19:704, 1978

10. Friedman J, VanTrain K, Maddahi J, et al: Upward creed of heart: Frequent source of false-positive reversible defects during ^{201}Tl stress redistribution SPECT. J Nucl Med 30:1718, 1989

11. Friedman J, Berman DS, VanTrain K, et al: Patient motion in ^{201}Tl myocardial SPECT imaging — an easily identified frequent source of artifactual defect. Clin Nucl Med 13:321, 1988

12. Garver PR, Wasnich RD, Shibuya AM, et al: Appearance of breast attenuation artifacts with thallium myocardial SPECT imaging. Clin Nucl Med 10:694, 1985

13. Gupta NC, Beauvais J: Physiologic assessment of coronary artery fistula. Clin Nucl Med 16:40, 1991

14. He ZX, Darcourt J, Benoliel J, et al: Major upward creep of heart during exercise ^{201}Tl myocardial SPECT in patient with chronic obstructive pulmonary disease. J Nucl Med 33:1846, 1992

16. Kipper MS, Grosshans C, Ashburn WL: False-positive ^{201}Tl SPECT studies in patients with left bundle branch block — frequency and clinical significance. Clin Nucl Med 17:890, 1992

17. McKillop JH: Thallium-201 scintigraphy (medical progress). West J Med 133:26, 1980

18. Makler PT, Lavine SJ, Denenberg BS, et al: Redistribution on the thallium scan in myocardial sarcoidosis: Concise communication. J Nucl Med 22:428, 1981

19. Maseri A, Severi S, de Nes M, et al: "Variant" angina: One aspect of a continuous spectrum of vasospastic myocardial ischemia — pathogenetic mechanisms, estimated incidence and clinical and coronary arteriographic findings in 138 patients. Am J Cardiol 42:1019, 1978

20. Massie B, Botvinick E, Arnold S, et al: Effect of contrast enhancement on the sensitivity and specificity of Tl-201 scintigraphic. Am J Cardiol 43:357, 1979

21. Matthews RJ, Lightfoote J, Grusd RS: Constrictive pericarditis causing a positive ^{201}Tl SPECT stress test for myocardial ischemia. Clin Nucl Med 15:548, 1990

22. Meller J, Goldsmith SJ, Rudin A, et al: Spectrum of exercise thallium-201 myocardial perfusion imaging in patients with chest pain and normal coronary angiograms. Am J Cardiol 43:717, 1979

23. Nakajima K, Taki J, Bunko H, et al: Demonstration of therapeutic effect in a patient with myocardial bridge by exercise — myocardial SPECT imaging. Clin Nucl Med 10:116, 1985

24. Okada RD, Boucher CA, Strauss HW, et al: Exercise radionuclide imaging approaches to coronary artery disease. Am J Cardiol 46:1188, 1980

25. Rubin KA, Morrison J, Padnick MB, et al: Idiopathic hypertrophic subaortic stenosis: Evaluation of anginal symptoms with thallium-201 myocardial imaging. Am J Cardiol 44:1040, 1979

26. Starksen NF, O'Connell W, Dae MW, Botvinick EH: Basal interventricular septal ^{201}Tl defects: Real or artifact? Clin Nucl Med 18:291, 1993

27. Verani MS, Marcus ML, Spoto G, et al: Thallium-201 myocardial perfusion scintigrams in the evaluation of aortocoronary saphenous bypass surgery. J Nucl Med 19:765, 1978

PERFUSION IMAGING

Reverse Redistribution

COMMON: Coronary artery disease
           Normal

UNCOMMON
AND RARE: Cardiomyopathy
           Incomplete infarction
           Recanalization of plaque
           Spasm
           Variability in postischemic hyperemic response
           Variability of exercise effort and physiologic
              response

REFERENCE

1. Candell-Riera J, Ortega-Alcalde D: Reverse redistribution pattern of thallium-201 stress test in subjects with normal coronary angiograms (letter to the editor). J Nucl Med 27:1377, 1986
2. Silberstein EB, DeVries DF: Reverse redistribution phenomenon in thallium-201 stress tests: Angiographic correlation and clinical significance. J Nucl Med 26:707, 1985

PERFUSION IMAGING

Global Decrease in Uptake

COMMON AND
UNCOMMON: Adriamycin cardiotoxicity
Cardioactive drugs (cardiac glycosides, propranolol, phenytoin)
Cardiomyopathy (e.g., congestive)
Hypoxia
Metabolic acidosis
Spasm of dominant left coronary system with hypotension
Transient myocardial ischemia of newborn
Triple-vessel disease

REFERENCES

1. Ahmad M, Merry SL, Haibach H: Thallium-201 scintigraphic evidence of ischemia in patients with myocardial bridges. Am J Cardiol 45:482, 1980

2. Costin JC, Zaret BL: Effect of propranolol and digitalis upon radioactive thallium and potassium uptake in myocardial and skeletal muscle. J Nucl Med 17:535, 1976

3. Finley JP, Howman-Giles RB, Gilday DL, et al: Transient myocardial ischemia of the newborn infant demonstrated by thallium myocardial imaging. J Pediatr 94:263, 1979

4. Forst D, Sorensen S, O'Rourke R, et al: Reversibility of Adriamycin-induced reduction in myocardial thallium-201 uptake by intravenous digoxin. Am J Cardiol 45:482, 1980

5. Goldman MR, Boucher CA: Value of radionuclide imaging techniques in assessing cardiomyopathy. Am J Cardiol 46:1232, 1980

6. Hamilton GW, Harahara KA, Yee H, et al: Myocardial imaging with thallium-201: Effect of cardiac drugs on myocardial images and absolute tissue distribution. J Nucl Med 19:10, 1978

7. McKillop JH: Thallium-201 scintigraphy (medical progress). West J Med 133:26, 1980

8. Schachner ER, Oster ZH, Cicale N, et al: The effect of diphenylhydantoin (Dilantin) on thallium-201 chloride uptake. J Nucl Med 21:57, 1980

9. Stolzenberg J, Pollack RH: Absent myocardial uptake of Tl-201 under stress in spite of anatomically normal coronary arteries. J Nucl Med 20:900, 1979

10. Weich HF, Strauss HW, Pitt B: The extraction of thallium-201 by the myocardium. Circulation 56:188, 1977

PERFUSION IMAGING

Myocardial Hot Spots

COMMON AND
    UNCOMMON: Ideopathic
                 Overlying visceral activity
                 Papillary muscles

REFERENCE

1. DePuey EG, Garcia EV: Optimal specificity of ^{201}Tl SPECT through recognition of imaging artifacts. J Nucl Med 30:441, 1989

PERFUSION IMAGING

Right Ventricular Visualization

COMMON: With exercise
Right ventricular overload, volume, pressure, or
both
Examples quoted in literature
Atrial septal defect
Chronic cor pulmonale
Congestive cardiomyopathy
Corrected transposition of the great vessels
Cystic fibrosis
Endocardial fibroelastosis
Following myocardial infarction
Hypertrophic cardiomyopathy
Primary pulmonary hypertension
Pulmonary hypertension secondary to left
ventricular dysfunction
Sarcoidosis
Tetralogy of Fallot
Valvular disease (aortic stenosis, pulmonic
stenosis, mitral stenosis, aortic insufficiency)
Ventricular septal defect with Eisenmenger's
complex
Newborns

UNCOMMON
AND RARE: Normals at rest

REFERENCES

1. Buckley BH, Bouleau JR, Whitaker JQ, et al: The use of [201]thallium for myocardial perfusion imaging in sarcoid heart disease. Chest 72:27, 1977

2. Cowley MJ, Voghlan HC, Logic JR: Visualization of atrial myocardium with thallium-291: Case report. J Nucl Med 18:984, 1977

3. Gottlieb SL, Siegel ME, Caldwell J, et al: Detection and follow-up of myocardial sarcoid involvement by Tl-201: Preliminary report. J Nucl Med 21:83, 1980

4. Kondo M, Kubo A, Yamazaki H, et al: Thallium-201 myocardial imaging for evaluation of right ventricular overloading. J Nucl Med 19:1197, 1978

5. McKillop JH: Thallium-201 scintigraphy (medical progress). West J Med 133:26, 1980

6. Nakajima K, Bunko H, Tonami N, et al: Congenitally corrected transposition of the great arteries associated with the preexcitation syndrome. Clin Nucl Med 11:564, 1986

7. Ohsuzu F, Handa S, Kondo M, et al: Thallium-201 myocardial imaging to evaluate right ventricular overloading. Circulation 61:620, 1980

8. Treves S: Detection and quantitation of cardiovascular shunts with commonly available radionuclides. Semin Nucl Med 10:16, 1980

PERFUSION IMAGING

Enlarged Heart without a Murmur in an Infant

COMMON: Aortic stenosis
Coarctation of the aorta
Endocardial fibroelastosis
Hypoxia (any cause)
Severe anemia

UNCOMMON
AND RARE: Cardiac tumor
Glycogen storage disease (Pompe's)
Hurler's syndrome

REFERENCE

1. Sty JR, Babbitt DP, Gallen WJ: Scintigraphy in endocardial fibroelastosis. Clin Nucl Med 3:476, 1978

PERFUSION IMAGING

Increased Thallium Lung Uptake

COMMON: Left ventricular dysfunction any cause (e.g., ischemic, valvular, cardiomyopathy, congenital)
Smoking

UNCOMMON
AND RARE: ARDS
Asphyxiated newborns
Hypertension
Injection in supine position
Kaposi's sarcoma
Pectoralis muscle uptake simulating lung uptake with arm exercise
Sarcoidosis
Simulation postmastectomy
Subcritical stenosis
Supine exercise

REFERENCES

1. Bingham JB, McKusick KA, Strauss HW, et al: Influence of coronary artery disease on pulmonary uptake of thallium-201. Am J Cardiol 46:821, 1980

2. Boucher CA, Zir LM, Beller GA, et al: Increased lung uptake of thallium-201 during exercise myocardial imaging: Clinical, hemodynamic and angiographic implications in patients with coronary artery disease. Am J Cardiol 46:189, 1980

3. Campeau RJ, Garcia OM, Correa OA, Mace JE: Pectoralis muscle uptake of ^{201}Tl after arm exercise ergometry — possible confusion with lung ^{201}Tl activity. Clin Nucl Med 15:303, 1990

4. Cook DJ, Bailey I, Strauss HW, et al: Thallium-201 for myocardial imaging: Appearance of the normal heart. J Nucl Med 17:583, 1976

5. Kushner FG, Okada RD, Kirshenbaum HD, et al: Lung thallium-201 uptake after stress testing in patients with coronary artery disease. Circulation 63:341, 1980

6. Lear JL: Effect of exercise position during stress testing on cardiac and pulmonary thallium kinetics and accuracy in evaluating coronary artery disease. J Nucl Med 27:788, 1986

7. Lee VW, Fuller JD, O'Brien MJ, et al: Pulmonary Kaposi sarcoma in patients with AIDS: Scintigraphic diagnosis with sequential thallium and gallium scanning. Radiology 180:409, 1991

8. Lee VW, Rosen MP, Baum A, et al: AIDS-related Kaposi sarcoma: Findings on ^{201}Tl scintigraphy. Am J Roentgenol 151:1233, 1988

9. Leppo JA, Scheuer J, Prohost GM, et al: The evaluation of ischemic heart disease thallium-201 with comments on radionuclide angiography. Semin Nucl Med 10:115, 1980

10. Liu P, Diess M, Okada RD, et al: Increased thallium lung uptake after exercise in isolated left anterior descending coronary artery disease. Am J Cardiol 55:1469, 1985

11. McKillop JH: Thallium-201 scintigraphy (medical progress). West J Med 133:26, 1980

12. Movahed A, Wait J: Radionuclide imaging in pulmonary edema (letter to the editor). J Nucl Med 26:97, 1985

13. Okada RD, Boucher CA, Strauss HW, et al: Exercise radionuclide imaging approaches to coronary artery disease. Am J Cardiol 46:1188, 1980

14. Prohost GM, Alpert NM, Ingall JS, et al: Thallium redistribution: Mechanisms and clinical utility. Semin Nucl Med 10:70, 1980

15. Ritchie JL, Hamilton GW, Wackers FJ (eds): Thallium-201 Myocardial Imaging. New York, Raven Press, 1978

16. Shih WJ, Mills BJA: Increased pulmonary radiothallium uptake during stress ^{201}Tl chloride myocardial imaging. Semin Nucl Med XXII:206, 1992

17. Stoffey RD, Leckie RG, Buckner AB: Incidental finding of pulmonary sarcoidosis during stress thallium imaging. Clin Nucl Med 17:910, 1992

18. Sty JR: Atlas of pediatric nuclear cardiology. Part II. Clin Nucl Med 5:424, 1980

19. Weizenberg A, Goodenday LS, Leighton RF: Scintigraphic detection of ventricular aneurysm with thallium-201. J Nucl Med 24:34, 1983

20. Wilson RA, Okada RD, Boucher CA, et al: Radionuclide-determined changes in pulmonary blood volume and thallium lung uptake in patients with coronary artery disease. Am J Cardiol 51:741, 1983

21. Yitzchak H, Gerson MC: Simulation of abnormal pulmonary thallium-201 activity following mastectomy. Clin Nucl Med 10:767, 1985

PERFUSION IMAGING

Increased Splanchnic Thallium Activity

COMMON AND
UNCOMMON: Injection while supine
             Recent meal

REFERENCES

1. Ritchie JL, Hamilton GW, Wackers FJ (eds): Thallium-201 Myocardial Imaging. New York, Raven Press, 1978
2. Sprengelmeyer J, Weisberger CL: Practical Nuclear Cardiology. Hagerstown, Harper and Row, 1979

PERFUSION IMAGING

Soft Tissue Thallium Uptake

COMMON: Tumor benign or malignant
Examples quoted in the literature
Breast adenoma
Breast carcinoma
Brown tumors of hyperparathyroidism
Esophageal carcinoma
Glioma
Hepatoma
Hodgkin's disease
Kaposi's sarcoma
Lung carcinoma
Malignant hemangioendothelioma
Mesothelioma
Parathyroid adenoma
Primary and metastatic cerebral tumors
Rhabdomyosarcoma
Thymoma
Thyroid adenoma
Thyroid carcinoma
Physiologic (e.g., gastrointestinal tract)
Subacute thyroiditis
Chronic thyroiditis
Multinodular goiter
Colloid cyst
Skeletal muscle with exercise

UNCOMMON
AND RARE: Abscess
Candidiasis
Epidermoid inclusion cyst
Pigmented villonodular synovitis
Primary hypothyroidism
Sarcoidosis
Sclerosing adenosis of the breast
Suppressed normal thyroid tissue
Transplanted parathyroid
Ulcers
Veins

REFERENCES

1. Arnstein NB, Juni JE, Sisson JC, et al: Recurrent medullary carcinoma of thyroid demonstrated by ^{201}Tl scintigraphy. J Nucl Med 27:1564, 1986

2. Atkins HL, Budinger TF, Lebowitz E, et al: Thallium-201 for medical use. Part 3. Human distribution and physical imaging properties. J Nucl Med 18:133, 1977

3. Bordlee RP, Ware RW: [201]Tl accumulation by epidermoid inclusion cyst. J Nucl Med 33:1857, 1992

4. Brendel AJ, Guyot M, Jeandot R, et al: [201]Tl imaging in followup of differentiated thyroid carcinoma. J Nucl Med 29:1515, 1988

5. Burt RW, Mullinix FM, Schauwecker DS, et al: Leg perfusion evaluated by delayed administration of thallium-201. Radiology 151:219, 1984

6. Caluser C, Healey J, Macapinlac H, et al: [201]Tl uptake in recurrent pigmented villonodular synovitis — correlation with 3-phase bone imaging. Clin Nucl Med 17:751, 1992

7. Campeau RJ, Ey EH, Varma DGK: Thallium-201 uptake in a benign thymoma. Clin Nucl Med 11:524, 1986

8. Davidson RM, Round ME, Lamki N, et al: [201]Tl chloride scan in multiple endocrine neoplasia Type 2A. Clin Nucl Med 17:406, 1992

9. Durak H, Aras T, Sungur CEM, et al: [201]Tl uptake in brown tumors of hyperparathyroidism. Clin Nucl Med 16:931, 1991

10. Eisenberg B, Velchik MG, DeVries DF: [201]Tl chloride uptake in lung tumor during routine stress thallium exam. Clin Nucl Med 13:215, 1988

11. El-Desouki M: [201]Tl thyroid imaging in differentiating benign from malignant thyroid nodules. Clin Nucl Med 16:425, 1991

12. El-Gazzar AH, Sahweil A, Abdel-Dayem HM, Kubasik H, et al: Experience with ^{201}Tl imaging in head and neck cancer. Clin Nucl Med 13:286, 1988

13. Fukuchi M, Hyodo K, Tachibana K, et al: Marked thyroid uptake of thallium-201 in patients with goiter: Case report. J Nucl Med 18:1199, 1977

14. Fukuchi M, Kido A, Hyodo K, et al: Uptake of thallium-201 in enlarged thyroid glands: Concise communication. J Nucl Med 20:827, 1979

15. Fukuchi M, Tachibana K, Kuwata K, et al: Thallium-201 imaging in thyroid carcinoma — appearance of a lymph node metastasis. J Nucl Med 19:195, 1978

16. Fukunaga M, Morita R, Yonekura Y, et al: Accumulation of ^{201}Tl chloride in parathyroid adenoma. Clin Nucl Med 4:229, 1979

17. Garcia MJ, Arbizu J, Ramirez JC, et al: Extracardiac activity with ^{201}Tl in pleural mesothelioma recurrence. Clin Nucl Med 16:595, 1991

18. Gruber ML, Hochberg FH: Systematic evaluation of primary brain tumors. J Nucl Med 31:969, 1990

19. Harada T, Ito Y, Chimaoka K, et al: Clinical evaluation of [201]thallium chloride scan for thyroid nodular. Eur J Nucl Med 5:125, 1980

20. Hisada K, Tonami N, Miyamae T, et al: Clinical evaluation of tumor imaging with ^{201}Tl chloride. Radiology 129:497, 1978

21. Hoefnagel CA, Delprat CC, Marcuse HR, deVijlder JJM: Role of ^{201}Tl total-body scintigraphy in follow up of thyroid carcinoma. J Nucl Med 27:1854, 1986

22. Ichiya Y, Nakashima T, Gunasekera R, et al: Coexistence of nonfunctioning thyroid nodule in Plummer's disease demonstrated by ^{201}Tl imaging. Clin Nucl Med 13:117, 1988

23. Iida Y, Kasagi K, Misaki T, et al: Visualization of suppressed normal thyroid tissue by ^{201}Tl in patients with toxic nodular goiter. Clin Nucl Med 13:283, 1988

24. Ikekubo K, Higa T, Hirasa M, et al: Evaluation of radionuclide imaging and echography in the diagnosis of thyroid nodules. Clin Nucl Med 11:145, 1986

25. Intenzo CM, Desai AG, Park CH: Thallium-201 uptake by the sternum. Clin Nucl Med 11:214, 1986

26. Kaplan WD, Takvorian T, Morris JH, et al: [201]Tl brain tumor imaging: Comparative study with pathologic correlation. J Nucl Med 28:47, 1987

27. Kida T, Hujita Y, Munaka S, et al: Malignant hemangioendothelioma demonstrated by thallium imaging. Clin Nucl Med 12:886, 1987

28. Kim KT, Black KL, Marciano D, et al: [201]Tl SPECT imaging of brain tumors: Methods and results. J Nucl Med 31:965, 1990

29. Kosuda S, Aoka S, Suzuki K, et al: Primary malignant lymphoma of central nervous system by ^{67}Ga and ^{201}Tl brain SPECT. Clin Nucl Med 17:961, 1992

30. Kox PH, Belfer AJ, van der Pompe WB: Thallium-201 chloride uptake in tumours, a possible complication in heart scintigraphy. Brit J Radiol 49:767, 1976

31. Lee VW, Chen H, Panageas E, et al: Subcutaneous Kaposi's sarcoma — thallium scan demonstration. Clin Nucl Med 15:569, 1990

32. Linde R, Basso L: Hodgkin's disease with hypercalcemia detected by ^{201}Tl scintigraphy. J Nucl Med 28:112, 1987

33. McKillop JH: Thallium-201 scintigraphy (medical progress). West J Med 133:26, 1980

34. Makler PT, Sherwin N, McCarthy DM, et al: Detection of sclerosing adenosis of the breast on a thallium scan. Clin Nucl Med 9:277, 1984

35. Nakano S, Hasegawa Y, Kuriyama K, et al: Visualization of jugular vein on ^{201}Tl scan for thyroid cancer. Clin Nucl Med 14:449, 1989

36. Nestico PF, Hakki A, Iskandrian AS, et al: Thallium-201 imaging in pericardial effusion. Clin Nucl Med 11:213, 1986

37. Sawa H, Fukuda T, Itami M, et al: Clinical evaluation of thallium-201 for breast tumors. Jap J Nucl Med 16:321, 1979

38. Segall GM, Lennon SE, Stevick CD: Exercise whole-body thallium scintigraphy in diagnosing and evaluating occlusive arterial disease in legs. J Nucl Med 31:1443, 1990

388 7. CARDIOVASCULAR

39. Siegel ME, Siemsen JK: A new noninvasive approach to peripheral vascular disease: Thallium-201 leg scans. AJR 131:827, 1978

40. Silberstein EB, Robbins PJ: Thallium-201 venography. J Nucl Med 21:34, 1980

41. Takebayashi S, Matsui K, Nozawa T, et al: Hyperplasia of autotransplanted parathyroid in forearm. Clin Nucl Med 15:354, 1990

42. Thrall J, Freitas J, Gross M, et al: Noncardiac organ perfusion imaging with thallium-201. J Nucl Med 19:708, 1978

43. Tonami N, Bunko H, Kuwajima A, et al: Increased localization of ^{201}Tl chloride in subacute thyroiditis. Clin Nucl Med 4:3, 1979

44. Tonami N, Bunko H, Michigishi T, et al: Clinical application of ^{201}Tl scintigraphy in patients with cold thyroid nodules. Clin Nucl Med 3:217, 1978

45. Tonami N, Hisada K: Clinical experience of tumor imaging with ^{201}Tl chloride. Clin Nucl Med 2:75, 1977

46. Tonami N, Hisada K: [201]Tl scintigraphy in postoperative detection of thyroid cancer: A comparative study with [131]I. Radiology 136:461, 1980

47. Tonami N, Matsuda H, Ooba H, et al: [201]Tl accumulation in cerebral candidiasis — unexpected finding on SPECT. Clin Nucl Med 15:397, 1990

48. Tonami N, Michigishi T, Bunko H, et al: Clinical tumor scanning with Tl-201 chloride. J Nucl Med 18:617, 1977

49. Tonami N, Shuke N, Yokoyama K, et al: [201]Tl single-photon emission computed tomography in evaluating suspected lung cancer. J Nucl Med 390:997, 1989

50. Tyson IB, Bough EW, Gandsman EJ: 201-thallium exercise scintigraphy of leg muscle — useful for evaluation of peripheral vascular disease? J Nucl Med 21:35, 1980

51. Waxman AD, Ramanna L, Memsic LD, et al: Thallium scintigraphy in evaluating mass abnormalities of breast. J Nucl Med 34:18, 1993

PERFUSION IMAGING

MIBI Uptake Outside the Heart

COMMON AND
UNCOMMON: Acoustic schwannoma
Astrocytoma
Aneurysmal bone cyst
Breast carcinoma
Burkitt's lymphoma
Chondrosarcoma
Choroid plexus
Diabetic osteoarthropathy
Ependymoma
Ewing's sarcoma
Fibrosing alveolitis
Glioma
Hepatocellular carcinoma
Lung carcinoma — squamous, adeno-, small-cell
Malignant thymoma
Medulloblastoma
Non-Hodgkin's lymphoma
Osteomyelitis
Osteosarcoma
Parathyroid adenomas and hyperplasia
Poststernotomy
Renal cell carcinoma
Thyroid adenoma
Thyroid cancer
Undifferentiated mesenchymal tumor

REFERENCES

1. Aktolun C, Bayham H, Kir M: Clinical experience with ^{99m}Tc MIBI imaging in patients with malignant tumors — preliminary results and comparison with ^{201}Tl. Clin Nucl Med 17:171, 1992

2. Caner B, Kitapci M, Erbengi G, et al: Increased accumulation of ^{99m}Tc MIBI in undifferentiated mesenchymal tumor and its metastatic lung lesions. Clin Nucl Med 17:144, 1992

3. Caner B, Kitapci M, Unlu M, et al: ^{99m}Tc MIBI uptake in benign and malignant bone lesions: Comparative study with ^{99m}Tc MDP. J Nucl Med 33:319, 1992

4. Hassan IM, Sahweil A, Constantinides C, et al: Uptake and kinetics of ^{99m}Tc hexakis 2-methoxy isobutyl isonitrile in benign and malignant lesions in lungs. Clin Nucl Med 14:333, 1989

5. O'Doherty MJ, Kettle AG, Wells P, et al: Parathyroid imaging with ^{99m}Tc sestamibi: Preoperative localization and tissue uptake studies. J Nucl Med 33:313, 1992

6. O'Tuama LA, Treves ST, Larar JN, et al: ^{201}Tl vs ^{99m}Tc MIBI Spect in evaluting childhood brain tumors: Within-subject comparison. J Nucl Med 34:1045, 1993

7. Park CH, Kim SM, Zhang J, et al: ^{99m}Tc MIBI brain SPECT of acoustic schwannoma. Clin Nucl Med 19:152, 1994

8. Piwnica-Worms D, Holman BL: Noncardiac applications of hexakis (alkylisonitrile) ^{99m}Tc complexes. J Nucl Med 31:1166, 1990

PERFUSION IMAGING

Delayed Thallium Clearance (Washout)

COMMON: Coronary artery disease
               Injection into veins other than medial antecubital

UNCOMMON
AND RARE: Normal
              Submaximal exercise
              Technical (repositioning errors, etc.)

REFERENCES

1. Brown KA, Benoit L, Clements JP, Wackers FJT: Fast washout of ^{201}Tl from area of myocardial infarction: Possible artifact of background subtraction. J Nucl Med 28:945, 1987

2. Datz FL, Gullberg G, Gabor FV, Morton KA: SPECT myocardial perfusion imaging update. Semin Ultrasound, CT, MR 12:28, 1991

3. Gal R, Port SC: Arm vein uptake of thallium-201 during exercise: Incidence and clinical significance. J Nucl Med 27:1353, 1986

4. Horowitz SF, Machac J, Levin H, et al: Effect of variable left ventricular vertical orientation on planar myocardial perfusion imaging. J Nucl Med 27:694, 1986

5. Kaul S, Chesler DA, Pohost GM, et al: Influence of peak exercise heart rate on normal thallium-201 myocardial clearance. J Nucl Med 27:26, 1986

6. Lancaster JL, Starling MR, Kopp DT, et al: Effect of errors in reangulation on planar and tomographic thallium-201 washout profile curves. J Nucl Med 26:1445, 1985

7. Leppo J: Thallium washout analysis: Fact or fiction? J Nucl Med 28:1058, 1987

8. Nordrehaug JE, Danielsen R, Vik-Mo H: Effects of heart rate on myocardial ^{201}Tl uptake and clearance. J Nucl Med 30:1972, 1989

9. Rabinovitch M, Suissa S, Elstein J, et al: Sex-specific criteria for interpretation of ^{201}Tl myocardial uptake and washout studies. J Nucl Med 27:1837, 1986

PERFUSION IMAGING

Cardiomyopathies

COMMON AND
UNCOMMON: Congestive Cardiomyopathy
    Primary
        Idiopathic
            Endocardial fibroelastosis (dilated type)
            Idiopathic
            Postpartum
        Toxic
            Alcohol
            Bleomycin
            Diptheria
            Heavy metals
        Inflammatory
            Chagas' disease
            Rheumatic
    Secondary
        Inflammatory
            Bacterial
            Lupus erythematosus
            Mycoplasmal
            Polyarteritis nodosa
            Rickettsial (e.g., Q fever)
            Sarcoidosis
            Viral
        Metabolic
            Acromegaly
            Thiamine deficiency
        Neuromuscular
            Friedreich's ataxia
            Muscular dystrophy
        Cardiac
            Congenital
            Ischemic
            Valvular
    Restrictive Cardiomyopathy
        Primary
            Idiopathic
                Davies' disease
                Endocardial fibroelastosis

Endomyocardial fibrosis
Loffler's disease
Secondary
Inflammatory
Scleroderma
Metabolic
Amyloidosis
Glycogen storage disease
Hemochromatosis
Cardiac
Constrictive (pericardial)
Hypertrophic cardiomyopathy
Primary
Idiopathic
Nonobstructive
Obstructive

REFERENCE

1. Strauss HW, Pitt B (eds): Cardiovascular Nuclear Medicine. St. Louis, C.V. Mosby, 1979

PERFUSION IMAGING

False-Negative Rest Study

COMMON AND
UNCOMMON: Increasing time postinfarction (scar retraction?)
Interobserver variability
Rest study rather than redistribution postexercise
Small size of infarct

REFERENCES

1. Botvinick EH, Dunn RF, Hattner RS: A consideration of factors affecting the diagnostic accuracy of thallium-201 myocardial perfusion scintigraphy in detecting coronary artery disease. Semin Nucl Med 10:157, 1980

2. Cohen MV, Steingart RM: Exercise thallium-201 scintigraphy in dogs: Effects of long-term coronary occlusion and collateral development on early and late scintigraphic images. Circulation 72:881, 1985

3. Hiess GS, Logic JR, Russell RO, et al: Usefulness and limitations of thallium-201 myocardial scintigraphy in delineating location and size of prior myocardial infarction. Circulation 59:1010, 1979

4. McKillop JH: Thallium-201 scintigraphy (medical progress). West J Med 133:26, 1980

5. Mueller TM, Marcus ML, Ehrhardt JC, et al: Limitations of thallium-201 myocardial perfusion scintigrams. Circulation 54:640, 1976

6. Schelbert HR, Henning H, Rigo P: Intravenous myocardial imaging performed serially early and late after acute myocardial infarction. Eur J Nucl Med 2:75, 1977

7. Trobaugh GB, Wackers FJ, Sokole EB, et al: Thallium-201 myocardial imaging: An interinstitutional study of observer variability. J Nucl Med 19:359, 1978

PERFUSION IMAGING

False-Negative Stress Study

COMMON AND
UNCOMMON: Balanced lesions involving all major vessels
(homogenous pattern)
Collateral vessels supplying Tl-201 to an area with
an obstructed vessel
Exercise not maintained minimum time
postinjection
Females
Increased background (e.g., thick chested male)
Interobserver variability
Location (lowest sensitivity for left circumflex)
Masked by areas with normal or supernormal uptake
Propranolol
Rapid redistribution
Size of ischemic zone
Submaximal stress

REFERENCES

1. Atwood JE, Jensen D, Froelicher V, et al: Agreement in human interpretation of analog thallium myocardial perfusion images. Circulation 64:601, 1981

2. Berman D, Maddahi J, Freeman H, et al: Variable time to redistribution in Tl-201 exercise myocardial scintigraphy: Inverse relationship to degree of coronary stenosis. J Nucl Med 20:688, 1979

3. Botvinick EH, Dunn RF, Hattner RS, et al: A consideration of factors affecting the diagnostic accuracy of thallium-201 myocardial perfusion scintigraphy in detecting coronary artery disease. Semin Nucl Med 10:157, 1980

4. Hung J, Gordon EP, Houston N, et al: Changes in rest and exercise myocardial perfusion and left ventricular function 3 to 25 weeks after clinically uncomplicated acute myocardial infarction: Effects of exercise training. Am J Cardiol 54:943, 1984

5. Jengo JA, Freeman R, Brizendine M, et al: Detection of coronary artery disease: Comparison of exercise stress radionuclide angiocardiography and thallium stress perfusion scanning. Am J Cardiol 45:535, 1980

6. Lenaers A, Block P, van Thiel E, et al: Segmental analysis of Tl-201 stress myocardial scintigraphy. J Nucl Med 18:509, 1977

7. Leppo J, Yipintsoi T, Blankstein R, et al: Thallium-201 myocardial scintigraphy in patients with triple-vessel disease and ischemic exercise stress tests. Circulation 59:714, 1979

8. McKillop JH: Thallium-201 scintigraphy (medical progress). West J Med 133:26, 1980

9. Massie BM, Botvinick EH, Brundage BH: Correlation of thallium-201 scintigrams with coronary anatomy: Factors affecting region by region sensitivity. Am J Cardiol 44:616, 1979

10. Mueller TM, Marcus ML, Ehrhardt JC, et al: Limitations of thallium-201 myocardial perfusion scintigrams. Circulation 54:640, 1976

11. Okada RD, Boucher CA, Krishenbaum HK, et al: Improved diagnostic accuracy of thallium-201 stress test using multiple observers and criteria derived from interobserver analysis of variance. Am J Cardiol 46:619, 1980

12. Prohost GM: Thallium-201 for myocardial imaging. Nuklearmedizin 17:149, 1978

13. Rigo P, Bailey IK, Griffith LSC, et al: Value and limitations of segmental analysis of stress thallium myocardial imaging for localization of coronary artery disease. Circulation 61:973, 1980

14. Rothendler JA, Okada RD, Wilson RA, et al: Effect of a delay in commencing imaging on the ability to detect transient thallium defects. J Nucl Med 26:880, 1985

15. Trobaugh GB, Wackers FJ, Sokole EB, et al: Thallium-201 myocardial imaging: An interinstitutional study of observer variability. J Nucl Med 19:359, 1978

PERFUSION IMAGING

False-Negative Dipyridamole or Adenosine Study

COMMON AND
UNCOMMON: Caffeine-containing foods — coffee, soft drinks,
chocolate, etc.
Causes listed under false-negative stress study
Drugs — xanthine derivatives such as theophylline
Infiltrated dose

REFERENCES

1. Smits P, Aengevaeren WRM, Corstens FHM, Thien T: Caffeine reduces dipyridamole-induced myocardial ischemia. J Nucl Med 30:1723, 1989
2. Smits P, Corstens FHM, Aengevaeren WRM, et al: False-negative dipyridamole ^{201}Tl myocardial imaging after caffeine infusion. J Nucl Med 32:1538, 1991

PERFUSION IMAGING

False-Positive Stress Study

COMMON: Idiopathic
Physiologic (e.g., prominent apex defect)
Rotation
Soft tissue attenuation by breast, arm, or adipose
tissue
Soft tissue attenuation by diaphragm
Left bundle branch block

UNCOMMON
AND RARE: Abnormal myocardial cell function without
disturbing coronary blood flow
Computer enhancement
Field nonuniformity
Interobserver variability
Propranolol

REFERENCES

1. Atwood JE, Jensen D, Froelicher V, et al: Agreement in human interpretation of analog thallium myocardial perfusion images. Circulation 64:601, 1981

2. Berger BC, Watson DD, Taylor GJ, et al: Effect of coronary collateral circulation on regional myocardial perfusion assessed with quantitative thallium-201 scintigraphy. Am J Cardiol 46:365, 1980

3. Brown KA, Osbakken M, Boucher CA, et al: Positive exercise thallium-201 test responses in patients with less than 50% maximal coronary stenosis: Angiographic and clinical predictors. Am J Cardiol 55:54, 1985

4. Collins S, Ehrhardt JC, Go RT, et al: Problems with the definition of a normal tomographic thallium-201 perfusion scintigram. Am J Cardiol 45:481, 1980

5. Cook DJ, Bailey I, Strauss HW, et al: Thallium-201 for myocardial imaging: Appearance of the normal heart. J Nucl Med 17:583, 1976

6. DePuey EG, Guertler-Krawczynska E, Robbins WL: ^{201}Tl SPECT in coronary artery disease patients with left bundle branch block. J Nucl Med 29:1479, 1988

7. Dunn RF, Wolff L, Wagner S, et al: The inconsistent pattern of thallium defects: A clue to the false-positive perfusion scintigram. Am J Cardiol 48:224, 1981

8. Gordon DG, Pfisterer M, Williams R, et al: The effect of diaphragmatic attenuation on ^{201}Tl images. Clin Nucl Med 4:150, 1979

9. Johnstone DE, Wackers FJ, Berger HJ, et al: Effect of patient positioning on left lateral thallium-201 myocardial images. J Nucl Med 20:183, 1979

10. McKillop JH: Thallium-201 scintigraphy (medical progress). West J Med 133:26, 1980

11. Massie B, Botvinick E, Arnold S, et al: Contrast enhancement of thallium-201 myocardial scintigrams: Improved sensitivity with diminished specificity in coronary disease detection. Am Heart J 102:37, 1981

12. Massie B, Botvinick E, Arnold S, et al: Effect of contrast enhancement on the sensitivity and specificity of Tl-201 scintigraphy. Am J Cardiol 43:357, 1979

13. Meller J, Goldsmith SJ, Rudin A, et al: Spectrum of exercise thallium-201 myocardial perfusion imaging in patients with chest pain and normal coronary angiograms. Am J Cardiol 43:717, 1979

14. Okada RD, Boucher CA, Kirshenbaum HK, et al: Improved diagnostic accuracy of thallium-201 stress test using multiple observers and criteria derived from interobserver analysis of variance. Am J Cardiol 46:619, 1980

15. Okada RD, Boucher CA, Strauss HW, et al: Exercise radionuclide imaging approaches to coronary artery disease. Am J Cardiol 46:1188, 1980

16. Stein MA, Friedenberg MJ: Elevation of a hemidiaphragm simulating posterior myocardial fibrosis. J Nucl Med 20:1103, 1979

17. Stolzenberg J, Kaminsky J: Overlying breast as cause of false-positive thallium scans. Clin Nucl Med 3:229, 1978

18. Trobaugh GB, Wackers FJ, Sokole EB, et al: Thallium-201 myocardial imaging: An interinstitutional study of observer variability. J Nucl Med 19:359, 1978

PERFUSION IMAGING

False-Positive Bull's-eye Display

COMMON AND
UNCOMMON: Apical variations
                        Displaced laterally or medially
                        Partial-volume
                        Thinning
                  Duodenogastric reflux
                  Gender differences
                  Myocardial hot spots (See Gamut)
                  Noncoronary disease
                        Dextro/levorotation
                        Left bundle branch block
                        Myocardial hypertrophy
                  Patient motion
                  Technical
                        Center-of-rotation errors
                        Floodfield nonuniformity
                        Reconstruction errors — SPECT and bull's-eye
                  Soft tissue attenuation
                        Breasts
                        Diaphragm
                        Lateral chest wall fat

REFERENCES

1. DePuey EG, Garcia EV: Optimal specificity of ^{201}Tl SPECT through recognition of imaging artifacts. J Nucl Med 30:441, 1989

2. Eisner R, Churchwell A, Noever T, et al: Quantitative analysis of tomographic ^{201}Tl myocardial bull's-eye display: Critical role of correcting for patient motion. J Nucl Med 29:91, 1988

3. Eisner RL, Tamas MJ, Cloninger K, et al: Normal SPECT ^{201}Tl bull's-eye display: Gender differences. J Nucl Med 29:1901, 1988

4. Hassan IM, Mohammad MMJ, Constantinides C, et al: Problems of duodenogastric reflux in ^{99m}Tc hexa MIBI planar, tomographic and bull's-eye display. Clin Nucl Med 14:286, 1989

PERFUSION IMAGING

Complications Associated with Dipyridamole Stress

COMMON: Blood pressure lability
Chest pain
Dizziness
Dyspnea
Flushing
Headaches
Nausea
ST-T wave changes
Tachycardia

UNCOMMON
AND RARE: Anaphylaxis
AV block
Bronchospasm
CVA
Frank hypo- or hypertension
Myocardial infarction
Supraventricular tachycardia
TIA
Ventricular fibrillation

REFERENCES

1. Beller GA: Dipyridamole ^{201}Tl imaging: How safe is it? Circulation 81:1425, 1990

2. DuPont Merck Pharmaceutical Co. I.V. Persantine (dipyridamole USP) product monograph 1990

3. Homma S, Gilliland Y, Guiney TE, et al: Safety of intravenous dipyridamole for stress testing with thallium imaging. Am J Cardiol 59:152, 1987

4. Laarman G, Niemeyer MG, van der Wall EE, et al: Dipyridamole thallium testing: Noncardiac side effects, cardiac effects, electrocardiographic changes and hemodynamic changes after dipyridamole infusion with and without exercise. Int J Cardiol 20:231, 1985

5. Lam JYT, Chairman BR, Glaenzer M, et al: Safety and diagnostic accuracy of dipyridamole-thallium imaging in the elderly. J Am Coll Cardiol 11:535, 1988

6. Lette J, Cerino M, Laverdier M, et al: Severe bronchospasm followed by respiratory arrest during thallium-dipyridamole imaging. Chest 95:1345, 1989

7. Ranhosky A, Kempthorne-Rawson J, et al: Safety of intravenous dipyridamole thallium myocardial perfusion imaging. Circulation 81:1205, 1990

8. Whiting JH, Datz FL, Gabor FV, et al: Cerebrovascular accident associated with dipyridamole ^{201}Tl myocardial imaging. J Nucl Med 34:128, 1993

MIBG IMAGING

Decreased Cardiac MIBG Uptake

COMMON AND
UNCOMMON: Cardiac denervation
Congestive heart failure
Diabetic autonomic neuropathy
Drugs (digoxin, amiodarone)
Extracardiac pheochromocytoma
Left ventricular hypertrophy secondary to aortic
stenosis
Myocardial infarction

REFERENCES

1. Dae M, Davis J, Bovinick E, et al: Scintigraphic assessment of regional cardiac adrenergic density. Circulation 72:444, 1985

2. Dae M, Herre J, Botvinick E, et al: Scintigraphic detection of denervated myocardium after infarction. J Nucl Med 27:949, 1986

3. Fagret D, Wolf JE, Vanzetto G, Borrel E: Myocardial uptake of metaiodobenzylguanidine in patients with left ventricular hypertrophy secondary to valvular aortic stenosis. J Nucl Med 34:57, 1993

4. Glowniak JV, Sisson JC, Shapiro B, et al: Scintigraphic mappings of autonomic neuropathy. Clin Res 32:730A, 1984

5. Glowniak JV, Turner FE, Gray LL, et al: [123]I metaiodobenzylguanidine imaging of heart in idiopathic congestive cardiomyopathy and cardiac transplants. J Nucl Med 30:1182, 1989

6. Merlet P, Valette H, Dubois-Randle JL, et al: Prognostic value of cardiac metaiodobenzylguanidine imaging in patients with heart failure. J Nucl Med 33:471, 1992

7. Nakajo M, Shapiro B, Glowniak JV, et al: Inverse relationship between cardiac accumulation of meta-[131]-I-iodobenzylguanidine (^{131}I MIBG) and circulating catecholamines: Observations in patients with suspected pheochromocytoma. J Nucl Med 24:1127, 1983

8. Schofer J, Spielman R, Schuchert A, Weber K: Meta-(123)iodobenzylguanidine (MIBG) scintigraphy in idiopathic dilated cardiomyopathy (icd): A noninvasive method to assess myocardial catecholamine depletion? Circulation 76:308, 1987

9. Sisson JC, Wieland DM, Sherman P, et al: Metaiodobenzylguanidine as an index of the adrenergic nervous system integrity and function. J Nucl Med 28:1620, 1987

GATED CARDIAC BLOOD POOL IMAGING

Enlarged Left Atrium

COMMON: Mitral insufficiency — any cause, congenital,
acquired, or secondary to another cardiac process
Mitral stenosis
Papillary muscle/chordae tendinae dysfunction or
rupture (e.g., myocardial infarction, rheumatic
fever)
Patent ductus arteriosus
Ventricular septal defect

UNCOMMON
AND RARE: Constrictive pericarditis
Coronary artery fistula
Endocardial fibroelastosis
Idiopathic
Left atrial myxoma
Myocardiopathy
Origin of both great vessels from the right ventricle
Transposition of the great vessels
Tricuspid atresia
Trilogy of Fallot
Truncus arteriosus

REFERENCES

1. Dilsizian V, Rocco TP, Bonow RO, et al: Cardiac blood pool imaging II: Applications in noncoronary heart disease. J Nucl Med 31:10, 1990

2. Reeder MM, Felson B: Gamuts in Radiology. Cincinnati, Audiovisual Radiology of Cincinnati, 1975

3. Sprengelmeyer J, Weisberger CL: Practical Nuclear Cardiology. Hagerstown, Harper and Row, 1979

GATED CARDIAC BLOOD POOL IMAGING

Enlarged Right Atrium

COMMON: Atrial fibrillation
Left-to-right shunt, atrial level (e.g., atrial septal
  defect, transposition, TAPVR, tricuspid atresia)
Pulmonary stenosis
Right heart failure, any cause (e.g., chronic
  obstructive pulmonary disease, left heart failure)
Right ventricular enlargement leading to right atrial
  enlargement (see enlarged right ventricle gamut)
Tricuspid insufficiency

UNCOMMON
AND RARE: Aneurysm of the right atrium
Aortic atresia
Constrictive pericarditis
Endocardial fibroelastosis
Idiopathic
Right atrial myxoma
Tricuspid stenosis

REFERENCES

1. Bingham JB, McKusick KA, Strauss HW: Right atrial enlargement — cardiac imaging. Semin Nucl Med 10:195, 1980

2. Meszaros WT: Cardiac Roentgenology. Springfield, Illinois, Charles C Thomas, 1969

3. Reeder MM, Felson B: Gamuts in Radiology. Cincinnati, Audiovisual Radiology of Cincinnati, 1975

4. Sprengelmeyer J, Weisberger CL: Practical Nuclear Cardiology. Hagerstown, Harper and Row, 1979

GATED CARDIAC BLOOD POOL IMAGING

Enlarged Left Ventricle

COMMON: Aortic insufficiency
Aortic stenosis
Atherosclerotic cardiovascular disease
Coarctation of the aorta
Cardiomyopathy
Congestive heart failure — any cause
Hypertension
Left ventricular aneurysm
Mitral insufficiency
Myocardial infarction
Patent ductus arteriosus
Ventricular septal defect

UNCOMMON
AND RARE: Anemia
Idiopathic hypertrophic subaortic stenosis
Origin of both great vessels from the right ventricle
Pulmonary atresia
Renal failure
Transposition of the great vessels
Tricuspid atresia or stenosis
Truncus arteriosus
Tumor

REFERENCES

1. Reeder MM, Felson B: Gamuts in Radiology. Cincinnati, Audiovisual Radiology of Cincinnati, 1975
2. Sprengelmeyer J, Weisberger CL: Practical Nuclear Cardiology. Hagerstown, Harper and Row, 1979

GATED CARDIAC BLOOD POOL IMAGING

Enlarged Right Ventricle

COMMON: Congestive cardiomyopathy
          Cor pulmonale
          Left-to-right shunt
          Mitral stenosis
          Pulmonary stenosis
          Right ventricular infarction
          Tetralogy of Fallot

UNCOMMON
AND RARE: Ebstein's anomaly
           Hypoplastic left heart
           Left atrial myxoma
           Origin of both great vessels from the right ventricle
           Pulmonary insufficiency
           Transposition of the great vessels
           Tricuspid insufficiency
           Trilogy of Fallot
           Truncus arteriosus

REFERENCES

1. Meszaros WT: Cardiac Roentgenology. Springfield, Illinois, Charles C Thomas, 1969
2. Reeder MM, Felson B: Gamuts in Radiology. Cincinnati, Audiovisual Radiology of Cincinnati, 1975
3. Sprengelmeyer J, Weisberger CL: Practical Nuclear Cardiology. Hagerstown, Harper and Row, 1979

GATED CARDIAC BLOOD POOL IMAGING

Decreased Wall Motion at Rest

COMMON AND
UNCOMMON: Abscess
Aneurysm (true and false)
Aortic insufficiency
Contusion
Endocarditis
Medial splenic tubercle
Mitral regurtitation
Myocardial contusion
Myocardial infarction
Myocardiopathy
Observer variance
Severe ischemic heart disease

REFERENCES

1. Arreaza N, Puigbo JJ, Acquatella H, et al: Radionuclide evaluation of left-ventricular function in chronic Chagas' cardiomyopathy. J Nucl Med 24:563, 1983

2. Bodenheimer MM, Banka VS, Fouche CM, et al: Radionuclide angiographic assessment of wall motion and regional ejection fraction at rest and during exercise to detect coronary artery disease. Am J Cardiol 43:431, 1979

3. Botvinick EH, Shames DM: Nuclear Cardiology: Clinical Applications. Baltimore, Williams and Wilkins, 1979

4. Boucher CA, Okada RD, Prohost GM: Current status of radionuclide imaging in valvular heart disease. Am J Cardiol 46:1153, 1980

5. Okada RD, Kirshenbaum HD, Kushner FG, et al: Observer variance in the qualitative evaluation of left ventricular wall motion and the quantitation of left ventricular ejection fraction using rest and exercise multigated blood pool imaging. Circulation 61:128, 1980

6. Pitt B, Strauss HW: Myocardial imaging in the noninvasive evaluation of patients with suspected ischemic heart disease. Am J Cardiol 37:797, 1976

7. Simon TR, Parkey RW, Lewis SE: Role of cardiovascular nuclear medicine in evaluating trauma and the postoperative patient. Semin Nucl Med 13:123, 1983

8. Sinusas AJ, Hardin NJ, Clements JP, et al: Pathoanatomic correlates of regional left ventricular wall motion assessed by equilibrium radionuclide angiocardiography: A postmortem correlation. Am J Cardiol 54:975, 1984

9. Strauss HW, Pitt B (eds): Cardiovascular Nuclear Medicine. St. Louis, C.V. Mosby, 1979

10. Vincent LM, McCartney WH, Hicks R, et al: Medial splenic tubercle: Potential radionuclide ventriculography pitfall. Clin Nucl Med 10:294, 1985

11. Winzelberg GG: Focal left ventricular dyskinesis. Semin Nucl Med 14:141, 1984

12. Winzelberg GG, Strauss HW, Bingham JB, et al: Scintigraphic evaluation of left ventricular aneurysm. Am J Cardiol 46:1138, 1980

GATED CARDIAC BLOOD POOL IMAGING

Paradoxical Septal Motion

COMMON: Coronary artery disease — stenosis or infarction
Following cardiac surgery — bypass, mitral or aortic valve replacement
Left bundle branch block
Right ventricular pacing

UNCOMMON: Anomalous pulmonary venous return
Atrial septal defect
Ebstein's anomaly
Pulmonary hypertension
Pulmonic regurgitation
Tricuspid regurgitation

RARE: Aortic regurgitation
Complete absence of the pericardium
Constrictive pericarditis
Large pericardial effusion
Mitral regurgitation
Normal variant
Partial atrioventricular canal
Pulmonary stenosis
Right ventricular tumor
Ventricular septal defect
Wolff-Parkinson-White syndrome

REFERENCES

1. Abbasi AS, Eber LM, MacAlpin RN, et al: Paradoxical motion of interventricular septum in left bundle branch block. Circulation 49:423, 1974

2. Bingham JB, McKusick KA, Boucher CA, et al: Paradoxical septal motion. Semin Nucl Med 11:165, 1981

3. Eslami B, Roitman D, Karp RB, et al: Paradoxical septal motion in a patient with pulmonic stenosis. Chest 67:244, 1975

4. Francis GS, Theroux P, O'Rourke RA, et al: An echocardiographic study of interventricular septal motion in the Wolff-Parkinson-White syndrome. Circulation 54:174, 1976

5. Gomes JA, Damato AN, Akhtar M, et al: Ventricular septal motion and left ventricular dimensions during abnormal ventricular activation. Am J Cardiol 39:641, 1977

6. Hearne MJ, Sherber HS, deLeon AC Jr: Paradoxical motion of the interventricular septum in a patient with normal right heart hemodynamics. Chest 69:125, 1976

7. Katdare AV, Vengsarkar AS, Nair KG: Echocardiographic features of the interventricular septal motion in constrictive pericarditis. J Postgrad Med 25:214, 1979

8. Kolibash AJ, Beaver BM, Fulkerson PK, et al: The relationship between abnormal echocardiographic septal motion and myocardial perfusion in patients with significant obstruction of the left anterior descending artery. Circulation 56:780, 1977

9. Meyer RA, Schwartz DC, Benzing G, et al: Ventricular septum in right ventricular volume overload. Am J Cardiol 30:349, 1972

10. Miller HC, Gibson DG, Stephens JD: Role of echocardiography and phonocardiography in diagnosis of mitral paraprosthetic regurgitation with Starr Edwards prostheses. Br Heart J 35:1217, 1973

11. Righetti A, Crawford MH, O'Rourke RA, et al: Interventricular septal motion and left ventricular function after coronary bypass surgery. Am J Cardiol 39:372, 1977

12. Sasse L, Lorentzen D, Alvarez H: Paradoxical septal motion secondary to right ventricular tumor. JAMA 234:955, 1975

GATED CARDIAC BLOOD POOL IMAGING

Decreased Left Ventricular Ejection Fraction at Rest

COMMON AND
UNCOMMON: Alcohol intoxication
Aortic regurgitation
Aortic stenosis or insufficiency
Cardiomyopathies (see Cardiomyopathies gamut)
Congenital heart disease
Congestive heart failure — any cause
Constrictive pericarditis
Contusion
Following aortic or mitral valve replacement (early)
Mitral stenosis or insufficiency
Pacing
Paradoxical pulse with cardiac tamponade
Premature ventricular contractions
Prior myocardial infarction
Prior myocarditis
Severe ischemic heart disease
Transplant rejection

REFERENCES

1. Berger HJ, Zaret BL: Nuclear cardiology (second of two parts). N Engl J Med 305:855, 1981

2. Borer JS, Bacharach SL, Green SL, et al: Exercise-induced left ventricular dysfunction in symptomatic and asymptomatic patients with aortic regurgitation: Assessment with radionuclide cineangiography. Am J Cardiol 42:351, 1978

3. Boucher CA, Bingham JB, Osbakken GD, et al: Early changes in left ventricular size and function after correction of left ventricular volume overload. Am J Cardiol 47:991, 1981

4. Boucher CA, Okada RD, Prohost GM: Current status of radionuclide imaging in valvular heart disease. Am J Cardiol 46:1153, 1980

5. Camargo EE, Harrison KS, Wagner HN Jr, et al: Noninvasive beat to beat monitoring of left ventricular function by a nonimaging nuclear detector during premature ventricular contractions. Am J Cardiol 45:1219, 1980

6. Das, SK, Brady TJ, Thrall JH, et al: Cardiac function in patients with prior myocarditis. J Nucl Med 21:689, 1980

7. Dennis JB, Winzelberg GG: Cardiac imaging — diminished resting left ventricular ejection fraction. Semin Nucl Med 13:290, 1983

8. Greenberg ML, Uretsky BF, Reddy PS, et al: Long-term hemodynamic follow-up of cardiac transplant patients treated with cyclosporine and prednisone. Circulation 71:487, 1985

9. Ikaheimo MJ, Niemela KO, Linnaluoto MM, et al: Early cardiac changes related to radiation therapy. Am J Cardiol 56:943, 1985

10. Kelbaek H, Gjørup T, Brynjolf I, et al: Acute effects of alcohol on left ventricular function in healthy subjects at rest and during upright exercise. Am J Cardiol 55:164, 1985

11. Keren A, Billingham ME, Weintraub D, et al: Mildly dilated congestive cardiomyopathy. Circulation 72:302, 1985

12. Narahara KA, Blettel ML: Effect of rate on left ventricular volumes and ejection fraction during chronic ventricular pacing. Circulation 67:323, 1983

13. O'Toole JD, Geiser EA, Reddy PS, et al: Effect of preoperative ejection fraction on survival and hemodynamic improvement following aortic valve replacement. Circulation 58:1175, 1978

14. Qureshi S, Wagner HN Jr, Alderson PO, et al: Evaluation of left ventricular function in normal persons and patients with heart disease. J Nucl Med 19:135, 1978

15. Ritchie JL, Singer JW, Thorning D, et al: Anthracycline cardiotoxicity: Clinical and pathologic outcomes assessed by radionuclide ejection fraction. Cancer 46:1109, 1980

16. Rosenbaum RC, Johnson GS: Posttraumatic cardiac dysfunction: Assessment with radionuclide ventriculography. Radiology 160:91, 1986

17. Vogel HJK, Horgan JA, Strahl CL: Left ventricular dysfunction in chronic constrictive pericarditis. Chest 59:484, 1971

18. Yeh EL: Varying ejection fractions of both ventricles in paradoxical pulses — demonstration by radionuclide study. J Nucl Med 20:1005, 1979

GATED CARDIAC BLOOD POOL IMAGING

Elevated Left Ventricular Ejection Fraction at Rest

COMMON AND
UNCOMMON: Aortic stenosis
Hypertrophic cardiomyopathy — both latent and
resting obstruction
Medications
Normal variant
Observer variation
Physical conditioning

REFERENCES

1. Boucher CA, Okada RD, Prohost GM: Current status of radionuclide imaging in valvular heart disease. Am J Cardiol 46:1153, 1980

2. Gibbons RJ, Lee KL, Cobb FR, et al: Ejection fraction response to exercise in patients with chest pain and normal coronary arteriograms. Circulation 64:952, 1981

3. Pollick C, Bar-Shlomo B, McLaughlin PR, et al: Hypertrophic cardiomyopathy: Ventricular function studied by radionuclide angiography. Circulation 62(III):302, 1980

4. Prohost GM, Vignola PA, McKusick KE, et al: Hypertrophic cardiomyopathy. Evaluation of gated cardiac blood pool scanning. Circulation 55:92, 1977

5. Shah PM, Taylor RD, Hecht HS, et al: Asymmetric left ventricular hypertrophy — a study of anatomy and function by cross-sectional echocardiography and radionuclide angiography. Am J Cardiol 45:491, 1980

6. Wacker FJ, Berger HJ, Johnstone DE, et al: Multiple gated cardiac pool imaging for left ventricular ejection fraction: Validation of the technique and assessment of variability. Am J Cardiol 43:1159, 1979

7. Williams RS, McKinnis RA, Cobb FR, et al: Effects of physical conditioning on left ventricular ejection fraction in patients with coronary artery disease. Circulation 70:69, 1984

GATED CARDIAC BLOOD POOL IMAGING

Decreased Wall Motion with Exercise

COMMON: Coronary artery disease

UNCOMMON
AND RARE: Beta blockers
Electrocardiogram abnormalities
Interobserver variance
Mitral valve prolapse

REFERENCES

1. Bodenheimer MM, Banka VS, Fouche CM, et al: Radionuclide angiographic assessment of wall motion and regional ejection fraction at rest and during exercise to detect coronary heart disease. Am J Cardiol 43:431, 1979

2. Borer JS, Bacharach SL, Green MV, et al: Sensitivity of stress radionuclide cineangiography and stress thallium perfusion scanning in detecting coronary disease. Am J Cardiol 43:431, 1979

3. Borer JS, Kent KM, Bacharach SL, et al: Sensitivity, specificity and predictive accuracy of radionuclide cineangiography during exercise in patients with coronary artery disease. Circulation 60:572, 1979

4. Boucher CA, Okada RD, Prohost GM: Current status of radionuclide imaging in valvular heart disease. Am J Cardiol 46:1153, 1980

5. Upton MT, Newman GE, Port S, et al: Left ventricular function during two levels of exercise in patients with coronary artery disease. Am J Cardiol 43:433, 1979

GATED CARDIAC BLOOD POOL IMAGING

Abnormal Response to Exercise, Left Ventricle

COMMON: Coronary artery disease

UNCOMMON
AND RARE: Adriamycin cardiotoxicity
Aging
Aortic regurgitation
Aortic stenosis
COPD
Complete heart block (congenital)
Congenital heart disease
Females
Hypertension
Hypertrophic cardiomyopathy — with resting
    obstruction and no obstruction
Intrinsic variation of patient
Mitral regurgitation
Mitral valve prolapse
Normal variant
Observer variance
Other cardiomyopathies
Postirradiation
Prior myocarditis
Propranolol
Region-of-interest selection
Sickle cell anemia
Supine exercise
Thyrotoxicosis

REFERENCES

1. Bar-Shlomo B, Druck M, Morch J, et al: Ventricular function in patients treated by mediastinal irradiation for Hodgkin's disease. Circulation 62(III):179, 1980

2. Bodenheimer MM, Banka VS, Fouche CM, et al: Radionuclide angiographic assessment of wall motion and regional ejection fraction at rest and during exercise to detect coronary artery disease. Am J Cardiol 43:431, 1979

3. Borer JS, Bacharach SL, Green MV, et al: Exercised-induced left ventricular dysfunction in symptomatic and asymptomatic patients with aortic regurgitation: Assessment with radionuclide cineangiography. Am J Cardiol 42:351, 1978

4. Borer JS, Bacharach SL, Green MV, et al: Real time radionuclide cineangiography in the non-invasive evaluation of global and regional left ventricular function at rest and during exercise in patients with coronary artery disease. N Engl J Med 296:839, 1977

5. Borer JS, Bacharach SL, Green MV, et al: Sensitivity of stress radionuclide cineangiography and stress thallium perfusion scanning in detecting coronary artery disease. Am J Cardiol 43:431, 1979

6. Borer JS, Kent KM, Bacharach SL, et al: Sensitivity, specificity and predictive accuracy of radionuclide cineangiography during exercise in patients with coronary artery disease. Circulation 60:572, 1979

7. Boucher CA, Kanarek DJ, Okada RD, et al: Exercise testing in aortic regurgitation: Comparison of radionuclide left ventricular ejection fraction with exercise performance at the anaerobic threshold and peak exercise. Am J Cardiol 52:801, 1983

8. Caldwell JH, Hamilton GW, Sorensen SG, et al: The detection of coronary artery disease with radionuclide techniques: A comparison of rest — exercise thallium imaging and ejection fraction response. Circulation 61:610, 1980

9. Covitz W, Eubig C, Balfour IC, et al: Exercise-induced cardiac dysfunction in sickle cell anemia: A radionuclide study. Am J Cardiol 51:570, 1983

10. Dennis JB, Winzelberg GG: Cardiac imaging — decrease in the left ventricular ejection fraction after exercise. Semin Nucl Med 13:292, 1983

11. Gibbons RJ, Lee KL, Cobb FR, et al: Ejection fraction response to exercise in patients with chest pain, coronary artery disease and normal resting ventricular function. Circulation 66:643, 1982

12. Greenberg B, Massie B, Thomas D, et al: Association between the exercise ejection fraction response and systolic wall stress in patients with chronic aortic insufficiency. Circulation 71:458, 1985

13. Higginbotham MB, Morris KG, Coleman RE, et al: Sex-related differences in the normal cardiac response to upright exercise. Circulation 70:357, 1984

14. Huxley RL, Gaffney FA, Corbett JR, et al: Early detection of left ventricular dysfunction in chronic aortic regurgitation as assessed by contrast angiography, echocardiography, and rest and exercise scintigraphy. Am J Cardiol 51:1542, 1983

15. Iskandrian AS, Rose L, Hakki A, et al: Cardiac performance in thyrotoxicosis: Analysis of 10 untreated patients. Am J Cardiol 51:349, 1983

16. Manno BV, Hakki A. Eshaghpour E, et al: Left ventricular function at rest and during exercise in congenital complete heart block: A radionuclide angiographic evaluation. Am J Cardiol 52:92, 1983

17. Okada RD, Kirshenbaum HD, Kushner FG, et al: Observer variance in the qualitative evaluation of left ventricular wall motion and the quantitation of left ventricular ejection fraction using rest and exercise multigated blood pool imaging. Circulation 61:128, 1980

18. Osbakken MD, Boucher CA, Okada RD, et al: Spectrum of global left ventricular responses to supine exercise: Limitations in the use of ejection fraction in identifying patients with coronary artery disease. Am J Cardiol 51:28, 1983

19. Palmeri ST, Bonow RO, Myers CE, et al: Prospective evaluation of doxorubicin cardiotoxicity by rest and exercise radionuclide angiography. Am J Cardiol 58:607, 1986

20. Pfisterer ME, Battler A, Swanson SM, et al: Reproducibility of ejection fraction determinations by equilibrium radionuclide angiography in response to supine bicycle exercise. Concise communication. J Nucl Med 20:491, 1979

21. Sorensen, SG, Caldwell J, Ritchie J, et al: "Abnormal" responses of ejection fraction to exercise, in healthy subjects, caused by region-of-interest selection. J Nucl Med 22:1, 1981

22. Sorensen SG, Ritchie JL, Caldwell JH, et al: Serial exercise radionuclide angiography. Validation of count-derived changes in cardiac output and quantitation of maximal exercise ventricular volume change after nitroglycerin and propranolol in normal men. Circulation 61:600, 1980

23. Upton MT, Newman GE, Port S, et al: Left ventricular function during two levels of exercise in patients with coronary artery disease. Am J Cardiol 43:433, 1979

24. Vered Z, Battler A, Segal P, et al: Exercise-induced left ventricular dysfunction in young men with asymptomatic diabetes mellitus (diabetic cardiomyopathy). Am J Cardiol 54:633, 1984

25. Wackers FJ, Berger HJ, Johnstone DE, et al: Multiple gated cardiac blood pool imaging for left ventricular ejection fraction. Validation of the technique and assessment of variability. Am J Cariol 43: 1159, 1979

GATED CARDIAC BLOOD POOL IMAGING

False-Negative Response to Exercise, Ejection Fraction

COMMON AND
   UNCOMMON: Hypercontractility of adjacent normal area
                  Lowered resting ejection fraction in patients with
                     coronary artery disease
                  Propranolol
                  Random variation in patient
                  Submaximal exercise
                  Technical error (underestimating resting or
                     overestimating maximal value)

REFERENCES

1. Brown JM, White CJ, Sobol SM, et al: Increased left ventricular ejection fraction after a meal: Potential source of error in performance of radionuclide angiography. Am J Cardiol 51:1709, 1983

2. Caldwell JH, Hamilton GW, Sorensen SG, et al: The detection of coronary artery disease with radionuclide techniques: A comparison of rest-exercise thallium imaging and ejection fraction response. Circulation 61:610, 1980

3. Okada RD, Kirschenbaum HD, Kushner FG, et al: Observer variance in the qualitative evaluation of left ventricular wall motion and the quantitation of left ventricular ejection fraction using rest and exercise multigated blood pool imaging. Circulation 61:128, 1980

4. Port S, McEwan P. Cobb FR, et al: Influence of resting left ventricular function on the ventricular response to exercise in patients with coronary artery disease. Circulation 63:856, 1981

5. Reduto LA, Wickemeyer WJ, Young JB, et al: Left ventricular diastolic performance at rest and during exercise in patients with coronary artery disease. Circulation 63:1228, 1981

6. Wackers FJ, Berger HJ, Johnstone DE, et al: Multiple gated cardiac blood pool imaging for left ventricular ejection fraction: Validation of the technique and assessment of variability. Am J Cardiol 43:1159, 1979

GATED CARDIAC BLOOD POOL IMAGING

Decreased Right Ventricular Ejection Fraction at Rest

COMMON: Chronic obstructive pulmonary disease (especially with cor pulmonale)

Inferior myocardial infarction involving the right ventricle

UNCOMMON
AND RARE: Aortic and mitral valve disease

Congenital heart disease

Congestive cardiomyopathy

Contusion

Cystic fibrosis

Essential hypertension

Isolated right ventricular infarction

Paradoxical pulse with cardiac tamponade

Pulmonary thromboembolism

Tricuspid regurgitation

REFERENCES

1. Berger HJ, Mathay RA, Loke J, et al: Assessment of cardiac performance with quantitative radionuclide angiocardiography: Right ventricular ejection fraction with reference to findings in chronic obstructive pulmonary disease. Am J Cardiol 41:897, 1978

2. Cohen M, Horowitz SF, Machae J, et al: Response of the right ventricle to exercise in isolated mitral stenosis. Am J Cardiol 55:1054, 1985

3. Garty I, Antonelli D, Barzilay J: The noninvasive diagnosis of isolated right ventricular infarction. Clin Nucl Med 9:712, 1984

4. Maddahi J, Berman DS, Matsuoka DT, et al: Right ventricular ejection fraction during exercise in normal subjects and in coronary artery disease patients: Assessment by multiple gated equilibrium scintigraphy. Circulation 62:133, 1980

5. Marmor A, Frankel A, Blondeheim DS, et al: Scintigraphic assessment of atrial function in patients with long-standing hypertension. Radiology 151:483, 1984

6. Olvey SK, Reduto LA, Stevens PM, et al: First pass radionuclide assessment of right and left ventricular ejection fraction in chronic pulmonary disease. Chest 78:4, 1980

7. Sprengelmeyer J, Weisberger CL: Practical Nuclear Cardiology. Hagerstown, Harper and Row, 1979

8. Sutherland GR, Driedger AA, Holliday RL, et al: Frequency of myocardial injury after blunt chest trauma as evaluated by radionuclide angiography. Am J Cardiol 52:1099, 1983

9. Winzelberg GG: Diminished right ventricular ejection fraction on radionuclide cardiography. Semin Nucl Med 12:304, 1982

GATED CARDIAC BLOOD POOL IMAGING

Abnormal Response to Exercise, Right Ventricle

COMMON AND
UNCOMMON: Chronic obstructive pulmonary disease
Coronary artery disease
Cystic fibrosis
Total correction of a tetralogy of Fallot
Valvular disease

REFERENCES

1. Berger HJ, Johnstone DE, Sands JM, et al: Response of right ventricular ejection fraction to upright bicycle exercise in coronary artery disease. Circulation 60:1292, 1979

2. Johnson LL, McCarthy DM, Sciacca RR, et al: Right ventricular ejection fraction during exercise in patients with coronary artery disease. Circulation 60:1284, 1979

3. Maddahi J, Berman DS, Matsuoka DT, et al: A new technique for assessing right ventricular ejection fraction using rapid multiple gated equilibrium cardiac blood pool scintigraphy. Circulation 60:581, 1979

4. Maddahi J, Berman DS, Matsuoak DT, et al: Right ventricular ejection fraction at rest and during exercise in normals and in coronary artery disease patients: Assessment by multiple gated equilibrium scintigraphy. J Nucl Med 20:625, 1979

5. Maddahi J, Berman DS, Matsuoka DT, et al: Right ventricular ejection fraction during exercise in normal subjects and in coronary artery disease patients: Assessment by multiple gated equilibrium scintigraphy. Circulation 62: 133, 1980

6. Olvey SK, Reduto LA, Stevens PM, et al: First pass radionuclide assessment of right and left ventricular ejection fraction in chronic pulmonary disease. Chest 78:4, 1980

7. Slutsky R, Hooper W, Gerber K, et al: Assessment of right ventricular function at rest and during exercise in patients with coronary heart disease: A new approach using equilibrium radionuclide angiography. Am J Cardiol 45:63, 1980

GATED CARDIAC BLOOD POOL IMAGING

Increased Regurgitant Fraction from Aortic Valve Disease

COMMON: Rheumatic heart disease

UNCOMMON: Aortitis (e.g., syphilis, Takayasu's)
Bacterial endocarditis
Congenital bicuspid aortic valve
Marfan's syndrome
Sinus of Valsalva aneurysm
Subvalvular aneurysm of left ventricle
Trauma
Ventricular septal defect with prolapsed aortic cusp

REFERENCES

1. Baxter RH, Becker LC, Alderson PO, et al: Quantification of aortic valvular regurgitation in dogs by nuclear imaging. Circulation 61:404, 1980

2. Bough EW, Gandsman EJ, North DL, et al: Gated radionuclide angiographic evaluation of valve regurgitation. Am J Cardiol 46:423, 1980

3. Konstam MA, Wynne J, Holman L, et al: Use of equilibrium (gated) radionuclide ventriculography to quantitate left ventricular output in patients with and without left-sided valvular regurgitation. Circulation 64:578, 1981

4. Reeder MM, Felson B: Gamuts in Radiology. Cincinatti, Audiovisual Radiology of Cincinatti, Inc., 1975

5. Sorensen SG, O'Rourke RA, Chaudhuri TK: Noninvasive quantitation of valvular regurgitation by gated equilibrium radionuclide angiography. Circulation 62:1089, 1980

GATED CARDIAC BLOOD POOL IMAGING

Increased Regurgitant Fraction from Mitral Valve Disease

COMMON;   Rheumatic heart disease
Secondary to other cardiac disease (e.g.,
hypertension, myocardiopathy, aortic
insufficiency)

UNCOMMON
AND RARE: Bacterial endocarditis
Congenital
Corrected transposition
Idiopathic hypertrophic subaortic stenosis
Marfan's syndrome
Ostium primum defect
Papillary muscle dyfunction (e.g. myocardial
infarction)

REFERENCES

1. Bough EW, Gandsman EJ, North DL, et al: Gated radionuclide angiographic evaluation of valve regurgitation. Am J Cardiol 46:423, 1980

2. Konstam MA, Wynne J, Holman L, et al: Use of equilibrium (gated) radionuclide ventriculography to quantitate left ventricular output in patients with and without left-sided valvular regurgitation. Circulation 64:578, 1981

3. Reeder MM, Felson B: Gamuts in Radiology. Cincinnati, Audiovisual Radiology of Cincinnatti, 1975.

4. Sorensen SG, O'Rourke RA, Chaudhuri TK: Noninvasive quantitation of valvular regurgitation by gated equilibrium radionuclide angiography. Circulation 62:1089, 1980

GATED CARDIAC BLOOD POOL IMAGING

Saccular Deformities of the Left Ventricle

COMMON: Aneurysm

UNCOMMON
AND RARE: Artifact due to nursing
Diverticulum
Ectopic spleen
Localized herniation through a partial pericardial
defect

REFERENCES

1. Baltaxe HA, Wilson WJ, Amiel M: Diverticulosis of the left ventricle. AJR 133:257, 1979

2. Cassidy DB, Goldstein RA, Wu DB, et al: Apparent left ventricular aneurysm due to unilateral secretion of ^{99m}Tc pertechnetate in nursing mother with breast cancer. Clin Nucl Med 15:264, 1990

3. Goldwag S, Campeau RJ, Agasala M, Karcioglu G: Pseudo-pseudoaneurysm — left ventricular pseudoaneurysm mimicked by ectopic spleen. Clin Nucl Med 19:69, 1994

4. Nicod P, Laird WP, Firth BG, et al: Congenital diverticula of the left and right ventricles: 3 cases. Am J Cardiol 53:342, 1984

5. Raipal R, Thomas J, Sty JR: Left ventricular diverticulum. A scintigraphic diagnosis. Pediatri Radiol 10:39, 1980

GATED CARDIAC BLOOD POOL IMAGING

True Aneurysm

COMMON: Myocardial infarction

UNCOMMON
AND RARE: Congenital defects
Erosive bacterial endocarditis
Myocardial abscess
Trauma

REFERENCES

1. Friedman ML, Cantor RE: Reliability of gated heart scintigrams for detection of left ventricular aneurysm: Concise communication. J Nucl Med 20:720, 1979
2. Winzelberg GG, Strauss HW, Bingham JB, et al: Scintigraphic evaluation of left ventricular aneurysm. Am J Cardiol 46:1138, 1980

GATED CARDIAC BLOOD POOL IMAGING

False Aneurysm

COMMON: Prior cardiac surgery
                        Transmural myocardial infarction

UNCOMMON: Bacterial endocarditis
                              Myocarditis
                              Trauma — blunt and penetrating

RARE: Syphilis
                  Tuberculosis

REFERENCES

1. Botvinick EH, Shames D, Hutchinson JC, et al: Noninvasive diagnosis of a false left ventricular aneurysm with radiosotope gated cardiac blood pool imaging. Am J Cardiol 37:1089, 1976

2. Breisblatt WM, Berger RB, Cabin HS, et al: Unsuspected left ventricular pseudoaneurysm. AJR 142:680, 1984

3. Dymond DS, Elliot AT, Banim S: Detection of a false left ventricular aneurysm by first pass radionuclide ventriculography. J Nucl Med 20:851, 1979

4. Higgins CB, Lipton MJ, Johnson AD, et al: False aneurysms of the left ventricle. Radiology 127:21, 1978

5. Katz RJ, Simpson A, DiBianco R, et al: Noninvasive diagnosis of left ventricular psuedoaneurysm: Role to two-dimensional echocardiography and radionuclide gated pool imaging. Am J Cardiol 44:372, 1979

6. Onik G, Recht L, Edwards JE, et al: False left ventricular aneurysm: Diagnosis by noninvasive means. J Nucl Med 21:177, 1980

7. Sweet SE, Sterling R, McCormick JR, et al: Left ventricular false aneurysm after coronary bypass surgery: Radionuclide diagnosis and surgical resection. Am J Cardiol 43:54, 1979

8. Winzelberg GG, Strauss HW, Bingham JB, et al: Scintigraphic evaluation of left ventricular aneurysm. Am J Cardiol 46:1138, 1980

GATED CARDIAC BLOOD POOL IMAGING

Square Left Ventricle

COMMON: Thrombus

REFERENCE

1. Goolsby J, Steele P, Kirch D, et al: The square left ventricle: An angiographic and radionuclide sign of left ventricular thrombus. Radiology 115:533, 1975

GATED CARDIAC BLOOD POOL IMAGING

Chamber Filling Defects

COMMON AND
UNCOMMON: Atrial myoma
Metastases
Other cardiac tumors (e.g., rhabdomyoma which is
the most common cardiac tumor in infants)
Prominent posterior papillary muscle or trabeculae
Thrombus

REFERENCES

1. Antico VF, Hands ME, Lloyd BL, et al: Metastatic uterine cervical cell carcinoma to myocardium. Clin Nucl Med 11:131, 1986
2. Bidula LP, Maurer AH, Denenberg BS, et al: Multiple scintigraphic findings in a patient with a primary myocardial sarcoma. Clin Nucl Med 8:474, 1983
3. Bunko H, Nakajima K, Tonami N, et al: Visualization of hypertrophied papillary muscle mimicking left ventricular mass on gated blood pool and T1-201 myocardial perfusion imaging. Clin Nucl Med 6:571, 1981
4. Dresser TP, Rao R, Winebright JW: Nuclear angiocardiogram to demonstrate right atrial myxoma. Clin Nucl Med 2:206, 1977
5. Gewirtz H, Wilner A, Garriepy S, et al: Diagnosis of left-ventricular mural thrombus by means of radionuclide ventriculography. J Nucl Med 22:610, 1981
6. Meyers SN, Shapiro JE, Barressi V, et al: Right atrial myxoma with right to left shunting and mitral valve prolapse. Am J Med 62:308, 1977
7. Novetsky GJ, Berlin L, Turner DA, et al: Left ventricular thrombus: Detection by ECG synchronized cineangiography. Clin Nucl Med 8:155, 1983
8. Parisi AF, Tow DE, Sasahara AA: Clinical appraisal of current nuclear and other noninvasive cardiac diagnostic techniques. Am J Cardiol 38:722, 1976
9. Prohost GM, Pastore JO, McKusick KA, et al: Detection of left atrial myxoma by gated radionuclide cardiac imaging. Circulation 55:88, 1977
10. Shih WJ, Stipp V: Intraventricular photon deficiency in gated cardiac blood pool imaging due to left ventricular metastases from renal cell carcinoma. Clin Nucl Med 16:754, 1991
11. Starshak RJ, Sty JR: Radionuclide angiocardiography: Use in the detection of myocardial rhabdomyoma. Clin Nucl Med 3:106, 1978
12. Stratton JR, Ritchie JL, Hammermeister KE, et al: Detection of left ventricular thrombi with radionuclide angiography. Am J Cardiol 48:565, 1981
13. Sullivan K, Park CH: Hypertrophied moderator band in atrial septal defect. Clin Nucl Med 9:458, 1984

14. Winzelberg GG, Rapoport F, Boucher CA, et al: Combined gated cardiac blood pool scintigraphy and ^{61}Ga-citrate scintigraphy for detection of cardiac lymphoproliferative disorders. Radiology 141:191, 1981

GATED CARDIAC BLOOD POOL IMAGING

Halo Sign

COMMON: Normal variant (especially between the cardiac and
           liver)
           Pericardial fluid (e.g., effusion, blood)

UNCOMMON
AND RARE: Ascites
           Mediastinal adenopathy, fat, or tumor
           Myocardial hypertrophy
           Pericardial cyst
           Pericardial tumor
           Pleural fluid (e.g., effusion, blood)
           Pneumopericardium

REFERENCES

1. Bonte FJ, Curry TS III: Blood pool scanning with Tc-99m human serum albumin. Radiology 85:1120, 1965

2. Datz FL, Lewis SE, Parkey RW, et al: Radionuclide evaluation of cardiac trauma. Semin Nucl Med 10:187, 1980

3. Gottschalk A, Potchen EJ (eds): Diagnostic Nuclear Medicine. Baltimore, Williams and Wilkins, 1976

4. Rothendler JA, Schick EC, Leppo J, et al: Diagnosis of pericardial effusions from routine gated blood pool imaging. J Nucl Med 18:1419, 1987

5. Weitzman LB, Tinker WP, Kronzon I, et al: The incidence and natural history of pericardial effusion after cardiac surgery — and echocardiographic study. Circulation 69:506, 1984

6. Winzelberg GG: Photon-deficient areas around the heart. Semin Nucl Med 13:174, 1983

7. Yuille DL: Cardiac blood pool imaging: A review. CRC Crit Rev Diagn Imaging 11:223, 1979

CARDIAC ANGIOGRAPHY

Lung Curve Indicating a Left-to-Right Shunt

COMMON: Atrial septal defect
Heart failure — any cause
Patent ductus arteriosus
Poor bolus injection
Ventricular septal defect

UNCOMMON: Aorticopulmonary window
Arteriovenous fistula
Coarctation — shunt group
Endocardial cushion defect
Palliative shunts
Partial anomalous pulmonary venous return
Ruptured sinus of Valsalva aneurysm
Truncus arteriosus
Ventricular septal defect with corrected
transposition

RARE: Origin of right pulmonary artery from the aorta
Single atrium
Single ventricle
Tetralogy of Fallot, acyanotic

REFERENCES

1. Alderson PO, Douglass KH, Mendenhall KG, et al: Deconvolution analysis in radionuclide quantitation of left-to-right shunts. J Nucl Med 20:502, 1979

2. Alderson PO, Guadiani VA, Watson DC: Quantitative radionuclide angiocardiography in animals with experimental atrial septal defects. J Nucl Med 19:364, 1978

3. Askenazi J, Ahnberg DS, Korngold E, et al: Quantitative radionuclide angiocardiography: Detection and quantitation of left-to-right shunts. Am J Cardiol 37:382, 1976

4. Bosnjakovic VB, Bennett LR, Greenfield LD, et al: Dual isotope method for diagnosis of intracardiac shunts. J Nucl Med 14:514, 1973

5. Buit GL, Kroom HM, Chon JG, et al: Radionuclide angiocardiography in the clinical evaluation of cardiac malpositions in situs solitus in adults. J Nucl Med 27:484, 1986

6. Edwards JE, Carey LS, Neufeld HN, et al: Congenital Heart Disease. Philadelphia, W.B. Saunders, 1965

7. Kriss JP, Enright LP, Hayden WG, et al: Radioisotopic angiocardiography. Wide scope of applicability in diagnosis and evaluation of therapy in diseases of the heart and great vessels. Circulation 43:792, 1971

8. McIlveen BM, Murray IPC, Giles RW, et al: Clinical application radionuclide quantitation of left-to-right cardiac shunts in children. Am J Cardiol 47:1273, 1981

9. Mishkin FS: Lung curve indicating a left-to-right shunt in an infant with a large heart. Semin Nucl Med 11:161, 1981

10. Reeder MM, Felson B: Gamuts in Radiology. Cincinnati, Audiovisual Radiology of Cincinnati, 1975

11. Treves S, Collins-Nakai R: Radioactive tracers in congenital heart disease. Am J Cardiol 38:711, 1976

12. Treves S, Fogle R, Lang P: Radionuclide angiography in congenital heart disease. Am J Cardiol 46:1247, 1980

CARDIAC ANGIOGRAPHY

Right-to-Left Shunt

COMMON: Left-to-right shunt with Eisenmenger's physiology
Tetralogy of Fallot
Transposition of the great vessels

UNCOMMON
AND RARE: Common atrium
Common ventricle
Cor biloculare
Ebstein's anomaly with atrial septal defect
Hepatic cirrhosis
Isolated hypoplasia of right ventricle with atrial
    septal defect
Origin of both great vessels from the right ventricle
Pentalogy of Fallot
Pulmonary arteriovenous fistula
Pulmonary atresia with atrial septal defect
Pulmonary telangiectasia
Right pulmonary artery to left atrium fistula
Systemic venous connection to the left atrium
Total anomalous pulmonary venous return
Triscuspid atresia
Trilogy of Fallot
Truncus arteriosus

REFERENCES

1. Bank ER, Thrall JH, Dantzker DR: Radionuclide demonstration of intrapulmonary shunting in cirrhosis. AJR 140:967, 1983

2. Bosnjakovic VB, Bennett LR, Greenfield LD, et al: Dual isotope method for diagnosis of intracardiac shunts. J Nucl Med 14:514, 1973

3. Chen NS, Barnett CA, Farrer PA: Reversibility of intrapulmonary arteriovenous shunts in liver cirrhosis documented by serial radionuclide perfusion lung scans. Clin Nucl Med 9:279, 1984

4. Edwards JE, Carey LS, Neufeld HN, et al: Congenital Heart Disease. Philadelphia, W.B. Saunders, 1965

5. Kriss JP, Enright LP, Hayden WG, et al: Radioisotopic angiocardiography. Wide scope of applicability in diagnosis and evaluation of therapy in diseases of the heart and great vessels. Circulation 43:792, 1971

6. Peter CA, Armstrong BE, Jones RH: Radionuclide quantitation of right-to-left intracardiac shunts in children. Circulation 64:572, 1981

7. Reeder MM, Felson B: Gamuts in Radiology. Cincinnati, Audiovisual Radiology of Cincinnati, 1975

8. Suzuki Y: Quantitation of right-to-left shunt ratio in patients with pulmonary telangiectasia by technetium-99m MAA lung perfusion imaging. Clin Nucl Med 11:84, 1986

9. Villaneueva-Meyer J, Marcus C. Thompson K, et al: Diagnosis and quantitation of pulmonary arteriovenous malformations by factor analysis. Clin Nucl Med 11:88, 1986

PYROPHOSHPATE IMAGING

Increased Uptake — Focal or Diffuse

COMMON: Acute myocardial infarction (transmural and
subendocardial)

UNCOMMON: Chest wall trauma (e.g., rib fracture)
Costal cartilage calcification
Delayed clearance (e.g., renal disease)
Following cardioversion
Left ventricular aneurysm
Myocardial contusion
Postsurgical
Previous myocardial infarction
Slight blool pool labeling
Stable angina pectoris
Unstable angina pectoris

RARE: Breast carcinoma
Calcified valves
Cardiomyopathy
Cardiotoxic drugs
Endocarditis
Metastases
Metastatic calcification (e.g., hyperparathyroidism)
Myocarditis (e.g., Chagas' disease, viral)
Normal breast
Penetrating wounds (e.g., knife or bullet injury)
Pericardial effusion
Pericarditis
Prosthetic valves
Radiation therapy
Skin lesions (e.g., pseudoxanthoma elasticum)
Transplant rejection

REFERENCES

1. Ahmad M, Dubiel JP, Logan KW, et al: Limited clinical diagnostic specificity of technetium-99m-stannous pyrophosphate myocardial imaging in acute myocardial infarction. Am J Cardiol 39:50, 1977

2. Ahmad M, Dubiel JP, Verdon TA, et al: Technetium-99m-stannous pyrophosphate myocardial imaging in patients with and without left ventricular aneurysm. Circulation 58:833, 1976

3. Berman DS, Amsterdam EA, Hines HH, et al: New approach to interpretation of technetium-99m-pyrophosphate scintigraphy in detection of acute myocardial infarction. Am J Cardiol 39:341, 1977

4. Berman DS, Amsterdam EA, Hines HH, et al: Problem of diffuse cardiac uptake of technetium-99m-pyrophosphate in the diagnosis of acute myocardial infarction: Enhanced scintigraphic accuracy by computerized selective blood pool subtraction. Am J Cardiol 40:768, 1977

5. Botvinick EH, Shames DM, Sharpe DN, et al: The specificity of pyrophosphate myocardial scintigrams in patients with prior myocardial infarction: Concise communication. J Nucl Med 19:1121, 1978

6. Burdine JA, DePuey EG, Orzan F, et al: Scintigraphic, electrocardiographic, and enzymatic diagnosis of perioperative myocardial infarction in patients undergoing myocardial revascularization. J Nucl Med 20:711, 1979

7. Chacko AK, Gordon DH, Bennett JM, et al: Myocardial imaging with Tc-99m-pyrophosphate in patients on Adriamycin treatment for neoplasia. J Nucl Med 18:680, 1977

8. Chaudhuri TK: Intense myocardial uptake of gallium-67 citrate and technetium-99m pyrophosphate in a uremic patient. Clin Nucl Med 10:728, 1985

9. Cowley MJ, Mantle JA, Rogers WJ, et al: Use of blood pool imaging in evaluation of diffuse activity patterns in technetium-99m-pyrophosphate myocardial scintigraphy. J Nucl Med 20:496, 1979

10. Curry RC, Jackman WM: Persistently positive ^{99m}Tc-pyrophosphate myocardial scintigram in a patient with a left ventricular aneurysm. Clin Nucl Med 1:91, 1976

11. Davison R, Spies SM, Przybylek J, et al: Technetium-99m-stannous pyrophosphate myocardial scintigraphy after cardiopulmonary resuscitation with cardioversion. Circulation 60:292, 1979

12. Di Cola VC, Freedman GS, Downing SE, et al: Myocardial uptake of technetium-99m-stannous phyrophosphate following direct current transthoracic counter shock. Circulation 54:980, 1976

13. Downey J, Chagrasulis R, Fore D, et al: Accumulation of technetium-99m stannous phyrophosphate in contused myocardium. J Nucl Med 18:1171, 1977

14. Duska F, Vizda J, Kubicek J, et al: The sensitivity of scintigraphic myocardial imaging by use of ^{99m}Tc-labeled pyrophosphate in the diagnosis of cardiomyopathy of various etiology. Eur J Nucl. Med 4:87, 1979

15. Holman BL, Chisholm RJ, Braunwald E: The prognostic implications of acute myocardial infarct scintigraphy with ^{99m}Tc-pyrophosphate. Circulation 57:320, 1978

16. Jaffe AS, Klein MS, Patel BR, et al: Abnormal technetium-99m pyrophosphate images in unstable angina: Ischemia verus infarction? Am J Cardiol 44:1035, 1979

17. Jengo JA, Mena I, Joe SH, et al: The significance of calcific valvular heart disease in Tc-99m-pyrophosphate myocardial infarction scanning: Radiographic, scintigraphic, and pathological correlation. J Nucl Med 18:776, 1977

18. Kadota K, Matsumori A, Kambara H, et al: Myocardial uptake of technetium-99m-stannous pyrophosphate in experimental viral myopericarditis. J Nucl Med 20:1047, 1979

19. Karunaratne HB, Walsh WF, Fill HR, et al: Technetium-99m-pyrophosphate myocardial scintigraphy in patients with chest pain — lack of diagnostic specificity. J Nucl Med 17:523, 1976

20. Kelly RJ, Cowan RJ, Maynard CD, et al: Localization of ^{99m}Tc-Sn-pyrophosphate in left ventricular aneurysms. J Nucl Med 18:342, 1977

21. Klein MS, Coleman RE, Roberts R, et al: False-positive ^{99m}TC-Sn-pyrophosphate myocardial infarct images related to delayed blood pool clearance. Clin Nucl Med 1:45, 1976

22. Klein MS, Weiss AN, Roberts R, et al: Technetium-99m-stannous pyrophosphate scintigrams in normal subjects, patients with exercise-induced ischemia and patients with a calcified valve. Am J Cardiol 39:360, 1977

23. Landgarten S: Uptake of Tc-99m-pyrophosphate by the lactating breast. J Nucl Med 18:943, 1977

24. Langarten S, Gordon R: Radionuclide demonstration of Adriamycin induced cardiac toxicity. Clin Nucl Med 2:429, 1977

25. Lyons KP, Olson HG, Aronow WS: Sensitivity and specificity of Tc-99m-pyrophosphate myocardial scintigraphy for the detection of acute myocardial infarction. Clin Nucl Med 5:8, 1980

26. Lyons KP, Olson HG, Brown WT, et al: Persistence of an abnormal pattern on ^{99m}Tc-pyrophosphate myocardial scintigraphy following acute myocardial infarction. Clin Nucl Med 1:253, 1976

27. Mason JW, Myers RW, Alderman EL, et al: Technetium-99m-pyrophosphate uptake in patients with stable angina pectoris. Am J Cardiol 40:1, 1977

28. Matsumori A, Kadota K, Kawai C: Technetium-99m-pyrophosphate uptake in experimental viral perimyocarditis. Circulation 61:802, 1980

29. McGregor CGA, Hatz R, Aziz S, et al: Technetium-99m pyrophosphate in diagnosis of acute cardiac rejection in the rat with effect of cyclosporine: Concise communication. J Nucl Med 25:870, 1984

30. Muz J, Wizenberg T, Samlowski W, et al: Myocardial uptake of technetium 99m-pyrophosphate in patients with amyloidosis. J Nucl Med 21:49, 1980

31. Parkey RW, Bonte FJ, Buja LM, et al (eds): Clinical Nuclear Cardiology. New York, Appleton-Century-Crofts, 1979

32. Perez LA, Hayt DB, Freeman LM: Localization of myocardial disorders other than infarction with ^{99m}Tc-labeled phosphate agents. J Nucl Med 17:241, 1976

33. Platt MR, Mills LJ, Parkey RW, et al: Perioperative myocardial infarction diagnosed by technetium-99m-stannous pyrophosphate myocardial scintigrams. Circulation 54(III):24, 1976

34. Riba AL, Downs J, Thakur ML, et al: Technetium-99m stannous pyrophosphate imaging of experimental infective endocarditis. Circulation 58:111, 1978

35. Rocha AF, Meguerian BA, Harbert JC: Tc-99m-pyrophosphate myocardial scanning in Chagas' disease. J Nucl Med 22:347, 1981

36. Seo I, Donoghue G: Tc-99m-pyrophosphate accumulation on prosthetic valves. Clin Nucl Med 5:367, 1980

37. Willerson JT, Parkey RW, Bonte FJ, et al: Acute subendocardial myocardial infarction in patients. Circulation 51:436, 1975

38. Yeh E, Thompson MA, Meade RC: Accumulation of Tc-99m-diphosphonate in pericardial effusion. J Nucl Med 20:1103, 1979

PYROPHOSPHATE IMAGING

Focal Uptake

COMMON: Acute transmural myocardial infarction

UNCOMMON: Cardioversion
Chest wall trauma (e.g., rib fractures)
Costal cartilage calcification
Left ventricular aneurysm
Myocardial contusion
Postsurgical
Previous myocardial infarction
Stable angina pectoris
Unstable angina pectoris

RARE: Breast carcinoma
Calcified valves
Cardiomyopathy
Cardiotoxic drugs (e.g., doxorubicin)
Metastases
Normal breast
Penetrating wounds (e.g., knife, bullet)
Pericardial effusion
Prosthetic valves
Skin lesions (e.g., pseudoxanthoma elasticum)

REFERENCES

1. Ahmad M, Dubiel JP, Verdon TA, et al: Technetium-99m-stannous pyrophosphate myocardial imaging in patients with and without left ventricular aneurysm. Circulation 53:833, 1976

2. Berman DS, Amsterdam EA, Hines HH, et al: Problem of diffuse cardiac uptake of technetium-99m-pyrophosphate in the diagnosis of acute myocardial infarction: Enhanced scintigraphic accuracy by computerized selective blood pool subtraction. Am J Cardiol 40:768, 1977

3. Botvinick EH, Shames DM, Sharpe DN, et al: The specificity of pyrophosphate myocardial scintigrams in patients with prior myocardial infarction: Concise communication. J Nucl Med 19:1121, 1978

4. Burdine JA, DePuey EG, Orzan F, et al: Scintigraphic, electrocardiographic, and enzymatic diagnosis of perioperative myocardial infarction in patients undergoing myocardial revascularization. J Nucl Med 20:711, 1979

5. Curry RC, Jackman WM: Persistently positive ^{99m}Tc-pyrophosphate myocardial scintigram in a patient with a left ventricular aneurysm. Clin Nucl Med 1:91, 1976

6. Davison R, Spies SM, Przybylek J, et al: Technetium-99m-stannous pyrophosphate myocardial scintigraphy after cardiopulmonary resuscitation with cardioversion. Circulation 60:292, 1979

7. DiCola VC, Freedman GS, Downing SE, et al: Myocardial uptake of technetium-99m-stannous pyrophosphate following direct current transthoracic countershock. Circulation 54:980, 1976

8. Downey J, Chagrasulis R, Fore D, et al: Accumulation of technetium-99m-stannous pyrophosphate in contused myocardium. J Nucl Med 18:1171, 1977

9. Duska F, Vizda J, Kubicek J, et al: The sensitivity of scintigraphic myocardial imaging by the use of ^{99m}Tc-labeled pyrophosphate in the diagnosis of cardiomyopathy of various etiology. Eur J Nuc Med 4:87, 1979

10. Holman BL, Chisholm RJ, Braunwald E: The prognostic implications of acute myocardial infarct scintigraphy with ^{99m}Tc-pyrophosphate. Circulation 57:320, 1978

11. Jaffe AS, Klein MS, Patel BR, et al: Abnormal technetium-99m-pyrophosphate images in unstable angina: Ischemia versus infarction? Am J Cardiol 44:1035, 1979

12. Jengo JA, Mena I, Joe SH, et al: The significance of calcific valvular heart disease in Tc-99m-pyrophosphate myocardial infarction scanning: Radiographic, scintigraphic, and pathological correlation. J Nucl Med 18:776, 1977

13. Karunaratne HB, Walsh WF, Fill HR, et al: Technetium-99m-pyrophosphate myocardial scintigraphy in patients with chest pain — lack of diagnostic specificity. J Nucl Med 17:523, 1976

14. Kelly RJ, Cowan RJ, Maynard CD, et al: Localization of ^{99m}Tc-Sn-pyrophosphate in left ventricular aneurysms. J Nucl Med 18:342, 1977

15. Klein MS, Weiss AN, Roberts R, et al: Technetium-99m-stannous pyrophosphate scintigrams in normal subjects, patients with exercise-induced ischemia and patients with a calcified valve. Am J Cardiol 39:360, 1977

16. Lyons KP, Olson HG, Aronow WS: Sensitivity and specificity of Tc-99m pyrophosphate myocardial scintigraphy for the detection of acute myocardial infarction. Clin Nucl Med 5:8, 1980

17. Lyons KP, Olson HG, Brown WT, et al: Persistence of an abnormal pattern on ^{99m}Tc-pyrophosphate myocardial scintigraphy following acute myocardial infarction. Clin Nucl Med 1:253, 1976

18. Mason JW, Myers RW, Alderman EL, et al: Technetium-99m-pyrophosphate myocardial uptake in patients with stable angina pectoris. Am J Cardiol 40:1, 1977

19. Parkey RW, Bonte FJ, Buja LM, et al (eds): Clinical Nuclear Cardiology. New York, Appleton-Century-Crofts, 1979

20. Platt MR, Mills LJ, Parkey RW, et al: Perioperative myocardial infarction diagnosed by technetium-99m-stannous pyrophosphate myocardial scintigrams. Circulation 54(III):24, 1976

21. Riba AL, Downs J, Thakur ML, et al: Technetium-99m-stannous pyrophosphate imaging of experimental infective endocarditis. Circulation 58:111, 1978

22. Seo I, Donoghue G: Tc-99m-pyrophosphate accumulation on prosthetic valves. Clin Nucl Med 5:367, 1980

23. Willerson JT, Parkey RW, Bonte FJ, et al: Acute subendocardial myocardial infarction in patients. Circulation 51:436, 1975

24. Yeh E, Thompson MA, Meade RC: Accumulation of Tc-99m-diphosphonate in pericardial effusion. J Nucl Med 20:1103, 1979

PYROPHOSPHATE IMAGING

Diffuse Uptake

COMMON: Acute subendocardial myocardial infarction
Delayed renal clearance
Slight blood pool labeling
Stable angina pectoris
Unstable angina pectoris

UNCOMMON: Cardiomyopathy
Cardiotoxic drugs (e.g., doxorubricin)
Idiopathic
Previous myocardial infarction

RARE: Calcified valves?
Enlarged left ventricle
Metastatic calcification
Myocarditis (e.g., Chagas' disease, viral)
Pericarditis
Radiation
Transplant rejection

REFERENCES

1. Ahmad M, Dubiel JP, Logan KW, et al: Limited clinical diagnostic specificity of technetium-99m-stannous pyrophosphate myocardial imaging in acute myocardial infarction. Am J Cardiol 39:50, 1977

2. Berman DS, Amsterdam EA, Hines HH, et al: New approach to interpretation of technetium-99m-pyrophosphate scintigraphy in detection of acute myocardial infarction. Am J Cardiol 39:341, 1977

3. Berman DS, Amsterdam EA, Hines HH, et al: Problem of diffuse cardiac uptake of technetium-99m-pyrophosphate in the diagnosis of acute myocardial infarction: Enhanced scintigraphic accuracy by computerized selective blood pool subtraction. Am J Cardiol 40:768, 1977

4. Botvinick EH, Shames DM, Sharpe DN, et al: The specificity of pyrophosphate myocardial scintigrams in patients with prior myocardial infarction: Concise communication. J Nucl Med 19:1121, 1978

5. Chacko AK, Gordon DH, Bennett JM, et al: Myocardial imaging with Tc-99m-pyrophosphate in patients on Adriamycin treatment for neoplasia. J Nucl Med 18:680, 1977

6. Cowley MJ, Mantle JA, Rogers WJ, et al: Use of blood pool imaging in evaluation of diffuse activity patterns in technetium-99m-pyrophosphate myocardial scintigraphy. J Nucl Med 20:496, 1979

7. Duska F, Vizda J, Kubicek J, et al: The sensitivity of scintigraphic myocardial imaging by the use of ^{99m}Tc-labeled pyrophosphate in the diagnosis of cardiomyopathy of various etiology. Eur J Nucl Med 4:87, 1979

8. Holman BL, Chisholm RJ, Braunwald E: The prognostic implications of acute myocardial infarct scintigraphy with ^{99m}Tc-pyrophosphate. Circulation 57:320, 1978

9. Jaffe AS, Klein MS, Patel BR, et al: Abnormal technetium-99m-pyrophosphate images in unstable angina: Ischemia versus infarction? Am J Cardiol 44:1035, 1979

10. Jengo JA, Mena I, Joe SH, et al: The significance of calcific valvular heart disease in Tc-99m-pyrophosphate myocardial infarction scanning: Radiographic, scintigraphic, and pathological correlation. J Nucl Med 18:776, 1977

11. Kadota K, Matsumori A, Kambara H, et al: Myocardial uptake of technetium-99m-stannous pyrophosphate in experimental viral myopericarditis. J Nucl Med 20:1047, 1979

12. Karunaratne HB, Walsh WF, Fill HR, et al: Technetium-99m-pyrophosphate myocardial scintigraphy in patients with chest pain — lack of diagnostic specificity. J Nucl Med 17:523, 1976

13. Klein MS, Coleman RE, Roberts R, et al: False-positive ^{99m}Tc-Sn-pyrophosphate myocardial infarct images related to delayed blood pool clearance. Clin Nucl Med 1:45, 1976

14. Klein MS, Weiss AN, Roberts R, et al: Technetium-99m-stannous pyrophosphate scintigrams in normal subjects, patients with exercise-induced ischemia and patients with a calcified valve. Am J Cardiol 39:360, 1977

15. Landgarten S: Uptake of Tc-99m-pyrophosphate by the lactating breast. J Nucl Med 18:943, 1977

16. Landgarten S, Gordon R: Radionuclide demonstrations of Adriamycin-induced cardiac toxicity. Clin Nucl Med 2:429, 1977

17. Lee VW, Galdarone AG, Falk RH, et al: Amyloidosis of heart and liver: Comparison of Tc-99m pyrophosphate and Tc-99m methylene diphosphonate for detection. Radiology 148:239, 1983

18. Li CK, Rabinovitch MA, Juni JE, et al: Scintigraphic characterization of amyloid cardiomyopathy. Clin Nucl Med 10:156, 1985

19. Lyons KP, Olson HG, Aronow WS: Sensitivity and specificity of Tc-99m pyrophosphate myocardial scintigraphy for the detection of acute myocardial infarction. Clin Nucl Med 5:8, 1980

20. Lyons KP, Olson HG, Brown WT, et al: Persistence of an abnormal pattern on ^{99m}Tc-pyrophosphate myocardial scintigraphy following acute myocardial infarction. Clin Nucl Med 1:253, 1976

21. Mason JW, Myers RW, Alderman EL, et al: Technetium-99m-pyrophosphate myocardial uptake in patients with stable angina pectoris. Am J Cardiol 40:1, 1977

22. Matsumori A, Kadota K, Kawai C: Technetium-99m-pyrophosphate uptake in experimental viral perimyocarditis. Circulation 61:802, 1980

23. Muz J, Wizenberg T, Samlowski W, et al: Myocardial uptake of technetium 99m-pyrophosphate in patients with amyloidosis. J Nucl Med 21:49, 1980

24. Parkey RW, Bonte FJ, Buja LM, et al (eds): Clinical Nuclear Cardiology. New York, Appleton-Century-Crofts, 1979

25. Perez LA, Hayt DB, Freeman LM: Localization of myocardial disorders other than infarction with ^{99m}Tc-labeled phosphate agents. J Nucl Med 17:241, 1976

26. Riba AL, Downs J, Thakur ML, et al: Technetium-99m-stannous pyrophosphate imaging of experimental infective endocarditis. Circulation 58:111, 1978

27. Rocha AF, Merguerian BA, Harbert JC: Tc-99m-pyrophosphate myocardial scanning in Chagas' disease. J Nucl Med 22:347, 1981

28. Willerson JT, Parkey RW, Bonte FJ, et al: Acute subendocardial myocardial infarction in patients. Circulation 51:436, 1975

PYROPHOSPHATE IMAGING

Biventricular Uptake

COMMON: Amyloidosis

REFERENCE

1. Schiff S, Bateman T, Moffatt R, et al: Diagnostic considerations in cardio-myopathy: Unique scintigraphic pattern of diffuse biventricular technetium-99m-pyrophosphate uptake in amyloid heart disease. Am Heart J 103:562, 1982

PYROPHOSPHATE IMAGING

Causes of Myocardial Infarction in Children

COMMON AND
UNCOMMON: Anomalous left coronary artery
Atherosclerosis (progeria)
Coronary calcinosis
Frederich's ataxia
Kawasaki's disease
Muscular dystrophy
Muscular subaortic stenosis
Myocarditis
Polyarteritis nodosa
Postoperative
Refsum's syndrome
Rubella
Sickle cell anemia
Supravalvular aortic stenosis
Tetralogy of Fallot
Transient myocardial ischemia
Trauma
Tumors

REFERENCES

1. Flemming JC, Pysher TJ, Leonard JC: Myocardial localization of technetium-99m MDP in an infant. Clin Nucl Med 11:369, 1986
2. Wells RG, Ruskin JA, Sty JR: Myocardial imaging: Coxsackie myocarditis. Clin Nucl Med 11:661, 1986

8

Hematology

BONE MARROW IMAGING

Focal Defect

COMMON AND
UNCOMMON: Acute leukemia
Age (femoral heads)
Compression fracture
Healed rib fractures
Hodgkin's disease
Infarction (e.g., sickle cell anemia, steroids)
Metastases
Mutiple myeloma
Myelofibrosis
Osteomyelitis
Other lymphomas
Other myeloproliferative disorders
Paget's disease
Radiation

REFERENCES

1. Alavi A, Bond JP, Kuhl DE, et al: Scan detection of bone marrow infarcts in sickle cell disorders. J Nucl Med 15:1003, 1974
2. Chafetz N, Slivka J, Taylor A, et al: Decreased ^{99m}Tc-sulfur colloid activity in healed rib fractures. Radiology 126:735, 1978

3. Datz FL, Taylor A Jr: The clinical use of radionuclide bone marrow imaging. Semin Nucl Med 15:239, 1985

4. Feigin DS, Strauss HW, James AE: Detection of osteomyelitis by bone marrow scanning. J Nucl Med 15:490, 1974

5. Fletcher JW, Butler RL, Henry RE, et al: Bone marrow scanning in Paget's disease. J Nucl Med 14:928, 1973

6. Gilbert EH, Earle JD, Goris ML, et al: The accuracy of [111]InCl$_3$ as a bone marrow scanning agent. Radiology 119:167, 1976

7. Gottschalk A, Potchen EJ (eds): Diagnostic Nuclear Medicine. Baltimore, Williams and Wilkins, 1976

8. Harbert JC, Rocha AF: Textbook of Nuclear Medicine: Clinical Applications. Philadelphia, Lea and Febiger, 1984

9. Henry RE, Fletcher JW, Solaric-George E, et al: Effect of granulocytopenia, marrow suppressive drugs, and infection on marrow reticuloendothelial patterns. J Nucl Med 15:343, 1974

10. Hoppin EC, Lewis JP, DeNardo SJ: Bone marrow scintigraphy in the evaluation of acute nonlymphocytic leukemia. Clin Nucl Med 4:296, 1979

11. Pinckney L, Parker BR: Myelosclerosis and myelofibrosis in treated histiocytosis-X. AJR 129:521, 1977

12. Shih WJ, Domstad PA, DeLand FH, et al: Incidental vertebral lesions identified during technetium-99m sulfur colloid liver-spleen imaging. Clin Nucl Med 11:585, 1986

13. Theros EG (ed): Nuclear Radiology Syllabus. Chicago, American College of Radiology, 1974

14. Williams AG Jr, Mettler FA: Vertebral hemangioma: Radionuclide, radiographic, and CT correlation. Clin Nucl Med 10:598, 1985

15. Wiseman J, McHenry C: Focal marrow replacement in intervertebral disc space infection: Demonstrated by Tc-99m sulfur colloid imaging. Clin Nucl Med 9:291, 1984

BONE MARROW IMAGING

Focally Increased Activity (Sulfur Colloid)

COMMON AND
UNCOMMON: Compression fractures
Degenerative joint disease

REFERENCES

1. Shook DR, Reinke DB: Increased uptake of ^{99m}Tc-sulfur colloid in vertebral compression fractures. J Nucl Med 16:92, 1975
2. Webber MM, Wagner J: Demonstration of vascularity of the femoral head using technetium-sulfur colloid. J Nucl Med 11:376, 1970

BONE MARROW IMAGING

Decreased Central Activity with and without Peripheral Expansion

COMMON AND
UNCOMMON: Acute leukemia
Aplastic anemia
Chronic myelogenous leukemia
Chronic renal disease
Extensive metastases
Hodgkin's disease
Multiple myeloma
Myelofibrosis
Osteopetrosis
Other lymphomas
Radiation and chemotherapy

REFERENCES

1. Alavi A, Bond JP, Kuhl DE, et al: Scan detection of bone marrow infarcts in sickle cell disorders. J Nucl Med 15:1003, 1974

2. Berna L, Torres G, Carrio I, et al: Antigranulocyte antibody bone marrow scans in cancer patients with metastatic bone superscan appearance. Clin Nucl Med 19:121, 1994

3. Datz FL, Taylor A Jr: The clinical use of radionuclide bone marrow imaging. Semin Nucl Med 15:239, 1985

4. Gottschalk A, Potchen EJ (eds): Diagnostic Nuclear Medicine. Baltimore, Williams and Wilkins, 1976

5. Harbert JC, Rocha AF: Textbook of Nuclear Medicine: Clinical Applications. Philadelphia, Lea and Febiger, 1984

6. Henry RE, Fletcher JW, Solaric-George E, et al: Effect of granulocytopenia, marrow suppressive drugs, and infection on marrow reticuloendothelial pattern. J Nucl Med 15:343, 1974

7. Hoppin EC, Lewis JP, DeNardo SJ: Bone marrow scintigraphy in the evaluation of acute nonlymphocytic leukemia. Clin Nucl Med 4:296, 1979

8. Kirchner PT (ed): Nuclear Medicine Review Syllabus. New York, Society of Nuclear Medicine, 1980

9. Najean Y, Le Danvic M, Le Mercier N, et al: Significance of bone marrow scintigraphy in aplastic anemia: Concise communication. J Nucl Med 21:213, 1980

10. Otsuka N, Fukunaga M, Ono S, et al: Bone marrow scintigraphy and MRI in patient with osteopetrosis. Clin Nucl Med 16:443, 1991

11. Sayle BA, Fawcett HD, Gardner FH: Indium-111 chloride bone marrow imaging in chronic renal disease. Clin Nucl Med 10:498, 1985

BONE MARROW IMAGING

Marrow Hyperplasia

COMMON AND
UNCOMMON: Hereditary spherocytosis
Hodgkin's disease
Infection
Iron deficiency anemia
Mastocytosis
Multiple myeloma
Other chronic hemolytic anemias
Other lymphomas
Pernicious anemia
Polycythemia vera
Sickle cell, S-C, S-Thal disease

REFERENCES

1. Alavi A, Bond JP, Kuhl DE, et al: Scan detection of bone marrow infarcts in sickle cell disorders. J Nucl Med 15:1003, 1974

2. Datz FL, Taylor A Jr: The clinical use of radionuclide bone marrow imaging. Semin Nucl Med 15:239, 1985

3. Gottschalk A, Potchen EJ (eds): Diagnostic Nuclear Medicine. Baltimore, Williams and Wilkins, 1976

4. Harbert JC, Rocha AF: Textbook of Nuclear Medicine: Clinical Applications. Philadelphia, Lea and Febiger, 1984

5. Henry RE, Fletcher JW, Solaric-George E, et al: Effect of granulocytopenia, marrow suppressive drugs, and infection on marrow reticuloendothelial pattern. J Nucl Med 15:343, 1974

6. Hoppin EC, Lewis JP, DeNardo SJ: Bone marrow scintigraphy in the evaluation of acute nonlymphocytic leukemia. Clin Nucl Med 4:296, 1979

7. Kirchner PT (ed): Nuclear Medicine Review Syllabus. New York, Society of Nuclear Medicine, 1980

8. Malley MJ, Holmes RA: Mastocytosis: Scintigraphic findings with bone involvement. Clin Nucl Med 13:673, 1988

9. Najean Y, Le Danvic M, Le Mercier N, et al: Significance of bone marrow scintigraphy in aplastic anemia: Concise communication. J Nucl Med 21:213, 1980

BONE MARROW IMAGING

Disparate Findings with Indium and Sulfur Colloid

COMMON AND
UNCOMMON: Aplastic anemia
Congenital red cell aplasia
Hodgkin's disease
Idiopathic hypoplastic anemia
Radiation
Refractory anemia with excess blasts

REFERENCES

1. Datz FL, Taylor A Jr: The clinical use of radionuclide bone marrow imaging. Semin Nucl Med 15:239, 1985

2. Harbert JC, Rocha AF: Textbook of Nuclear Medicine: Clinical Applications. Philadelphia, Lea and Febiger, 1984

3. Lilien DL, Berger HG, Anderson DP, et al: ^{111}In-chloride: A new agent for bone marrow imaging. J Nucl Med 14:184, 1973

4. McIntyre PA, Larson SM, Eikman EA, et al: Comparison of the metabolism of iron-labeled transferrin (Fe-TF) and indium-labeled transferrin (In-TF) by the erythropoietic marrow. J Nucl Med 15:856, 1974

5. Najean Y, Le Danvic M, Le Mercier N, et al: Significance of bone marrow scintigraphy in aplastic anemia: Concise communication. J Nucl Med 21:213, 1980

6. Theros EG (ed): Nuclear Radiology Syllabus. Chicago, American College of Radiology, 1974

BLOOD VOLUME

Elevated Red Cell Mass

COMMON: Polycythemia rubra vera
Secondary polycythemia (COPD, AV fistulae,
  Pickwickian syndrome)
Smoker's polycythemia

UNCOMMON
AND RARE: Cobalt toxicity
Congenital heart disease
Cushing's disease
Familial erythrocytosis
Erythropoietin producing lesions
  Cerebellar hemangioblastoma
  Hepatic carcinoma
  Renal — carcinoma, cysts, hydronephrosis
  Uterine leiomyoma
High altitude
Hemoglobinopathies

REFERENCES

1. Harbert J, Rocha AF (eds): Textbook of Nuclear Medicine. Volume II. Philadelphia, Lea and Febiger, 1984
2. Itoh H, Kanamori M, Takahashi N: Dissociation between ^{111}In chloride and ^{99m}Tc colloid bone marrow scintigraphy in refractory anemia with excess blasts. Clin Nucl Med 15:124, 1990

BLOOD VOLUME

Normal Red Cell Mass and Decreased Plasma Volume

COMMON AND
UNCOMMON: Burns
Dehydration
Diarrhea
Stress polycythemia
Vomiting

REFERENCES

1. Harbert J, Rocha AF (eds): Textbook of Nuclear Medicine, Volume II. Philadelphia, Lea and Febiger, 1984
2. Silberstein EB: Nuclear hematology: The erythron. In Freeman LM, Weissman HS (eds): Nuclear Medicine Annual 1984. New York, Raven Press, 1984, p. 163

RED CELL SURVIVAL

Shortened CR-51 Red Cell Survival

COMMON AND
UNCOMMON: Anemia of chronic disease (cancer, inflammatory
bowel disease, hepatitis, uremia)
Artificial heart valve
Autoantibodies
Disseminated intravascular coagulation
Drugs (alpha-methyldopa, penicillin, phenacetin,
quinidine)
Gastrointestinal bleeding during test
Hereditary spherocytosis, elliptocytosis
Hemoglobinopathies
Infection (bacterial, malaria)
Iron deficiency
Leukemia
Paroxysmal nocturnal hemoglobinuria
Toxins (arsenic, benzene, lead, toluene, etc.)
Transfusion during test
Vasculitis
Vitamin deficiency (B_{12}, folate)

REFERENCES

1. Harbert J, Rocha AF (eds): Textbook of Nuclear Medicine, Volume II. Philadelphia, Lea and Febiger, 1984
2. Silberstein EB: Nuclear hematology: The erythron. In Freeman LM, Weissmann HS (eds): Nuclear Medicine Annual 1984. New York, Raven Press, 1984, p. 163

SEQUESTRATION STUDY

Rising Splenic Activity

COMMON: Hereditary spherocytosis

UNCOMMON
AND RARE: Acquired hemolytic anemia
Felty's syndrome
Gaucher's disease
Hodgkin's disease
Leukemia
Multiple myeloma
Myelofibrosis
Paroxysmal nocturnal hemoglobinuria
Sickle-thalessemia

REFERENCES

1. Harbert J, Rocha AF (eds): Textbook of Nuclear Medicine, Volume II. Philadelphia, Lea and Febiger, 1984
2. Silberstein EB: Nuclear hematology: The erythron. In Freeman LM, Weissmann HS (eds): Nuclear Medicine Annual 1984. New York, Raven Press, 1984, p. 163

SEQUESTRATION STUDY

Increased Liver Activity

COMMON: Sickle cell disease

UNCOMMON: Alcoholic liver disease

REFERENCES

1. Harbert J, Rocha AF (eds): Textbook of Nuclear Medicine, Volume II. Philadelphia, Lea and Febiger, 1984

SCHILLING'S TEST

Abnormal Stage I (B_{12} Only)

COMMON: Atrophic gastritis
Gastrectomy
Incomplete urine collection
Pernicious anemia

UNCOMMON
AND RARE: Bacterial overgrowth (blind loop, diverticula,
stricture)
Drugs (calcium chelating agents, neomycin, PAS)
Fish tape worm (*Diphyllobothrium latum*)
Lymphoma of ileum
Pancreatitis insufficiency
Radiation ileitis
Short bowel syndrome (surgical resection)
Small bowel fistula
Sprue
Transcobalamin II deficiency
Vitamin B_{12} deficiency-induced malabsorption
Zollinger-Ellison syndrome

REFERENCES

1. Harbert J, Rocha AF (eds): Textbook of Nuclear Medicine, Volume II. Philadelphia, Lea and Febiger, 1984
2. Silberstein EB: Nuclear hematology: The erythron. In Freeman LM, Weissmann HS (eds): Nuclear Medicine Annual 1984. New York, Raven Press, 1984, p. 163

SCHILLING'S TEST

Abnormal Stage II (B$_{12}$ and IF)

COMMON: Causes of intestinal malabsorption (See Stage I
Gamut)
Transcobalamin II deficiency
Vitamin B$_{12}$

REFERENCES

1. Harbert J, Rocha AF (eds): Textbook of Nuclear Medicine, Volume II.
Philadelphipa, Lea and Febiger, 1984
2. Silberstein EB: Nuclear hematology: The erythron. In Freeman LM, Weissmann
HS (eds): Nuclear Medicine Annual 1984. New York, Raven Press, 1984,
p. 163

SCHILLING'S TEST

Falsely Normal

COMMON AND
UNCOMMON: Fecal contamination of urine
Recent radiopharmaceutical administration

REFERENCES

1. Harbert J, Rocha AF (eds): Textbook of Nuclear Medicine, Volume II. Philadelphia, Lea and Febiger, 1984

2. Silberstein EB: Nuclear hematology: The erythron. In Freeman LM, Weissmann HS (eds): Nuclear Medicine Annual 1984. New York, Raven Press, 1984, p. 163

INDIUM LEUKOCYTE IMAGING

Increased Uptake

COMMON: Abscess
Adult respiratory distress syndrome
Cellulitis
Emphysema
Idiopathic
Indwelling enteric tubes
Intravenous sites, noninfected
Ostomies
Phlegmon
Pneumonia
Postarthroplasty
Swallowed leukocytes (e.g., sinusitis, rhinitis,
     endotracheal tube, nasogastric tube)
Wound infection

UNCOMMON: Accessory spleen
Acute pyelonephritis
Aspiration
Atelectasis
Bowel infarction
Colonic fistulas with pericolonic abscess
Congestive heart failure
Crohn's disease
Cystic fibrosis
Decubitus ulcers
Gastrointestinal bleeding
Gingivitis
Graft infection
Hematoma
Infected necrotic tumor
Injection site
Ischemic colitis
Multiple enemas
Neuropathic osteoarthropathy
Osteomyelitis
Septic arthritis
Sinusitis
Transplant with or without rejection
Tumor (noninfected)

Ulcerative colitis
Wound, noninfected

RARE: Acute cholecystitis
Cerebrovascular accident
Chemical cystitis
Deep venous thrombosis
Hartmann's pouch abscess
Hepatitis
Herpes esophagitis
Heterotopic bone
Hyperostosis frontalis
Idiopathic pseudoobstruction
Intramuscular injection sites
Lumbar puncture site
Lymph nodes draining infected site
Lymphocele
Myocardial infarction
Myocarditis
Nonseptic pulmonary embolism
Pancreatitis
Pseudoaneurysm
Rheumatoid arthritis
Sjögren's syndrome
Submandibular gland — children
Vaginitis
Vasculitis

REFERENCES

1. Alavi JB, Alavi A, Staum MM: Evaluation of infection in neutropenic patients with indium-111-labeled donor granulocytes. Clin Nucl Med 5:397, 1980

2. Anderson JR, Spence RAJ, Laird JD, et al: Indium-111 autologous leukocyte imaging in pancreatitis. J Nucl Med 27:345, 1986

3. Brown ML, Fitzgerald RH, Dewanjee MK, et al: Indium-111 leukocyte imaging in low grade osteomyelitis. J Nucl Med 23:65, 1982

4. Bushnell DL: Detection of pseudomembranous colitis with indium-111-labeled leukocyte scintigraphy. Clin Nucl Med 9:294, 1984

5. Coleman RE, Black RE, Welch DM, et al: Indium-111-labeled leukocytes in the evaluation of suspected abdominal abscesses. Am J Surg 139:99, 1980

6. Coleman RE, Welch D: Possible pitfalls with clinical imaging of indium-111 leukocytes: Concise communication. J Nucl Med 21:122, 1980

7. Collier BD, Isitman AT, Kaufman HLM, et al: Concentration of In-111-oxine-labeled autologous leukocytes in noninfected and nonrejecting renal allografts: Concise communication. J Nucl Med 25:156, 1984

8. Crass JR, L'Heureux P, Loken M: False-positive ^{111}In-labeled leukocyte scan in cystic fibrosis. Clin Nucl Med 4:291, 1979

9. D'Alonzo WA, Alavi A: Detection of deep venous thrombosis by indium-111 leukocyte scintigraphy. J Nucl Med 27:631, 1986

10. Doherty PW, Fawcett D, Goodwin DA, et al: Clinical evaluation of indium-111 leukocyte scans in diagnosis of inflammatory disease. Clin Nucl Med 20:659, 1979

11. Dudiak CM, Ali A, Dickerson M, et al: Acute tentorial subdural hematoma as a false-positive in indium-111 leukocyte scintigraphy. Clin Nucl Med 10:513, 1985

12. Dutcher JP, Schiffer CA, Johnston GS: Rapid migration of indium-labeled granulocytes to sites of infection. N Engl J Med 304:586, 1981

13. Dries DJ, Alazraki N, Lawrence PF, et al: Detection of acute synthetic vascular graft infection with ^{111}In-labeled leukocyte scanning: An animal study. AJR 145:1053, 1985

14. Fisher MF, Rudd TG: In-111-labeled leukocyte imaging: False-positive study due to acute gastrointestinal bleeding. J Nucl Med 24:803, 1983

15. Floyd JL, Jackson DE Jr, Carretta R: Appearance of hyperostosis frontalis interna on indium-111 leukocyte scans: Potential diagnostic pitfall. J Nucl Med 27:495, 1986

16. Fortner A, Datz FL, Taylor A Jr, et al: Uptake of ^{111}In-labeled leukocytes by tumor. AJR 146:621, 1986

17. Gilbert BR, Cerqueira MD, Vea HW, et al: Indium-111-labeled leukocyte uptake: False-positive results in noninfected pseudoaneurysms. Radiology 158:761, 1986

18. Gray HW, Cuthbert I, Richards JR: Clinical imaging with indium-111 leukocytes: Uptake in bowel infarction. J Nucl Med 22:701, 1981

19. Knochel JQ, Koehler PR, Lee TG, et al: Diagnosis of abdominal abscesses with computed tomography, ultrasound, and ^{111}In leukocyte scans. Radiology 137:425, 1980

20. Luers PR, Datz FL, Christian PE, et al: Causes of bowel uptake with [111]Indium leukocyte scanning. Las Vegas, Scientific exhibit, Society of Nuclear Medicine, 28th annual meeting, June, 1981

21. McAfee JG, Samin A: In-111-labeled leukocytes: A review of problems in image interpretation. Radiology 155:221, 1985

22. Martin WR, Gurevich N, Goris ML, et al: Detection of occult abscesses with ^{111}In-labeled leukocytes. AJR 133:123, 1979

23. Oates E, Staudinger K, Gilbertson V: Significance of nodal uptake on ^{111}In-labeled leukocyte scans. Clin Nucl Med 14:282, 1989

24. Rose JG, Serota AI, Wilson SE, et al: Detection of prosthetic graft infection with radiolabeled leukocytes. J Nucl Med 22:56, 1981

25. Stein DT, Paldi JH, Goodwin DA: In-111 leukocyte scan in "diversion" colitis. Clin Nucl Med 8:1, 1983

26. Taylor DW, Walz DJ, Babchuk WI, McGinnis KD: Positive ^{111}In leukocyte scintigraphy in vaginitis. Clin Nucl Med 12:477, 1987

27. Thakur ML, Coleman RE, Mayhall CG, et al: Preparation and evaluation of ^{111}In-labeled leukocytes as an abscess imaging agent in dogs. Radiology 119:731, 1976

28. Thakur ML, Coleman RE, Welch MJ: Indium-111-labeled leukocytes for the localization of abscesses: Preparation, analysis, tissue distribution, and comparison with gallium-67 citrate in dogs. J Lab Clin Med 89:217, 1977

29. Thakur ML, Lavender JP, Arnot RN, et al: Indium-111-labeled autologous leukocytes in man. J Nucl Med 18:1014, 1977

30. Thakur ML, Zaret BL, Gottschalk A: Indium-111-labeled leukocytes for imaging acute myocardial infarction: Influence of regional myocardial blood flow and age of infarct in canine models. J Nucl Med 19:744, 1978

31. Uno K, Matsui N, Nohira K, et al: Indium-111 leukocyte imaging of patients with rheumatoid arthritis. J Nucl Med 27:339, 1986

32. Williamson SL, Williamson MR, Siebert JJ, Boyd CM: Submandibular uptake on ^{111}In leukocyte scans in children. Clin Nucl Med 12:27, 1987

33. Williamson MR, Williamson SL, Siebert JJ: Indium-111 leukocyte scanning localization for detecting early myocarditis in Kawasaki disease. AJR 146:255, 1986

34. Wilson DG, Lieberman LM: Gastrointestinal bleeding in leukocyte scintigraphy. Clin Nucl Med 8:214, 1983

35. Wing VW, van Sonnenberg E, Kipper S, et al: Indium-111-labeled leukocyte localization in hematomas: A pitfall in abscess detection. Radiology 152:173, 1984

INDIUM LEUKOCYTE IMAGING

Intracranial Uptake

COMMON AND
UNCOMMON: Abscess
Bacterial meningitis
Cerebral infarction
Metastatic lesions
Primary brain tumor — glioma, glioblastoma,
astrocytoma

REFERENCES

1. Bauman JM, Osenbach R, Hartshorne MF, et al: Positive ^{111}In leukocyte scan in nocardia brain abscess. J Nucl Med 27:60, 1986

2. Bedont RA, Datz FL: ^{111}In-labeled leukocyte scan demonstrating septic meningitis complicating spinal epidural abscess. Clin Nucl Med 10:112, 1985

3. Coleman RE, Welch D: Possible pitfalls with clinical imaging of ^{111}In leukocytes. J Nucl Med 21:122, 1980

4. Palestro CJ, Swyer AJ, Kim CK, et al: Role of ^{111}In-labeled leukocyte scintigraphy in diagnosis of intracerebral lesions. Clin Nucl Med 16:305, 1991

5. Rehncrona S, Brisman J, Holtas S: Diagnosis of brain abscess with ^{111}In-labeled leukocytes. Neurosurg 16:23, 1985

6. Schmidt KG, Rasmussen JW, Frederiksen PB, Pedersen NT: [111]In granulocyte scintigraphy in brain abscess: Limitations and pitfalls. J Nucl Med 31:1121, 1990

7. Spieth ME, Kim HH, Ford PV: Unsuspected meningitis diagnosed by ^{111}In-labeled leukocytes. Clin Nucl Med 17:627, 1992

INDIUM LEUKOCYTE IMAGING

Head and Neck Uptake

COMMON: Cellulitis
Intravenous catheter — noninfected
Osteomyelitis
Periodontal disease
Sinusitis
Tracheostomy site

UNCOMMON
AND RARE: Hyperostosis frontalis
Intracranial uptake (See Gamut)
Sjögren's syndrome
Submandibular gland — children
Wound — noninfected

REFERENCES

1. Donnal JF, Baytas EM: [111]In WBC activity in salivary and lacrimal glands of a patient with Sjögren's syndrome. Clin Nucl Med 14:694, 1989

2. Park CH, Kim SM, Zhang JJ, McEwan J: Nonpustular psoriatic lesions detected by ^{99m}Tc HMPAO labeled granulocytes. Clin Nucl Med 17:657, 1992

3. Paulson E, Datz FL: False-positive calvarial uptake of ^{111}In leukocytes in patient with hyperostosis frontalis interna. Clin Nucl Med 13:68, 1988

INDIUM LEUKOCYTE IMAGING

Cardiac Uptake

COMMON AND
UNCOMMON: Endocarditis
Kawasaki disease
Myocarditis
Myocardial infarction
Pericarditis
Valve ring abscess

REFERENCES

1. Borst U, Becker W, Maisch B, et al: Clinical and prognostic effect of positive granulocyte scan in infective endocarditis. Clin Nucl Med 18:35, 1993

2. Cerqueira MD, Jacobson AF: [111]In leukocyte scintigraphic detection of myocardial abscess formation in patients with endocarditis. J Nucl Med 30:703, 1989

3. Coupland DB, Terriff B, Fung AYF, Sartori C: Hot halo sign — pyogenic pericarditis on ^{111}In leukocyte scintigraphy. Clin Nucl Med 17:579, 1992

4. Kao CH, Hsieh KS, Wang YL, et al: [99m]Tc HMPAO labeled WBC scan for detection of myocarditis in different phases of Kawasaki disease. Clin Nucl Med 17:185, 1992

5. Kao CH, Hsieh KS, Wang YL, et al: [99m]Tc HMPAO WBC imaging to detect carditis and evaluate results of high-dose gamma globulin treatment in Kawasaki disease. Clin Nucl Med 17:623, 1992

6. Kao CH, Wang SJ, Yeh SH: Detection of myocarditis with ^{111}In-labeled leukocytes. Clin Nucl Med 17:678, 1992

7. Oates E, Sarno RC: Detection of bacterial endocarditis with ^{111}In-labeled leukocytes. Clin Nucl Med 13:691, 1988

8. Schmidt U, Rebarber IF: Tuberculosis pericarditis identified with ^{67}Ga and ^{111}In leukocyte imaging. Clin Nucl Med 19:146, 1994

INDIUM LEUKOCYTE IMAGING

Disparity of Leukocyte and Sulfur Colloid Scan of Liver

COMMON: Abscess

UNCOMMON
AND RARE: Hepatic necrosis

REFERENCES

1. Davidson RM, Dhekne RD, Moore WH: [111]In WBC scan in acute toxic centrilobular hepatic necrosis. Clin Nucl Med 14:877, 1989

INDIUM LEUKOCYTE IMAGING

Increased Uptake, Abdomen

COMMON: Abscess
          Gastrointestinal activity (See Gamut)
          Phlegmon
          Wound infection

UNCOMMON
AND RARE: Accessory spleen
           Acute cholecystitis
           Acute pyelonephritis
           Chemical cystitis
           Graft infection
           Hematoma
           Hepatitis
           Infected tumor
           Lymphocele
           Pancreatitis
           Pseudoaneurysm
           Transplant (rejecting and nonrejecting)
           Tumor (noninfected)
           Unusual liver anatomy
           Wound — noninfected

REFERENCES

1. Budde RB, DeLong SR: False-positive ^{111}In WBC image secondary to unusual configuration of right hepatic lobe. Clin Nucl Med 14:64, 1989

2. Coleman RE, Black RE, Welch DM, et al: Indium-111-labeled leukocytes in the evaluation of suspected abdominal abscesses. Am J Surg 139:99, 1980

3. Coleman RE, Welch D: Possible pitfalls with clinical imaging of indium-111-leukocytes: Concise communication. J Nucl Med 21:122, 1980

4. Collier BD, Isitman AT, Kaufman HM, et al: Concentration of In-111-oxine-labeled autologous leukocytes in noninfected and nonrejecting renal allografts: Concise communication. J Nucl Med 25:156, 1984

5. Cutcher JP, Schiffer CA, Johnston GS: Rapid migration of indium-labeled granulocytes to sites of infection. N Engl J Med 304:586, 1981

6. Datz FL: Utility of indium-111-labeled leukocyte imaging in acute alcalculous cholecystitis. AJR 147:813, 1986

7. Doherty PW, Fawcett D, Goodwin DA, et al: Clinical evaluation of indium-111-leukocyte scans in diagnosis of inflammatory disease. J Nucl Med 20:659, 1979

8. Fortner A, Datz FL, Taylor A Jr, et al: Uptake of ^{111}In-labeled leukocytes by tumor. AJR 146:621, 1986

9. Gilbert BR, Cerqueira MD, Vea HW, et al: Indium-111-labeled leukocyte uptake: False-positive results in noninfected pseudoaneurysms. Radiology 158:761, 1986

10. Knochel JQ, Koehler PR, Lee TG, et al: Diagnosis of abdominal abscesses with computed tomography, ultrasound, and ^{111}In-leukocyte scans. Radiology 137:425, 1980

11. Martin WR, Gurevich N, Goris ML, et al: Detection of occult abscesses with ^{111}In-labeled leukocytes. AJR 133:123, 1979

12. Palestro CJ, Cohen IR, Goldsmith SJ: Labeled leukocyte imaging in chemical cystitis. Clin Nucl Med 18:75, 1993

13. Rose JG, Serota AI, Wilson SE, et al: Detection of prosthetic graft infections with radiolabeled leukocytes. J Nucl Med 22:56, 1981

14. Thakur ML, Coleman RE, Mayhall CG, et al: Preparation and evaluation of ^{111}In-labeled leukocytes as an abscess imaging agent in dogs. Radiology 119:731, 1976

15. Thakur ML, Coleman RE, Welch MJ: Indium-111-labeled leukocytes for the localization of abscesses: Preparation, analysis, tissue distribution, and comparison with gallium-67 citrate in dogs. J Lab Clin Med 89:217, 1977

16. Thakur ML, Lavender JP, Arnot RN, et al: Indium-111-labeled autologous leukocytes in man. J Nucl Med 18:1014, 1977

17. Wing VW, van Sonnenberg E, Kipper S, et al: Indium-111-labeled leukocyte localization in hematomas: A pitfall in abscess detection. Radiology 152:173, 1984

INDIUM LEUKOCYTE IMAGING

Gastrointestinal Activity

COMMON: Abscess communicating with bowel
Gastrointestinal bleeding
Idiopathic
Indwelling enteric tubes (e.g., Dobhoff, gastrostomy, jejunostomy)
Ostomies
Swallowed leukocytes (e.g., sinusitis, rhinitis, endotracheal tube, nasogastric tubes)

UNCOMMON
AND RARE: Behçet's disease
Bowel infarction
Crohn's disease
Cystic fibrosis
Diverticulitis
Gastroenteritis
Hartmann's pouch abscess
Herpes esophagitis
Idiopathic pseudoobstruction
Infected necrotic tumor
Ischemic colitis (e.g., rheumatoid vasculitis, polyarteritis nodosa)
Multiple enemas
Multiple interloop abscesses
Pseudomembranous colitis
Tumor (noninfected)
Typhlitis
Ulcerative colitis
Vasculitis

REFERENCES

1. Coleman RE, Welch D: Possible pitfalls with clinical imaging of indium-111-leukocytes: Concise communication. J Nucl Med 21:122, 1980
2. Crass JR, L'Heureux P, Loken M: False-positive ^{111}In-labeled leukocyte scan in cystic fibrosis. Clin Nucl Med 4:291, 1979
3. Datz FL: Utility of indium-111-labeled leukocyte imaging in acute acalculous cholecystitis. AJR 147:813, 1986

4. Datz FL, Thorne DA: Gastrointestinal tract radionuclide activity on In-111-labeled leukocyte imaging: Clinical significance in patients with fever of unknown origin. Radiology 160:635, 1986

5. Doherty PW, Fawcett D, Goodwin DA, et al: Clinical evaluation of indium-111-leukocyte scans in diagnosis of inflammatory disease. J Nucl Med 20:659, 1979

6. Fortner A, Datz FL, Taylor A Jr, et al: Uptake of ^{111}In-labeled leukocytes by tumor. AJR 146:621, 1986

7. Froelich JW, Field SA: Role of ^{111}In white blood cells in inflammatory bowel disease. Semin Nucl Med XVIII:300, 1988

8. Froelich J, Swanson D, Singer D, et al: In-111-labeled leukocytes in the diagnosis and management of granulomatous and ulcerative colitis. J Nucl Med 23:74, 1982

9. Gray HW, Cuthbert I, Richards JR: Clinical imaging with indium-111-leukocytes: Uptake in bowel infarction. J Nucl Med 22:701, 1981

10. Harre RG, Conrad GR, Seabold JE: Colonic localization of ^{111}In-labeled leukocytes in active Behçet's disease. Clin Nucl Med 13:459, 1988

11. Knochel JQ, Koehler PR, Lee TG, et al: Diagnosis of abdominal abscess with computed tomography, ultrasound, and ^{111}In-leukocyte scans. Radiology 137:425, 1980

12. Luers PR, Datz FL, Christian PE, et al: Causes of bowel uptake with [111]indium leukocyte scanning. Las Vegas, Scientific exhibit, Society of Nuclear Medicine, 28th annual meeting, June, 1981

13. Martin WR, Gurevich N, Goris ML, et al: Detection of occult abscesses with ^{111}In-labeled leukocytes. AJR 133:123, 1979

14. McAfee JG, Samin A: In-111 labeled leukocytes: A review of problems in image interpretation. Radiology 155:221, 1985

INDIUM LEUKOCYTE IMAGING

Failure of Liver to Visualize

COMMON AND
UNCOMMON: Alcoholic liver disease
Neutropenia

REFERENCE

1. Segall GM, Goodwin DA: Nonvisualization of the liver by indium-111-oxine-labeled leukocytes in alcoholic liver disease. Clin Nucl Med 11:79, 1986

INDIUM LEUKOCYTE IMAGING

Halo Sign in Gallbladder Fossa

COMMON: Acute cholecystitis (calculous and acalculous)

REFERENCES

1. Bauman JM, Boykin M, Hartshorne MF, et al: "Halo" sign on indium-111 leukocyte scan in gangrenous cholecystitis. Clin Nucl Med 11:136, 1986
2. Datz FL: Utility of indium-111-labeled leukocyte imaging in acute acalculous cholecystitis. AJR 147:813, 1986

INDIUM LEUKOCYTE IMAGING

Musculoskeletal and Skin Uptake

COMMON: Cellulitis
Intravenous sites — noninfected
Osteomyelitis
Postarthroplasty
Wound infection

UNCOMMON
AND RARE: Arthritis — rheumatoid, gout
Fracture
Hyperostotis frontalis
Injection site
Heterotopic bone
Lumbar puncture site
Myocardial infarction
Neuropathic osteoarthropathy
Paget's disease
Pigmented villonodular synovitis
Pseudogout
Pyoderma gangrenosum
Radiation
Septic arthritis
Sickle cell disease
Sinusitis
Wound — noninfected

REFERENCES

1. Alavi JB, Alavi A, Staum MM: Evaluation of infection in neutropenic patients with indium-111-labeled donor granulocytes. Clin Nucl Med 5:397, 1980
2. Callcott F, Gordon L, Schabel SI, Friedman R: [111]In WBC imaging — false-positive in a simple fracture. J Nucl Med 29:571, 1988
3. Chung CJ, Wilson AA, Melton JW, et al: Uptake of ^{111}In-labeled leukocytes by lymphocele — a cause of false-positive vascular graft infection. Clin Nucl Med 17:368, 1992
4. Coleman RE, Welch D: Possible pitfalls with clinical imaging of indium-111-leukocytes: Concise communication. J Nucl Med 21:122, 1980
5. Doherty PW, Fawcett D, Goodwin DA, et al: Clinical evaluation of indium-111-leukocyte scans in diagnosis of inflammatory disease. J Nucl Med 20:659, 1979

6. Dutcher JP, Schiffer CA, Johnson GS: Rapid migration of indium-labeled granulocytes to sites of infection. N Engl J Med 304:586, 1981

7. Esterhai JL, Silfen D: Indium white blood cell scan in evaluating osteomyelitis. J Nucl Med 31:2029, 1990

8. Floyd JL, Jackson DE Jr, Carretta R: Appearance of hyperostosis frontalis interna on indium-111 leukocyte scans: Potential diagnostic pitfall. J Nucl Med 27:495, 1986

9. Herrmann T, Granjon D, Loboguerrero A, Decousus M: ^{99m}Tc HMPAO leukocyte uptake in articular gout. Clin Nucl Med 16:457, 1991

10. Johnson MA, Wells J, Frankel A, et al: The role of in-111 leukocyte scanning in pyoderma gangrenosum. Clin Nucl Med 6:491, 1981

11. Martin WR, Gurevich N, Goris ML, et al: Detection of occult abscesses with ^{111}In-labeled leukocytes. AJR 133:123, 1979

12. Miron SD, Minotti AJ, Crass JR: Accumulation of ^{111}In-tagged white blood cells in heterotopic new bone. Clin Nucl Med 17:972, 1992

13. Oswald SG, VanNostrand D, Savory CG, Callaghan JJ: Three-phase bone scan and indium white blood cell scintigraphy following porous coated hip arthroplasty: A prospective study of the prosthetic tip. J Nucl Med 30:1321, 1989

14. Palestro CJ, Roumanas P, Kim CK, Goldsmith SJ: Early and late skeletal effects of radiation therapy on ^{111}In-labeled leukocyte imaging. Clin Nucl Med 16:128, 1991

15. Palestro CJ, Cohen IR, Goldsmith SJ: Wound dressing activity mimicking infection on labeled leukocyte imaging. Clin Nucl Med 17:711, 1992

16. Palestro CJ, Goldsmith SJ: ^{111}In-labeled leukocyte imaging in a case of pseudogout. Clin Nucl Med 17:366, 1992

17. Palestro CJ, Kim CK, Swyer AJ, et al: Total-hip athroplasty: Periprosthetic ^{111}In-labeled leukocyte activity and complementary ^{99m}Tc-sulfur colloid imaging in suspected infection. J Nucl Med 31:1950, 1990

18. Palestro CJ, Lee SO, Kim CK, Goldsmith SJ: Lumbar puncture — potential pitfall in ^{111}In-labeled leukocyte scintigraphy. Clin Nucl Med 16:58, 1991

19. Palestro CJ, Vega A, Kim CK, et al: Appearance of acute gouty arthritis on ^{111}In-labeled leukocyte scintigraphy. J Nucl Med 31:682,1990

20. Schauwecker DS, Park HM, Burt RW, et al: Combined bone scintigraphy and ^{111}In-leukocyte scans in neuropathic foot disease. J Nucl Med 29:1651, 1988

21. Schmidt KG, Rasmussen JW, Wedebye IM, Frederiksen PB: Accumulation of ^{111}In-labeled granulocytes in malignant tumors. J Nucl Med 29:479, 1988

22. Seabold JE, Flickinger FW, Kao SCS, et al: ^{111}In-leukocyte/^{99m}Tc-MDP bone and magnetic resonance imaging: Difficulty diagnosing osteomyelitis in patients with neuropathic osteoarthropathy. J Nucl Med 31:549, 1990

23. Stadalnik RC: Skeletal uptake of ^{111}In-labeled white blood cells. Semin Nucl Med XIX:152, 1989

24. Thakur ML, Zaret BL, Gottschalk A: Indium-111-labeled leukocytes for imaging acute myocardial infarction: Influence of regional myocardial blood flow and age of infarct in canine models. J Nucl Med 19:744,1978

25. Uno K, Matsui N, Nohira K, et al: Indium-111 leukocyte imaging in patients with rheumatoid arthritis. J Nucl Med 27:339, 1986

26. VanNostrand D, Abreu SH, Callaghan JJ, et al: ¹¹¹In-labeled white blood cell uptake in noninfected closed fracture in humans: Prospective study. Radiology 167:495, 1988

27. Williamson SL, Williamson MR. Seibert JJ, et al: ¹¹¹In leukocyte accumulation in submandibular gland saliva as cause for false-positive gut uptake in children. Clin Nucl Med 12:868, 1987

INDIUM LEUKOCYTE IMAGING

Decreased Osseous Activity

COMMON AND
UNCOMMON: Advanced age (femoral heads)
Avascular necrosis (e.g., following fracture, steroids)
Disc space infection following surgery
Fibrous dysplasia
Fracture
Idiopathic
Leukemia
Myelofibrosis
Paget's disease
Postsurgical
Prosthesis
Radiation
Treated osteomyelitis
Tumor involving bone

REFERENCES

1. Skeletal photopenic appearance of Paget's disease with ^{111}In white blood cell imaging. Clin Nucl Med 12:783, 1987

2. Coleman RE, Welch D: Possible pitfalls with clinical imaging of indium-111 leukocytes: Concise communication. J Nucl Med 21:122, 1980

3. Cooper JA, Elmendorf SL, Teixeira JP, et al: Diagnosis of sternal wound infection by ^{99m}Tc leukocyte imaging. J Nucl Med 33:59, 1992

4. Datz FL, Thorne DA: Cause and significance of cold bone defects on ^{111}In-labeled leukocyte imaging. J Nucl Med 28:820, 1987

5. Datz FL, Thorne DA, Taylor A: Cold bone defects on In-111-labeled leukocyte scans. J Nucl Med 27:977, 1986

6. Dunn EK, Vaquer RA, Strashun AM: Paget's disease: A cause of photopenic skeletal defect in ^{111}In WBC scintigraphy. J Nucl Med 29:561, 1988

7. Oliverio R, Oates E: Intraosseous hemorrhage of the sacrum — another cause of a photopenic lesion on ^{111}In-labeled leukocyte scintigraphy. Clin Nucl Med 15:578, 1990

8. Palestro CJ, Kim CK, Vega A, Goldsmith SJ: Acute effects of radiation therapy on ^{111}In-labeled leukocyte uptake in bone marrow. J Nucl Med 30:1889, 1989

9. Swyer AJ, Palestro CJ, Kim CK, Goldsmith SJ: Appearance of fibrous dysplasia on ^{111}In-labeled leukocyte scintigraphy. Clin Nucl Med 16:133, 1991

INDIUM PLATELET IMAGING

Uptake

COMMON: Abscess
Accessory spleen
Aneurysm, pseudoaneurysm
Arteriosclerosis
Autoimmune thrombocytopenic purpura (spleen)
Cyclosporin nephrotoxicity
Following artery catheterization
Gastrointestinal bleeding
Grafts
Hematoma
Lymph nodes
Prosthetic valves
Status — postsurgery
Subacute bacterial endocarditis
Thrombosis
Transplant rejection

REFERENCES

1. Catafau AM, Lomena FJ, Ricart MJ, et al: ^{111}In-labeled platelets in monitoring human pancreatic transplants. J Nucl Med 30:1470, 1989

2. Desir G, Lang R, Smith E, et al: The value of indium-111 platelet scintigraphy in the management of renal transplants. J Nucl Med 27:983, 1986

3. Ezekowitz MD, Pope CF, Sostman HD, et al: Indium-111 platelet scintigraphy for the diagnosis of acute venous thrombosis. Circulation 73:668, 1986

4. Fawwaz RA: Clinical utility of labeled cells for detection of allograft rejection and myocardial infarction. Semin Nucl Med 14:198, 1984

5. Forstrom L: Thrope P, Weir EK, et al: Detection of an abdominal aneurysm by indium-111 platelet imaging. Clin Nucl Med 10:683, 1985

6. Goodgold HM, Samuels LD: False-positive ^{111}In platelet scintigraphy. J Nucl Med 30:267, 1989

7. Isaka Y, Kimura K, Yoneda S, et al: Platelet accumulation in carotid atherosclerotic lesions: Semiquantitative analysis with indium-111 platelets and technetium-99m human serum albumin. J Nucl Med 25:556, 1984

8. Jurewicz WA, Buckels JAC, Dykes JGA, et al: Indium-111-labeled platelets in monitoring pancreatic transplants in humans. Transplantation Proc 16:720, 1984

9. Jurewicz WA, Buckels JAC, Dykes JGA, et al: 111-Indium platelets in monitoring pancreatic allografts in man. Br J Surg 72:228, 1985

10. Kuippers EJ, Brouwers TM, Hazenberg HJA: Renal trapping of ^{111}In troponolate-labeled platelets in thrombotic thrombocytopenic purpura. Clin Nucl Med 16:506, 1991

11. Marcus CS, Koyle MA, Darcourt J: In-111 platelet imaging in renal transplant patients on cyclosporin A. J Nucl Med 27:984, 1986

12. Moser KM, Fedullo PF: Imaging of venous thromboemboli with labeled platelets. Semin Nucl Med 14:188, 1986

13. Sollinger HW, Lieberman LM, Kamps D, et al: Diagnosis of early pancreas allograft rejection with indium-111-oxine-labeled platelets. Transplantation Proc 16:785, 1984

14. Straus E, Smith EO, Morse S, et al: The use of indium-111 oxine labeled platelets in symptomatic patients with suspected deep vein thrombosis. J Nucl Med 27:1036, 1986

INDIUM PLATELET IMAGING

Renal Transplant Uptake

COMMON: Rejection

UNCOMMON
AND RARE: Acute cyclosporin nephrotoxicity
Hematoma
Iliac vein thrombosis
Renal artery or vein thrombosis
Scanning immediately postsurgery

REFERENCES

1. Martin-Comin J, Roca M, Grino JM, et al: In-111 oxine autologous labeled platelets in the diagnosis of kidney graft rejection. Clin Nucl Med 8:7, 1983
2. Tisdale PL, Collier BD, Kauffman HM, et al: Early diagnosis of acute postoperative renal transplant rejection by indium-111-labeled platelet scintigraphy. J Nucl Med 27:1266, 1986

INDIUM PLATELET IMAGING

Cardiac Uptake

COMMON: Left ventricular thrombus

UNCOMMON
AND RARE: Arterial thrombus
Coronary bypass graft
Prosthetic valve
Transplant rejection

REFERENCE

1. Datz FL, Taylor AT Jr: Section II: Radiolabeled platelets. In Freeman and Johnson's Clinical Radionuclide Imaging. Orlando, Grune and Stratton, 1986

INDIUM PLATELET IMAGING

Vascular Uptake

COMMON AND
UNCOMMON: Aneurysm, pseudoaneurysm
Arteriosclerotic plaque
Following catheterization
Graft
Thrombosis (arterial or venous)

REFERENCE

1. Datz FL, Taylor AT Jr: Section II: Radiolabeled platelets. In Freeman and Johnson's Clinical Radionuclide Imaging. Orlando, Grune and Stratton, 1986

INDIUM PLATELET IMAGING

Shortened Survival

COMMON AND
UNCOMMON: Arterial grafts
Atherosclerotic coronary heart disease
Diabetes mellitus
Eisenminger's syndrome
Hepatic cirrhosis
Hyperlipidemia
Idiopathic thrombocytopenia purpura
Infection
Other antiplatelet antibody diseases
Peripheral vascular disease
Primary pulmonary hypertension
Prosthetic heart valves
Renal transplantation

REFERENCE

1. Datz FL, Taylor AT Jr: Section II: Radiolabeled platelets. In Freeman and Johnson's Clinical Radionuclide Imaging. Orlando, Grune and Stratton, 1986

VENOGRAPHY

Positive I-125 Fibrinogen Study

COMMON: Acute thrombophlebitis of deep system

UNCOMMON
AND RARE: Arthritis
Cellulitis
Extravascular clot
Hematoma
Injection sites
Massive edema
Postoperative
Previous contrast venogram
Previous lymphangiogram
Previous arthrogram
Recent fracture
Room background
Superficial thrombophlebitis
Tumor
Ulcers
Varicose veins

REFERENCES

1. Charkes ND, Dugan MA, Maier WP, et al: Scintigraphic detection of deep vein thrombosis with ^{131}I-fibrinogen. J Nucl Med 15:1163, 1974

2. Freeman LM (ed): Nuclear Medicine Annual 1980. New York, Raven Press, 1980

3. Prescott SM, Tikoff G, Coleman RE: ^{131}I-labeled fibrinogen in the diagnosis of deep vein thrombosis of the lower extremities. AJR 131:451, 1978

4. Tow DE: Thrombus detection: Here and now. J Nucl Med 18:91, 1977

INTRAPERITONEAL IMAGING

Focal Intraperitoneal Collection Prior to Therapy

COMMON: Loculation

UNCOMMON
AND RARE: Low volume of injected material

REFERENCE

1. Tulchinsky M, Eggli DF: Intraperitoneal distribution imaging prior to chromic phosphate (P-32) therapy in ovarian cancer patients. Clin Nucl Med 19:43, 1994